Pharmacology - Research, Safety Testing and Regulation

nova
Medicine & Health
New York

Pharmacology - Research, Safety Testing and Regulation

Clinical Pharmacist Tools to Deliver Rational Medication Use
Mohamed Emam Abdelmobdy Abdelrahim (Editor)
2023. ISBN: 979-8-88697-857-5 (Hardcover)
2023. ISBN: 979-8-88697-927-5 (eBook)

The Biochemical Guide to Antibiotics
David Aebisher and Dorota Bartusik-Aebisher (Editors)
2022. ISBN: 979-8-88697-193-4 (Softcover)
2022. ISBN: 979-8-88697-242-9 (eBook)

Essence of Clinical Pharmacy
Majid Khan, M.Phil (Editor)
2022. ISBN: 979-8-88697-056-2 (Hardcover)
2022. ISBN: 979-8-88697-240-5 (eBook)

An Introduction to P-Glycoprotein
M. Wahajuddin, PhD, FHEA, FRSB, FRSC (Editor),
Rahul Dev Jayant, PhD (Editor), Ravindra Varma Alluri, PhD (Editor)
2021. ISBN: 978-1-53619-488-3 (Hardcover)
2021. ISBN: 978-1-53619-728-0 (eBook)

A Pharmacological Guide to Non-Steroidal Anti-Inflammatory Medications
Pugazhenthan Thangaraju, MBBS, MD, DNB MNAMS,PGD Diab, MBA (Editor)
2021. ISBN: 978-1-53619-836-2 (Hardcover)
2021. ISBN: 978-1-53619-905-5 (eBook)

More information about this series can be found at https://novapublishers.com/product-category/series/pharmacology-research-safety-testing-and-regulation/

Mohamed Emam Abdelmobdy Abdelrahim
Editor

Clinical Pharmacist Tools to Deliver Rational Medication Use

nova
Medicine & Health
New York

DOI: https://doi.org/10.52305/XLXJ5358

Library of Congress Cataloging-in-Publication Data

Names: Abdelrahim, Mohamed E. A., editor.
Title: Clinical pharmacist tools to deliver rational medication use /
Mohamed Emam Abdelmobdy Abdelrahim (editor), Faculty of Pharmacy,
Department of Clinical Pharmacy, Beni-Suef University, Beni-Suef, Egypt.
Description: New York : Nova Science Publishers, [2023] | Series:
Pharmacology--research, safety testing and regulation | Includes
bibliographical references and index. |
Identifiers: LCCN 2023023406 (print) | LCCN 2023023407 (ebook) | ISBN
9798886978575 (hardcover) | ISBN 9798886979275 (adobe pdf)
Subjects: LCSH: Clinical pharmacology. | Clinical pharmacology--Vocational
guidance.
Classification: LCC RM301.28 .C55 2023 (print) | LCC RM301.28 (ebook) |
DDC 615.1--dc23/eng/20230703
LC record available at https://lccn.loc.gov/2023023406
LC ebook record available at https://lccn.loc.gov/2023023407

Published by Nova Science Publishers, Inc. † New York

Contents

Preface

The clinical pharmacy offers personalized patient care services that improve pharmaceutical use and advance wellness, good health, and disease prevention. In hospitals and clinics, the clinical pharmacy movement first got started. Clinical pharmacists provide patient care across the board of medical facilities. They frequently work along with doctors and other healthcare professionals to enhance pharmaceutical care in numerous fields of medicine and surgery. The interdisciplinary approach to patient care now includes them as a crucial component. They frequently take part in decisions regarding drug products and rounds of patient treatment. Clinical pharmacists are in charge of dosing and managing the potentially harmful medications that need close supervision in the majority of hospitals. According to the American College of Clinical Pharmacy, pharmacists will be responsible for ensuring that patients receive the best possible drug therapy for illness prevention and treatment during the next 10 to 15 years. The industry must guarantee that there will be a sufficient supply of clinical pharmacists who are suitably trained and skilled to realize this aim. This book makes an effort to offer such important education. It is broken up into various chapters. The most prevalent diseases are covered in each chapter and how they are treated by various medical specializations. We hope that clinical pharmacists all over the world will use this book as a set of guidelines or specific recommendations.

Chapter 1

Introduction

Hadeer Harb[*]
and Mohamed Emam Abdelmobdy Abdelrahim

Clinical Pharmacy Department, Faculty of Pharmacy,
Beni-Suef University, Beni Suef, Egypt

Learning Objectives

After completing this chapter, the reader would be able to:

- Recognize the responsibilities and function of the recent clinical pharmacist.
- Be aware of the many clinical pharmacy services offered throughout clinical pharmacy practice to increase the therapeutic advantages and reduce potential therapeutic dangers.
- Offer a thorough primer on techniques for therapy optimization using various clinical pharmacy interventions.
- Evaluate the clinical and financial advantages of various clinical pharmacy interventions in hospital and primary care settings.

Clinical Pharmacy Overview

The provision of pharmacological treatment must include a clinical pharmacy. Participation in physician rounds, drug reconciliation at admission or release, and the provision of pharmacist services specialized to a given drug class are just a few examples of clinical pharmacy interventions that might be used. The clinical pharmacist will be a crucial member of the medical care team thanks to these treatments, which can enhance clinical and financial results in both hospital and primary care settings. Clinical pharmacy interventions are used to enhance medical treatment cost-effectively in terms of quality, safety, and efficiency.

[*] Corresponding Author's Email: Hadeersafwat@pharm.bsu.edu.eg.

In: Clinical Pharmacist Tools to Deliver Rational Medication Use
Editor: Mohamed Emam Abdelmobdy Abdelrahim
ISBN: 979-8-88697-857-5

Clinical Pharmacists and Pharmacists

Pharmacists are knowledgeable about drugs and can offer pertinent medical advice. Community pharmacists carry out specific duties including filling prescriptions for out-patients, recommending over-the-counter medications, and carrying out various other related services. In recent years, the pharmaceutical industry has changed from being a task- or product-oriented (dispensing) profession to one that is patient-oriented (providing care, counseling, and advice). This is an effort to comprehend various illness states and the appropriate medical care for them better [1]. In addition to delivering pharmaceuticals, the function of the pharmacist has expanded to include a variety of duties, such as counseling patients and healthcare professionals [2].

In the United States, clinical pharmacy practice first appeared in the 1960s [3]. In the United Kingdom, hospital pharmacy activity has increasingly included clinical pharmacy practice over the past 30 years [4]. The provision of pharmacological treatment must include a clinical pharmacy. The technical caliber of pharmaceutical care can also be enhanced by knowing clinical pharmacy services [5]. Clinical pharmacists possess specialized training in therapeutics, comprehensive drug management for patients, and counseling for healthcare professionals (all members of the healthcare team) [6].

The Clinical Pharmacy Definition

Clinical pharmacy is described as "a health science specialty that includes the application, by pharmacists, of the scientific concepts of pharmacology, toxicology, pharmacokinetics, and therapeutics to the care of patients" by the American College of Clinical Pharmacy (ACCP) [7].

Clinical pharmacy is described as "services done by pharmacists on behalf of the patient to identify, resolve and prevent drug-related problems" in a draught report by the US Department of Health and Human Services on the clinical role of community pharmacies [8].

Clinical pharmacy is described as a health specialty that "describes the actions and services of the clinical pharmacist to create and promote the rational and appropriate use of medical products and technologies" by the European Society of Clinical Pharmacy [5].

Clinical pharmacy is described as "the contribution of hospital pharmacists and their assistants to drug therapy as a part of the overall care provided to patients, in cooperation with physicians and nursing staff, to optimize the efficiency, effectiveness, and safety of drug therapy" in a hospital setting [9].

All of these definitions that have been put forth focus on the contributions made by pharmacists to the development of effective and logical drug therapy.

Pharmaceutical Services for Patients

To optimize therapeutic benefits and reduce potential treatment hazards, many clinical pharmacy services could be offered during clinical pharmacy practice. These consist of [2]:

Therapeutic drug monitoring (TDM), pharmacokinetic analysis, manufacture of intravenous (IV) mixtures, total parenteral nutrition (TPN), dissemination of drug information, dispensing of drugs, drug selection, management of pharmaceutical therapy, and patient counseling are all included.

Clinical Pharmacist Interventions

Through participation in physician rounds, medication reconciliation at admission or release, and provision of pharmacist services tailored to certain drug classes, a variety of clinical pharmacy interventions could be used, including [6, 9]

1. Modifying doses to account for renal and hepatic clearance
2. Recommending the start, stop, or modification of therapies
3. Physicochemical and pharmacologic interactions detection and prevention
4. Finding and avoiding prescription and transcribing mistakes
5. Recognizing, monitoring, and avoiding adverse medication occurrences (ADEs)
6. Giving doctors, nurses, and patients pharmacological information
7. Evaluating drug use
8. Examining drug use history
9. Monitoring the antibiogram and results of microbiological laboratory tests
10. Implementing and monitoring the application of prescription drug usage guidelines
11. Using a formulary
12. Questioning and advising patients on admission and discharge medications
13. Improving posology and dose
14. Changing prescription medications based on the formulary, contraindications, allergies, or price
15. Changing the method of administration

Clinical Pharmacy Interventions' Advantages

Clinical pharmacy interventions can enhance both clinical and financial results in primary and hospital care settings, making the clinical pharmacist a crucial member of the healthcare team [10–13]. Inpatient clinical pharmacy interventions improve patient outcomes by reducing adverse drug events (ADEs), adverse drug reactions (ADRs), and medication errors, as well as by increasing medication appropriateness, patient adherence, satisfaction, and knowledge about their medications, according to a recent literature review [6].

"An injury resulting from medical intervention related to a drug," is how an ADE is defined [6].

While an adverse drug reaction (ADR) is described as "an unpleasant and unexpected result that occurs at levels utilized in man for prevention, diagnosis, or therapy" [6].

According to Kucukarslan et al., [14], adding a clinical pharmacist to the healthcare team decreased avoidable adverse drug events (ADEs) by 78%, but the number of occurrences was low (2 vs. 9; P=0.02). Another example is Smythe et al., [15], who evaluated 131 patients over the course of 8 weeks using a clinical pharmacist-structured examination and reported fewer adverse drug reactions (1 vs. 8 occurrences; P=.03) than they had at baseline. In another study, the inpatient physician's discharge letter to the patient's primary care physician was compared to normal release planning with pharmacist discharge counseling. With no difference in readmission rates, there has been a significant improvement in the relationship between discharge and home medications 10 to 14 days after discharge, as well as in awareness of drug name, dosage, and frequency [16].

Clinical pharmacy interventions also have a positive financial impact based on predicted cost avoidance and direct cost reductions from ADE prevention and shorter hospital stays (LOS). These savings were greater for particular measures (such as preventing ADEs and moving from intravenous to oral medicine), as well as for certain medical specialties (such as the intensive care unit versus geriatrics) [9, 17, 18]. Additionally, hospital and pharmacy expenditures were decreased as a result of pharmacist inclusion on general medical teams [19–21]. In comparison to the more conventional role of centralized pharmacy medication monitoring, one of the first intervention trials by clinical pharmacists in patient care units by Clapham et al., [21] entailed routine interaction with doctors, patients, and nurses. The intervention resulted in non-significant decreases in LOS and drug costs and decreased the overall average cost ($1293; P.05). Additionally, pharmacists discovered that working in the patient-care sector is more gratifying professionally.

Generally speaking, using clinical pharmacy treatments in hospital and primary care settings enhances the quality, safety, and effectiveness of medical care while being cost-effective.

References

[1] Inoue, Y., Y. Morita, M. Takikawa, K. Takao, I. Kanamoto, and K. Sugibayashi, Future expectations for Japanese pharmacists as compared to the rest of the world. *Research in Social and Administrative Pharmacy*, 2015. 11(3): p. 448-458.

[2] Abdel-Latif, M .M. and K. Sabra, Clinical pharmacy practice in Egyptian hospitals. *American Journal of Health-System Pharmacy*, 2016. 73(1): p. e63-e66.

[3] Miller, R. R., History of clinical pharmacy and clinical pharmacology. *The Journal of Clinical Pharmacology*, 1981. 21 :(4)p. 195-197.

[4] Cotter, S. M., N. D. Barber, and M. McKee, Survey of clinical pharmacy services in United Kingdom National Health Service hospitals. *American Journal of Health-System Pharmacy*, 1994. 51(21): p. 2676-2684.

[5] Hepler, C. D., Clinical pharmacy, pharmaceutical care, and the quality of drug therapy. *Pharmacotherapy: The Journal of Human Pharmacology and Drug Therapy*, 2004. 24(11): p. 1491-1498.

[6] Kaboli, P. J., A. B. Hoth, B. J. McClimon, and J. L. Schnipper, Clinical pharmacists and inpatient medical care: a systematic review. *Archives of internal medicine*, 2006. 166(9): p. 955-964.

[7] Cipolle, R. J., Strand, L. M., Morley, P. C. *Pharmaceutical Care Practice*. Capítulo, 1998. 8: p. 265-276.

[8] Kusserow, R. P., *The clinical role of the community pharmacist* USHHS Office of the Inspector General, Washington, DC, November, 1990.

[9] De Rijdt, T., L. Willems, and S. Simoens, Economic effects of clinical pharmacy interventions: a literature review. *American Journal of Health-System Pharmacy*, 2008. 65(12): p. 11.1172-61

[10] Kopp, B. J., M. Mrsan, B. L. Erstad, and J. J. Duby, Cost implications of and potential adverse events prevented by interventions of a critical care pharmacist. *American Journal of Health-System Pharmacy*, 2007. 64(23): p. 2483-2487.

[11] Bond, C. and C. L. Raehl, Clinical and economic outcomes of pharmacist-managed antimicrobial prophylaxis in surgical patients. *American Journal of Health-System Pharmacy*, 2007. 64(18): p. 1935-1942.

[12] Haumschild, M. J., T. L. Karfonta, M. S. Haumschild, and S. E. Phillips, Clinical and economic outcomes of a fall-focused pharmaceutical intervention program. *American Journal of Health-System Pharmacy*, 2003. 60(10): p. 1029-1032.

[13] Finley, P. R., H. R. Rens, J. T. Pont, S. L. Gess, C. Louie, S. A. Bull, and L. A. Bero, Impact of a collaborative pharmacy practice model on the treatment of depression in primary care. *American Journal of Health-System Pharmacy*, 2002. 59(16): p. 1518-1526.

[14] Kucukarslan, S. N., M. Peters, M. Mlynarek, and D. A. Nafziger, Pharmacists on rounding teams reduce preventable adverse drug events in hospital general medicine units. *Archives of Internal Medicine*, 2003. 163(17): p. 2014-2018.

[15] Smythe, M. A., P. P. Shah, T. L. Spiteri, R. L. Lucarotti, and R. L. Begle, Pharmaceutical care in medical progressive care patients. *Annals of Pharmacotherapy*, 1998. 32(3): p. 294-299.

[16] Bolas, H., K. Brookes, M. Scott, and J. McElnay, Evaluation of a hospital-based community liaison pharmacy service in Northern Ireland. *Pharmacy World and Science,* 2004. 26 :(2)p. 114-120.

[17] Doloresco, F., J. Hoffman, and P. Meek, Economic evaluations of clinical pharmacy services: 2001–2005. *Pharmacotherapy*, 2008. 28(11): p. 285e-323e.

[18] Willett, M. S., K. E. Bertch, D. S. Rich, L. Ereshefsky, and R. M. Elenbaas, Prospectus on the economic value of clinical pharmacy services: a position statement of the American College of Clinical Pharmacy. *Pharmacotherapy: The Journal of Human Pharmacology and Drug Therapy*, 1989. 9(1): p. 45-56.

[19] Haig, G. M. and L. A. Kiser, Effect of pharmacist participation on a medical team on costs, charges, and length of stay. *American Journal of Hospital Pharmacy*, 1991. 48(7): p. 1457-1462.

[20] Boyko Jr, W. L., P. J. Yurkowski, M. F. Ivey, J. A. Armitstead, and B. L. Roberts, Pharmacist influence on economic and morbidity outcomes in a tertiary care teaching hospital. *American Journal of Health-System Pharmacy*, 1997. 54(14): p. 1591-1595.

[21] Clapham, C. E., C. D. Hepler, T. P. Reinders, M. E. Lehman, and L. Pesko, Economic consequences of two drug-use control systems in a teaching hospital. *American Journal of Hospital Pharmacy*, 1988. 45(11): p. 2329-2340.

Chapter 2

First Aid

Amira abo Youssef*

Pharmacology and Toxicology Department, Faculty of Pharmacy,
Beni-Suef University, Beni Suef, Egypt

Learning Objectives

After completing this chapter, students will be able to:

- Define what is first aid
- Identify different types of injuries
- Outline the appropriate first aid measures for different types of injuries
- Understand the main role and responsibilities of the first aider
- Identify components of the first aid kits

Overview

The first few minutes following any physical injury or medical emergency are extremely crucial. It is highly recommended to stay tranquil and start an action to help the victim. Any knowledge regarding first aid will be of great importance in dealing with any sudden situation.

First aid is defined as providing basic medical care to a victim who suffers from sudden injury or illness. In general, it should be performed by a trained person to help the victim survive till professional medical help is reachable. It typically comprises a group of simple and sometimes life-saving procedures that an individual can be prepared to perform with the simplest minimal equipment.

Occasionally, the appropriate first aid measures are adequate such as, applying a Band-Aid on a cut or ice on a burn.

It is very crucial to clarify that the job of the first aid provider is completely different from that of a physician. His job is only restricted to the period between the accident and the appearance of the doctor and/or the ambulance.

---

* Corresponding Author's Email: amira.aboyoussef@gmail.com.

In: Clinical Pharmacist Tools to Deliver Rational Medication Use
Editor: Mohamed Emam Abdelmobdy Abdelrahim
ISBN: 979-8-88697-857-5

The main objectives of first aid include: lifesaving, prevention of any further harm, for example, transferring the victim away from the danger and stopping bleeding by applying pressure on the wound, and starting and speeding up recovery. Additionally, the first aid provider should also call the Emergency Medical Service (EMS), and alarm the surroundings regarding the danger. Keep him safe and away from any harm and comfort the victim. An ambulance is required in certain situations such as dyspnea, severe bleeding, shock……etc. Generally, the fastest method for providing emergency is to transport the victim using the car to the closest hospital unless it is dangerous to move the victim or the traffic may cause a delay in reaching the hospital. [1]

Many Medical Conditions Necessitate First Aid Including: Altitude sickness, anaphylaxis, bone fracture, burns, choking, near-drowning or asphyxiation, insect and animal bites, stings, etc.

History-taking questions are summarized using the acronym **CHAMPION**

C: Chief complain.
H: History of chief complaints.
A: Allergies.
M: Medical history and medications.
P: Pain assessment.
I: Important Information (Name, date of birth, age, address….).
O: Onset.
N: Next of Kin (who to contact?).

First aid steps include:

1. Field inspection to ensure the safety of both the victim and the first aid provider. This also may provide a quick clue for the cause of the injury and the diagnosis. For example, if you find the victim lying under a tree. The first thing to suspect is falling from the tree and suffering from fractures and internal bleeding.
2. History taking is very important and may help in providing the proper first aid help. History taking can be provided from the victim himself if conscious or from the spectators who had witnessed the accident.

What Are the Main Essential First Aid Skills?

ABCs, i.e., Airway, Breathing, and circulation. These three are very crucial and must be inspected before any interventions.

Airways: kept open by using the "*head tilt-chin lift*" technique. Usually, the unconscious victim can swallow their tongue. This may lead to airway obstruction.

Head tilt-chin lift is performed by putting your palm on the victim's forehead and gently pushing down then with the other hand; gently lifting the chin forward to open the airway.

Breathing: an examination of breathing usually takes place by look listen and feeling steps. Firstly, put your ear next to the victim's mouth and nose and ***look*** if the chest is rising or not. Listen carefully if there are any abnormal breathing sounds and finally ***feel*** for air movement on your cheek. *After* 5-10 seconds if you do not see, hear or feel normal signs of breathing you should immediately start mouth-to-mouth or mouth-to-nose breathing (in case of mouth injury).

Circulation: Pulse can be checked using radial or carotid arteries in the case of adults and brachial artery in the case of infants. You can count the pulse by using a watch. The normal pulse rate for adults is 60-80 beats/min while in children is about 80-140 beats/min. A carotid pulse can be determined by keeping a head-tilt position with one hand and then spotting the victim's Adam's apple with two fingers using the other hand. Move your fingers into the groove between Adam's apple and the muscle on the neck side where the carotid pulse can be detected. Radial pulse can be determined by pressing on the radial artery using the middle two fingers. In infants, the pulse is to be detected by pressing on the brachial artery between the elbow and shoulder.

Temperature recording: It is essential to measure the temperature whenever possible. The normal temperature ranges between 36.6ºC-37.2ºC. The thermometer is to be placed under the tongue, in the rectum, or under the armpit. The rectal temperature is higher than the oral by a half degree while that under the armpit is lower by a half degree. It is not allowed to use mouth thermometers if the victim is unconscious, or with an injured nose or mouth. An oral thermometer is not suitable for young children. [2]

Self-Assessment Questions

1. First aid means:
   a. Taking the victim to the hospital immediately
   b. The provision of initial and simple care for an illness or injury
   c. Medical treatment of an injured person
   d. Checking the vital signs of the victim

2. Duties of the first aid provider include:
   a. Notifying emergency medical service
   b. Giving alarm to others in the area
   c. Comforting the victim
   d. All of the above

3. If the victim is unconscious, what should you manage first?
   a. Bleeding
   b. Airway and breathing
   c. Spinal injury
   d. Fracture

4. When performing basic life support, how do we check for normal breathing?
   a. By holding a mirror up to the victim's mouth
   b. By looking for chest movement, listening, and feeling for normal breathing
   c. By putting our ear to their chest
   d. By looking and listening for any signs of movement

Cardio-Pulmonary-Resuscitation (CPR)

CPR is a technique for keeping someone alive until emergency services or an ambulance arrives. It is a combination of mouth-to-mouth breathing and chest compressions. The main objective is to keep blood flow to the brain and other vital organs. Firstly, assess if the victim is conscious or unconscious. If he is unconscious have someone call the emergency medical service (EMS) and instantly, start CPR. If you are alone, start CPR for two minutes and then call the EMS.

Steps of CPR For Adults and Children > 8

1. Start CPR with 30 chest compressions by clasping your hands together and placing them in the center of the casualty's chest in between the nipples. You should keep your elbows in a straight position and your shoulders above your hands. By using your upper body weight, push fast to compress the chest 1.5 to 2 inches (nearly 2 compressions per second).
2. Once you have delivered 30compressions, tilt the head back and lift the chin and then start to give the casualty two breaths. Make sure to close the nostrils and then take a deep breath and then put your lips on the victim's mouth and breath into it. A breath should last a second and you should notice the chest rise.
3. Carry on CPR until the casualty shows any signs of responsiveness or until the arrival of the ambulance.

Steps of CPR in children (1-8 years): Similar except we use only ***one hand*** to perform chest compressions.

Steps in infants (<1 year age): Use only *two fingers* for chest compressions down about only 1 inch. Give smaller rescue breaths enough only to raise the chest. [3]

Self-Assessment Questions

1. The following is true about CPR EXCEPT
   a. Pinch the nostrils shut for mouth-to-mouth breathing
   b. Use your arms only to compress the chest
   c. After 30 compressions tilt the head back and lift the chin up to open the airway
   d. Continue CPR until there are signs of movement

2. Which is the correct ratio of chest compressions to mouth breathing for use in CPR of an adult victim?
   a. 2 compressions: 30 breaths
   b. 5 compressions:1 breath
   c. 15 compression:2 breaths
   d. 30 compressions:2 breaths

The Recovery Position

This is a technique approved to treat unresponsive adults who breathe normally except for those suspected to have a spinal injury. Unconscious causality lying on his back (face upwards) can suffer from two major risks that 5rends up leading to suffocation. Firstly, fluids such as blood or vomitus can gather in the back of the throat leading to lungs and respiratory obstruction. Secondly, when a person is lying face up, the esophagus bends down slightly from the stomach toward the throat. This may lead to passive regurgitation (the stomach contents pass into the throat) leading to airway obstruction and aspiration pneumonia. The recovery position will allow the drainage of any fluids, and the chest is raised above the ground thus breathing will be easier. [4]

First Aid Steps to Put Causality in the Recovery Position

1. Kneel beside the victim lying on his back and takes any glasses and any objects from his pocket.
2. Make sure that both legs of the casualty are straight. Place his arm closest to you at right angles to his body with his elbow bent and palm facing upwards.
3. Place the casualty's other arm across his chest and put his hand against his face on the cheek nearest you.
4. Pull the patient's furthest knee up and keep his foot on the ground.
5. Keep the casualty's hand pressed on his cheek and then pull the far leg
6. towards you and roll the casualty onto his side.
7. Move the casualty's upper leg to make his hip and knee bent at right angles.
8. Secure the airways by tilting the casualty's head back.
9. Keep observing the casualty's breathing, pulse, and level of consciousness until the arrival of the ambulance.

N.B. If the casualty stays in the recovery position for more than 30 minutes, you should roll him on his back and then roll him to his other side.

Self-Assessment Questions

1. The recovery position is a first-aid technique recommended for assisting someone who is _______
   a. Unconscious and not breathing
   b. Conscious and not breathing
   c. Unconscious and breathing
   d. Conscious and breathing

2. If the casualty stays in the recovery position for more than _______, you should roll him on his back and then roll him to his other side.
   a. 10 minutes
   b. 20 minutes
   c. 30 minutes
   d. 60 minutes'

Effects of Temperature

Hypothermia

Hypothermia is when your body temperature is less than 35 ℃ due to exposure to cold temperature for a long period. Hypothermia occurs when there is more heat lost than heat generated by your body. It is usually caused by wet or insufficient clothes, falling in cold water, due to some medical conditions such as malnutrition and hypothyroidism. The main symptoms of hypothermia include pale and cold skin, slow breathing, shivering, slurred speech, fatigue, and confusion. [5]

First Aid Steps

1. Call EMS and move the victim immediately out of the cold if possible and if this is not feasible try to protect the person from winds by covering his head and insulating his body from the cold.
2. Replace wet clothes with a warm dry covering.
3. While waiting for the ambulance, monitor the casualty's breathing, and if there is no breathing start CPR instantly.

Heatstroke

Heatstroke is one of the most serious forms of heat-related problems. It usually results from over-exercise or heavy work in a hot environment combined with inadequate fluid intake. People with high risk for heat stroke include young children, the elderly, obese people, pregnant and breastfeeding females, people with poor cardiovascular fitness or with diabetes or kidney diseases, and people with an impaired ability to sweat. Symptoms include raised body temperature (40 >), confusion, dizziness, fainting, rapid heartbeat, breathing, and headache. The skin may become hot and dry.

First Aid Management

1. Immediately, remove the victim from exposure to extreme heat to a shady or cooled air -conditioner space.
2. Remove layers of clothes and loosen anything tightening the casualty.
3. Lay the person down and elevate the legs and feet slightly.
4. Cover the casualty with wet sheets or spray or sponge him with cold water to cool him.
5. Call EMS.
6. Offer him to drink cool water if the casualty is conscious and able to swallow.

Fever

Hypothalamus controls temperature and keeps normal body temperature via heating mechanisms such as shivering and via cooling mechanisms such as sweating. Fever occurs when body temperature is greater-than-normal body temperature (> 37°C). It is one of the body's reactions to infection. The main causes of fever include infections, poisons, heat exposure, some medications (thyroxine, amphetamine, ...), and some diseases (cancer, HIV,....). [6]

Fever might be dangerous and needs immediate medical help, if it occurs in babies and rectal temperature is > 38.0 °C, it lasts for longer than 3 days in adults or children. If it is associated with dehydration, febrile seizures, headache, skin rash, swelling of the throat, mental confusion, lack of appetite, ...

Adults

1. It can be reduced using NSAID s such as ibuprofen or acetaminophen. It is much better to alternate between both drugs to reduce overdose side effects.
2. The casualty should drink lots of water to avoid dehydration.
3. Any other therapies mainly depend on the main causes of the fever.

Children

1. Reduce the temperature by using alternating doses of acetaminophen and ibuprofen. Never use aspirin as it may cause Reye syndrome.
2. Avoid keeping children overdressed indoors.
3. Use cold packs to reduce temperature (Never use alcohol in a bath or rub it on the skin as it is poisonous to children).
4. Make the child drink fluids such as non-carbonated decaffeinated drinks or juice (water is not enough as it doesn't contain the necessary electrolytes and glucose).
5. Never give the child tea or caffeinated drinks as it will increase water loss by increasing urination.
6. In case of vomiting, give the child an antiemetic drug either by injection or by rectal suppository.

Febrile Seizures

Usually, occur in children (3 months-5years) with fever. They last for a few minutes. Seizures happen when the brain is highly sensitive to fever. They are not harmful and do not cause brain damage or epilepsy. It is very important to seek medical care if seizures predominate for more than five minutes, no breathing or cyanosis. Main causes include viral or bacterial infections and CNS infections such as meningitis. They are mostly generalized and may include any of the following symptoms; stiffening of the body, Jerking of the arms and legs, urinary incontinence, lack of response to any stimuli, and noisy or slow breathing. [7]

First Aid Measures

1. Maintain breathing by protecting the airways.
2. Clear the mouth by removing any food or pacifier.

3. Place the child on his side.
4. In case of vomiting try to clear your mouth. Use a suction pump if available.
5. Perform a chin-lift maneuver if there is labored breathing.
6. Never try to stop seizure movements by restraining the child.
7. To control the seizures, apply cold compresses on the face and neck and sponge the whole body with cold water.
8. Lower the fever by giving medications such as acetaminophen suppository.

Self-Assessment Questions

1. Symptoms of heat stroke include all the following EXCEPT:
   a. Markedly elevated body temperature, generally greater than 40ºC.
   b. Changes in mental status
   c. Slow heartbeat
   d. The skin may be hot and dry

2. Which of the following statement is not true regarding the management of heat stroke?
   a. Move the person out of the sun
   b. Lay the person down and with the legs and feet below the level of the heart
   c. Cool the person by covering him or her with damp sheets
   d. Loosen or remove the person's clothing

3. When to seek medical help in case of fever?
   a. In babies with rectal temperature > 40.0 °C .
   b. In children and adults with fever longer than four days.
   c. If febrile seizures develop in children
   d. All of the above

4. When to seek medical care in case of febrile seizures?
   a. The seizure lasts more than 5 minutes
   b. The child has serious troubled breathing
   c. The child develops cyanosis
   d. All of the above

Respiratory and Circulatory Emergencies

Choking

Choking is defined as the inability to breathe effectively due to the blockage of the upper airway. It may only cause simple coughing fits, but if complete obstruction of the airways occurs, it can lead to brain death within 3-5 min. Anyone can choke; however, it is more common in children than in adults. It is a true medical emergency and requires fast intervention. It is mainly caused by: *eating without improper chewing or quickly, eating large pieces of food at one time or large hard candies, talking or laughing while chewing, and putting small objects in the mouth such as pins, marbles, or coins.*

Symptoms include; coughing or gagging, universal choking signs (clutching the throat with hands), sudden loss the ability of to talk, cyanosis, and difficulty breathing. It may also lead to loss of consciousness. [8]

First-Aid Measures

1. If you have someone, make him call the ambulance and you immediately start first aid. If you are alone start first measures before dialing the emergency number.
2. If the victim is not cyanosed but coughing, ask him the following question *"Are you choking?"*. If it is only a partial obstruction, the casualty will be able to answer your question by talking. In such a condition, ask him to cough continuously until the obstruction is cleared.
3. Never offer the casualty anything to drink as fluids may fill up the space for air passage.
4. If the victim is cyanosed and there is no breathing, *five and five* approaches should be started. Firstly, *start* five back blows between the person's shoulder blades using the heel of your hand. Secondly, perform five sub-diaphragmatic thrusts *(Heimlich maneuver).*
5. Alternate between the five blows and five sub-diaphragmatic thrusts until the blockage is cleared.

How to Perform the Heimlich Maneuver

In Adults and Children (>1 year):

1. Stand behind the person. Wrap your arms around his waist.
2. Make a fist with one hand just above the victim's navel.
3. Clutch the fist with your other hand and press hard on the abdomen (quick, *inward, and upward* thrust, as if trying to lift the person).
4. Complete a total of five abdominal thrusts and repeat the *five and five* cycles as long as it is needed to clear the blockage.

In Babies (<1 year):

1. Sit and hold the infant face down on your forearm and make him rest on your thigh. Support the infant's head and neck by using your hand, and place the head lower than the trunk.
2. Deliver up to five gentle but firm back blows forcefully between the infant's shoulder blades by using the heel of your hand. Both combination of the gravity and the black blows should clear the blockage.
3. Turn the infant faceup on your forearm, resting on your thigh with the head lower than the trunk if the infant still not breathing. Use two fingers placed at the center of the

infant's breastbone, give five quick chest compressions Press down about 1 1/2 inches, and let the chest rise again in between each compression.

4. Repeat the back blows and chest thrusts if breathing doesn't resume. Call EMS.
5. If one of the two techniques opens the airway but the infant still not breathing, begin infant CPR.
6. Give only abdominal thrusts, if the child is older than age 1 and conscious.

Do not use too much force to avoid damage to the ribs or internal organs.

In unconscious persons:

1. Place the person on his back onto the floor.
2. If you see a visible blockage in the throat, clear the airway by reaching a finger into the mouth and removing the object. You should be careful not to push the object deeper into the airway
3. Bow beside the victim's hips and put the heel of one of your hands on the victim's abdomen *slightly above the navel. Place the other hand on the first.*
4. Press both hands into the abdomen and perform five quick upward thrusts.
5. Start CPR if the airways are still blocked. Chest compressions used in CPR may clear the blockage.

In pregnant/obese people:

In a pregnant female or an obese person, abdominal thrusts will not be effective so instead, chest thrusts are used.

Alone and Choking

1. If you are choking and there is no one around to help. Place your hand as if you are performing the maneuver on another person and deliver an inward and upward abdominal thrust to yourself.
2. Alternatively, bend your belly over a firm object like the back of the chair and perform the thrust.

Shock

Shock is a critical condition that occurs due to a sudden drop in blood flow through the body. It may lead to organ failure and death. It can be caused by many conditions such as trauma, heatstroke hemorrhage, allergic reaction, severe infection, poisoning, and severe burns. Symptoms of shock include; cold, clammy pale skin, bluish lips or fingernails, nausea and vomiting, dizziness or fainting, fast breathing and pulse, lethargy, mydriasis, and alteration in mental status.

First-Aid Measures

1. Call EMS then start the following steps.
2. Place the victim down and raise his legs and feet slightly (skip this if it may cause pain or further injury).
3. Start CPR if the victim is not breathing.
4. Lose any tight clothes and if necessary, cover him with a blanket.
5. Do not allow the victim to eat or drink anything.
6. If you suspect that the cause of the shock is an allergic reaction, use an epinephrine autoinjector, if the victim has one with him
7. If the victim is bleeding, hold pressure over the bleeding area, using a towel.
8. If the victim is vomiting and no spinal injury is suspected, roll the victim on his side (the recovery position).

Self-Assessment Questions

1. You are having lunch with a friend and he begins to choke on some food. He can not speak, or breathe what should you do first?
   a. Encourage him to cough
   b. Put your fingers down his throat to try to dislodge the obstruction
   c. The Heimlich manoeuvre
   d. Give up to five back blows between his shoulder blade

2. Choking may be caused by
   a. Poor dental fitting
   b. Chewing food improperly
   c. Parkinsonism
   d. All of the above

3. The universal choking sign is:
   a. Gagging
   b. The sudden inability of talking
   c. Hand signals, panic, and clutching the throat
   d. Cyanosis

4. When helping an unconscious choking victim you would give an adult ______ thrust and for an infant, you would give _____ back blows and _____ chest thrusts
   a. 3,3,3
   b. 5,3,3
   c. 5,5,5
   d. 3,5,5

5. First-aid of shock includes:
   a. Keeping the victim warm
   b. Putting the victim in the recovery position
   c. Help the victim to walk around
   d. All of the above

6. Shock is a condition where:
   a. The respiratory system fails to deliver air to the lung
   b. The cardiovascular system fails to deliver blood to the heart
   c. The circulatory system fails to deliver blood to all parts of the body
   d. All of the above

Surgical Emergencies

Fractures and Dislocations

Fracture	Dislocation
A fracture is a partial or complete break in a bone. It can occur crosswise, lengthwise, in several places, or in many pieces. It usually happens when a bone is impacted by more force or pressure than it can support. Fractures usually occur due to car accidents, falls, or sports injuries. It may also be due to low bone density and osteoporosis.	*A dislocation* occurs when the bones in a joint become knocked out of their usual positions. It can be very painful and lead to uneasiness in the movement of the affected joint area. It can also lead to tears in the surrounding muscles, tendons, or nerves. It can take place in any joint in the body, although they usually affect: Jaw, hip, elbow, shoulder, knee, and finger. Car accidents fall, and contact sports such as football are the main usual causes of dislocation
Symptoms of fractures include: *1. Intense pain.* *2. Deformity, tenderness, swelling, and discoloration of the bone.* *3. If the bone cracks the skin, bleeding can occur.* *4. If there is a nerve injury, loss of sensation may occur.*	*Symptoms of dislocations include:* *1. Swelling and bruising.* *2. Pain and instability of the joint.* *3. Inability to move the joint.* *4. Bone can appear out of its place.*

First Aid Steps

1. If there is bleeding, use a clean cloth or gauze and apply pressure on the source of the bleeding. Yet, never press the bone if it is visible. Take off any clothing around the injured area.
2. Try to leave the injured bone in its position and keep it immobilized. Movement may lead to further shock.
3. Apply ice packs to the affected area to reduce swelling. To avoid frost biting, never directly apply ice to the skin. Put it in a cloth or a bag and then use it.
4. To immobilize the injured bone and support it, splinting is used. A splint can be made from any basic household items such as rolled newspapers, cardboard, aluminum, sticks, or a backpack frame. You can use the splint with a cloth or belt.
5. Splinting means immobilization of the joint just above and below the broken bone without affecting the circulation; e.g., for a broken arm from the middle splint the elbow and the wrist.
6. In case of rib fracture, if the victim suffers from difficulty in breathing, advise him to take a shorter breath.
7. Inspect the limb near the fracture or dislocation, for any loss of sensation (nerve injury) or decreased temperature and pulse (arterial injury).

8. If the person faints or breathes in short- rapid breaths lay the person down with the head slightly lower than the trunk and, if possible, elevate the legs.
9. Immediately, if the bone penetrates the skin, if the extremity is cold, or if the pulse or sensation declines.

Very important: if you suspect a fracture of the neck or the backbone, NEVER try to move the victim

Sprain

A sprain means the tearing of a ligament on or near a joint. It occurs when soft tissues surrounding bones are overstretched due to a sudden movement. Most commonly, these ligaments, muscles, and tendons are injured in sports activities. [9]

First Aid Steps

1. Get the casualty to sit or lie down. Raise his injured limb and support it in a comfortable position.
2. Apply an ice pack to the injured part to reduce pain, bruising, and swelling.
3. Surround the area with some cotton wool or soft padding.
4. Keep the injured limb in its place by applying a bandage. Apply the bandage as far as the next joint. For example, if the injury is in the ankle, apply the bandage from the toes to the knees.
5. Elevate the injured part and comfortably support it using cushions or pillows.
6. Monitor the casualty's circulation every 10 minutes and if the bandage is affecting the circulation, take it off and reapply it more loosely.
7. Encourage the casualty to rest his injured limb and seek advice from a doctor if needed.
8. If the casualty suffers from severe pain or can not use his limb immediately seek medical care r take him to the hospital.

Always remember the **RICE** procedure:

R Rest the injured part.
I Apply ice packs or cold compresses.
C Provide comfortable support.
E Elevate the injured part.

Self-Assessment Questions

1. Which of the following is not true about dislocation?
   a. It may occur in major joints
   b. It may occur in your toe
   c. It is a crack in the bone
   d. May cause injury to nerves and blood vessels

2. The following is not true about fractures
   a. Not to move the injured area
   b. Support the broken limb with a splint
   c. Apply ice directly to the skin above the fractured bone
   d. If there is a wound cover it with a dry dressing

Burns

Medical Treatment for Burns

For minor burns, an antiseptic spray is usually used followed by a topical anti-burn ointment or an ointment with silver content and dressings. Severe burns may need surgery to clean the wounds or even skin grafting. Eye injuries require an examination by an ophthalmologist.

Electrical Burns

The risk from electrical shock leans mainly on the path and voltage of current through the body, the overall, health, and how quickly the person is first aided. Strong electrical shock can lead to internal damage, permanent seizures, depression, anxiety, and fractures. Death in hospitalized patients after electric shock usually occurs due to infection. Symptoms include; dysrhythmia, cardiac arrest, respiratory failure, loss of consciousness, numbness, and seizures.

First Aid Steps

1. Dial The EMS.
2. Inspect the place first and be careful never to touch the victim as he might be in still in touch with the electrical source.
3. Search for the electricity source and turn it off if feasible. If this is not possible, use a nonconducting tool (something made of wood, plastic, or cardboard) to move the source of electricity away from you and the victim.
4. Check up the ABCs and if breathing is a
5. Check for ABCs (breathing, coughing, or movement). If breathing is not present, instantly start CPR.
6. Prevent shock. Lay the victim on his back and if possible, put the head in a position lower than that of the trunk and elevate his legs to avoid shock.
7. Cover any burned areas with a sterile gauze bandage, if accessible. If not use a clean dry cloth. Avoid using any material with loose fibers such as a blanket or towel as they may stick to the burn.
8. Support the neck especially if you suspect that the victim has fallen from a height.

Immediately seek medical care if:

1. Apparent burn in the skin that is not healing well.
2. Increased redness, or drainage from the burn.

3. The victim is a pregnant woman.
4. There is a loss of consciousness.
5. There are any hearing, speech, or vision problems.
6. Apparent numbness, tingling, or paralysis.

Thermal Burns

They are very popular, especially with children. The number of skin layers affected determines the severity and the type of the burn. They are classified as superficial, partial, and full based on their thickness and are usually caused by injury from steam, fire, flame, and molten liquid.

Minor Burns

1. If possible, get rid of any hot or burned clothes.
2. To cool down the burnt area, put it under cold running water for a minimum of 5 minutes. If this is unfeasible bathe the burn in cold water compresses. Never use ice directly on the skin to avoid frostbite.
3. Cover the burn with burn cream, then with a bandage. Avoid cotton as it can irritate the skin.
4. To relieve pain, you can take an over-the-counter pain reliever such as acetaminophen or ibuprofen.
5. Seek medical help if any signs of infections such as elevated pain, redness, fever, swelling, or oozing appear.
6. If blisters are present, do not break them as this may increase the risk of infection.

Major Burns

1. Immediately, seek medical care.
2. If there is no breathing or circulation, start CPR.
3. Raise body parts above the heart level.
4. Never remove burnt clothes. Make sure that the victim is not still in contact with the smoke or the heat.
5. Never immerse the burn if it is large or severe in cold water as this may lead to shock.
6. Use a sterile gauze bandage to cover the burnt area
7. Instantly seek medical care if the burn affects genitals, eyes, ears, hands, feet, or major joints, it is a full-thickness burn and it is painless, it is a large partial-thickness burn (more than twice palms size) and there are severe uncontrolled pain and breathing difficulties.

Chemical Burns

The most common chemicals that cause chemical burns mainly include strong acids and strong bases (bleaching agents, chlorinated pools, and metal cleaners). Symptoms of chemical burns include irritation, redness, pain and numbness, blisters or charred skin, shortness of breath, and some visual changes if the chemical reaches the eye.

First Aid Measures

1. Wash the chemical off the skin using cool running water for at least twenty minutes. Flush the chemicals on the skin surface with cool, running water for 20 minutes or more. If it is a powder-like substance, brush it off the skin before washing it.
2. Take off any jewelry or clothes contaminated with the chemical agent.
3. To relieve pain, use a cool wet cloth or towel.
4. Apply a burn cream and use a dry sterile bandage or a clean cloth to cover the burnt area loosely.
5. Minor chemical burns do not usually require any further treatment and heal rapidly.
6. In some cases, IV fluids may be required to adjust blood pressure and heart rate.
7. If applicable, an antidote can be used to counteract the chemical.
8. Seek medical help for any signs of shock or uncontrolled severe pain, a second-degree burn that is large than 7.5 cm in diameter, and for eye, hands, feet, face, or a major joint burn.

Sunburns

Sunburns are very common when you visit the beach, go fishing, or work directly under the sun. Light-skinned and fair-haired people are usually at higher risk of sunburn injury. Mild sunburns can result in minor skin redness and irritation while severe and untreated sunburns can cause shock and even death. They are usually caused by exposure to Ultraviolet radiation from the sun. Symptoms of mild sunburns include red irritated skin and pain. This usually occurs 2-6 hours after exposure. Symptoms of severe cases include blisters, severe skin burning, dehydration, electrolyte imbalance, and, a high risk of infection.

First-Aid Steps

1. Use cool compresses soaked in equal parts of milk and water or aloe-based lotions several times a day.
2. Cool (not ice cold) baths may help. Adding 1/2 cup of cornstarch or baking soda to your bath water may also help.
3. Never puncture blisters and leave them intact to decrease the risk of infection.
4. Evade scrubbing or shaving the skin and avoid using perfumes or bath oils.
5. do not rub your skin and only use soft towels to dry yourself Use soft towels to gently dry yourself. do not rub.
6. Only apply fragrance-free skin moisturizer and never use any lotions that contain topical anesthetics.
7. Stay as much as possible out of the sun and take plenty of fluids to avoid dehydration.
8. If necessary, take an over-the-counter pain reliever.
9. Silver sulfadiazine cream can be used to treat mild sunburns and in severe cases, with appropriate cautions about use on the face. In severe cases, oral steroid therapy might be used for several days.
10. Immediately seek medical care if there is; severe pain, severe blistering, headache, nausea or vomiting, and loss of consciousness.

Self-Assessment Questions

1. The following is true regarding first aid management of major burns EXCEPT:
   a. Check for ABCs
   b. Remove the burnt clothes
   c. Elevate the burned body part
   d. Use a cool moist sterile bandage to cover the burn

2. Why burns should be covered with a clean or sterile dressing?
   a. To prevent infection
   b. To cool the burned area
   c. To keep the burned area warm
   d. Both a and c

3. When you care for a victim who has a large burn on their forearm, you ....
   a. Immerse in cold water or use ice
   b. Remove any cloth that has stuck to the burn
   c. Use running cool water to cool the burn
   d. All of the above

4. What should your first action be when treating an electrical burn?
   a. Ensure the victim is still breathing
   b. Wash the burn with cold water
   c. Ensure that contact with the electrical source is broken
   d. Check for level of response

5. What degree of burn causes a large amount of damage but minimal pain?
   a. Superficial burn
   b. Partial-thickness superficial burns
   c. Partial-thicknesses deep burns
   d. All of the above

6. Which of the following is the first measure in case of electric shock?
   a. Touch the victim and move him away
   b. Cover the victim with a blanket
   c. Lay the person down with the head slightly higher than the trunk

7. In chemical burns seek medical care in case of the following EXCEPT;
   a. The victim has signs of shock
   b. It resulted in uncontrolled pain
   c. It leads to a first-degree pain
   d. It occurred in the eye

8. Symptoms of sunburns include:
   a. Flu-like syndrome
   b. Nausea and vomiting
   c. Skin loss
   d. All of the above

Blisters

Blisters are commonly caused by friction and burns. Generally, if it is not painful, keep it intact if possible as the unbroken skin over a blistering acts as a natural barrier from bacteria and decreases any risk of infection. Small blisters are covered with an adhesive bandage while large blisters are covered with a porous, plastic-coated gauze pad that absorbs moisture and allows the wound to breathe. If a blister is painful or averts you from walking or using one of your hands include the following first aid tips to puncture it without damaging the overlying intact skin.

First Aid Steps

1. Clean your hands and the blister with warm water and soap.
2. Wipe the blister with rubbing alcohol.
3. Sanitize a sharp needle using rubbing alcohol.
4. Start to puncture the blister in several spots near the blister's edge using the needle. Allow the fluid to drain.
5. Cover the blister with a bandage or gauze pad.
6. After several days, cut all the dead skin, using alcohol sterilized tweezers and scissors sterilized then apply more ointment and recover with a bandage.
7. If any signs of infection appear around the blister (pus, redness, warmth....) immediately call your doctor.
8. To avoid having blisters, use gloves, socks, or a bandage to protect the area being rubbed. Additionally, special athletic socks with extra padding can be used.

Self-Assessment Questions

1. In case of minor burns, it is better to break blisters
   a. True
   b. False

2. In blisters:
   a. Wash your hands and the blister with soap and warm water
   b. Swab the blister with iodine or rubbing alcohol
   c. Use the needle to puncture the blister near its edges
   d. All of the above

Animal Bites

Dogs, cats, hamsters, and squirrels are common animals that can bite adults and children. Dogs bite humans more than cats. However, cat bites are more likely to cause infection. A high risk of rabies occurs in domestic animals that are non-immunized or bite is from wild animals. Any animal bites must be evaluated by a physician for the following reasons: Risk of infection, embedded broken teeth or any other foreign material, rabies, nerve or blood vessel damage, and severe bleeding. [10]

First Aid Management Steps

1. If the bite only causes a superficial cut (minor wound) there is no risk of rabies and you will only need to wash it with soap and water and cover it with a bandage.
2. If the bites cause a deep wound in the skin (major wound) or the skin is badly torn and bleeds, apply pressure using a clean dry cloth to stop bleeding and then seek medical help.
3. If there are any signs of infection (severe pain, edema, redness, warmth at the site, and fever), immediately see a doctor.
4. For pain control, the doctor may prescribe an OTC drug such as ibuprofen or acetaminophen.
5. The doctor might also prescribe an antibiotic such as amoxicillin for heavily contaminated bites.
6. If the bite is caused by an animal that might carry rabies, the doctor will recommend a tetanus shot.

> ✓ Doctors usually recommend a tetanus shot every 10 years
> ✓ However, if your last shot is less than 5 years ago and the bite is deep or highly contaminated, the doctor may recommend a booster sot within 48 hours.

Snake Bites

Snake venom is a combination of many substances with various actions namely, cytotoxins (local tissue damage), hemotoxins (c internal bleeding), neurotoxins (affect the nervous system), and cardiotoxins (affect the heart). Symptoms of snake bite include pain, swelling tenderness, and bleeding (local effect), internal organs bleeding such as the brain, effects on the nervous system (vision, speaking,.... problems), and multiple muscle death.

First Aid Management

1. Try to keep calm as possible.
2. Never try to catch the snake as it might bite you.
3. To retard the absorption of the venom, immobilize the bitten arm or leg.
4. Remove any jewelry as edema might progress and can cut off the blood flow.
5. To reduce the movement of the affected area, apply a loose (doesn't restrict blood flow).
6. Never use a tourniquet as it might increase tissue damage.
7. It is not recommended to apply ice as it doesn't deactivate the venom and may cause frostbite.

8. do not cut the wound or suck the venom as you might increase the risk of damage to the underlying organs or infection.
9. Never use alcohol. Although it might decrease pain it can cause vasodilatation and increase venom absorption.
10. Giving the ant venom to the victim is lifesaving so seek medical attention as soon as possible.

Insect Bites

A bee, wasp, mosquito, etc., sting usually causes a mild but sudden sharp pain as well as mild swelling that disappears soon. Symptoms include pain, redness, itching, and swelling. The delayed reaction might include fever and swollen glands and few people might develop anaphylaxis.

First Aid Steps

1. Firstly, calm the casualty and try to move him to a safer area to avoid more stings.
2. If you can see the stinger, scrape it out using a hard straight edge such as a bank card or a fingernail.
3. Do not try to pinch the stinger with your fingers, as you may spread the venom.
4. Clean the affected area with soap and water.
5. To minimize the swelling raise the area where the casualty has been stung and apply a cold compress and an ice pack for at least 10 minutes.
6. Loosen any tight clothing and use a blanket to cover the victim
7. Do not try to give him something to drink or to eat.
8. Check, the ABCs and if there is no breathing, commence CPR.
9. Turn the casualty on his side if you notice vomiting or bleeding from the mouth to avoid choking.
10. Keep monitoring the casualty for any severe reactions such as wheezing or difficulty breathing, a swollen face, mouth, or throat, rapid heart rate, dizziness or feeling faint, difficulty swallowing, or becoming unresponsive. If so, immediately call EMS

Self-Assessment Questions

1. If a girl was bitten by a snake
   a. Apply ice to the wound
   b. Keep the injured area lower than the heart level
   c. Cut an x at the site of injury and suck the blood
   d. All of the above

2. The snake venom usually contains:
   a. Endotoxins
   b. Hemotoxins
   c. Cardiotoxins
   d. All of the above

3. In case of an insect bite, you shouldn't not:
   a. Brush off the stinger with the back of the knife
   b. Try to pull out the stinger
   c. Apply a cold pack
   d. Wash the affected area with soap and water

4. Signs of infection after animal bites include the following EXCEPT:
   a. Redness
   b. Pain
   c. Hypothermia
   d. Oozing

Anaphylaxis

Anaphylaxis is a life-threatening respiratory distress condition of severe allergic reaction that may lead to shock. After exposure to the allergic causing agent; anaphylaxis can develop in sensitive people within a few minutes or up to several hours. Substances causing allergy include insect venom, pollen, dust, some foods, and drugs. Symptoms of anaphylaxis include hives, swelling of the eyes, lips, and throat, difficulty in breathing, shock, mental confusion, nausea and vomiting, diarrhea, and muscle cramping. Sensitive persons who had suffered before from an anaphylactic reaction in the past must carry their medications all the time (e.g., epinephrine, antihistaminics).

First Aid Management

1. Call your local EMS.
2. Assess ABCs, if there are no signs of circulation, start CPR.
3. Check if the casualty is carrying a special medication for allergic reaction treatment such as EpiPen (auto-injector of epinephrine). If it is present, press the autoinjector directly in the thigh and hold it in its place for several seconds and then massage the injection site to increase absorption.
4. After epinephrine administration, give him an antihistaminic pill.
5. Assist the casualty to lie down on his back, and lift and support his legs above the level of his heart.
6. Untighten any clothing; cover the casualty with a blanket.
7. Turn the casualty on his side if you notice vomiting or bleeding from the mouth to avoid choking.

Self-Assessment Questions

1. The following is true about anaphylaxis EXCEPT:
    a. Can be a life-threatening condition
    b. Occur after several hours
    c. Some people have anaphylactic reactions from unknown causes
    d. Can cause abdominal cramping

2. What should a victim with anaphylaxis carry all the time?
    a. Insulin
    b. Paracetamol
    c. Adrenaline
    d. Aspirin

3. First aid management of anaphylaxis includes
    a. Call the emergency medical number
    b. Give the victim cold water
    c. Make the victim lie on his face
    d. All of the above

Asthma Attack

In an asthma attack, the casualty will suffer from muscles spasm in their air passage. This leads to narrowing of the airways and difficulty in breathing. As a first aider, your main priority is to comfort the casualty and ease his breathing. It is a necessity to keep casualties away from any smoke in order not to worsen the case. [11]

First Aid Steps

1. Calm the casualty and encourage him the usual dose of his inhaler and deeply and slowly breathe.
2. Make the casualty sit down in a comfortable position.
3. In the case of mild asthma, the casualty should be better within a few minutes.
4. In severe attacks, make the casualty take one or two puffs from the inhaler every couple of minutes (Maximum 10 puffs) or until he feels better.
5. If the asthma attack is very severe and does not respond to treatment with the inhaler and the casualty becomes exhausted, immediately call EMS.
6. While waiting for the ambulance, keeps monitoring his breathing, pulse, and response level.

Self-Assessment Questions

1. In an asthma attack, you should do all the following EXCEPT:
   a. Make the casualty sit down in a comfortable position
   b. Make the casualty take one or two puffs from the inhaler every couple of minutes in case of mild and severe attacks
   c. If the casualty looks tired and exhausted immediately call the ambulance.
   d. Keep monitoring him till the arrival of the ambulance

2. As a first aider, your main priority is to comfort the casualty and ease his breathing
   a. True
   b. False

Motion Sickness

In some persons, any means of transportation can lead to motion sickness. This can happen all of the sudden and the person starts to feel uncomfortable with increased sweating, nausea, and vomiting. Normally, motion sickness ceases once the motion stops.

Motion sickness can be avoided if you plan well for your trip as follows:

1. If you traveling by ship reserve a cabinet in the front of the middle of the ship.
2. By plane, reserve a seat over the front edge of a wing.
3. By train, request a seat in the front and next to the window.
4. By car, sit in the front passenger's seat or drive by yourself.

First Aid Steps

If you're susceptible to motion sickness, first aid steps includes:

1. Never read and keep your head comfortable and still against your seat back,
2. Always try to focus on the horizon or a far stationary object.
3. Do not smoke or sit beside a smoker.
4. Before or during the trip do not eat any spicy foods or drink alcohol. You can eat dry crackers or drink a carbonated beverage (help settle your stomach).
5. Before you feel sick take an over-the-counter antihistaminic drug such as meclizine (Drowsiness may happen).
6. Applying a scopolamine adhesive patch behind your ear several hours before traveling will provide good protection from motion sickness for around 72 hours.

Self-Assessment Questions

1. The following is true about Motion sickness EXCEPT:
   a. Can be caused by any type of transportation
   b. It can strike suddenly
   c. May quiet down as soon as the motion stops.
   d. The more you travel, the more uneasiness you find

2. You can skip motion sickness by:
   a. Taking a seat near the front and next to a window in the train
   b. Taking a seat in the middle of the airplane
   c. Requesting a cabin in the back of the ship
   d. All of the above

Food Poisoning

Food poisoning usually arises when you consume food containing detrimental germs including viruses, bacteria, or parasites. The most common causes of food poisoning include eating raw or undercooked meat or poultry and consuming unpasteurized dairy products, raw shellfish, and unwashed fruits and vegetables. Food poisoning symptoms can start hours to days and this is mainly due to the cause of poisoning and the amount of food or drink consumed by the casualty. Symptoms include Abdominal cramps or pain, nausea, vomiting, loss of appetite, diarrhea, fever, and weakness.

People at high risk for food poisoning include: children, pregnant females and the elderly, people with chronic medical conditions (liver, kidney diseases....), or weakened immune systems or have recently traveled to areas outside your country where you may have had greater exposure to germs that can cause food poisoning.

First Aid Management

1. Generally, food poisoning cases are mild and can cease within a few days. In such cases, the main objective is to avert dehydration (loss of fluids and electrolytes).
2. Prevent any solid foods or dairy products till vomiting and diarrhea stop
3. When you feel better, ease into eating and drinking again. Only consume easy digested and light food such as toast and bananas boiled potatoes or carrots.
4. Avoid consuming high fat or sugary, spicy fried foods and dairy products.
5. Try to drink plenty of fluids. Avoid milk, caffeinated beverages, and sports drinks.
6. If you noticed any signs of mild dehydration (dry mouth, fatigue, dizziness, headache, confusion......etc.), do the following: take multiple sips of water, soups, or clear sodas, and do not drink any dark sodas, coffee or tea, give children with mild dehydration oral rehydration solution which can help n replacing lost body fluids as it contains a mixture of sugar, salt potassium, and other nutrients.

7. In case of severe dehydration, the casualty may require intravenous fluids and electrolytes and thus should be hospitalized.

How to Elude Food Poisoning

1. Completely and intensively, wash fruits and vegetables.
2. Knives countertops, cutting boards, and other tools should be carefully cleaned before usage.
3. Regularly, wash your hands and different tools.
4. Never mix raw and cooked meats on the same plate.
5. Do not reuse different tools that have been used in cutting raw meat to cut any ingredients that will not be cooked.
6. Meat to be cooked to a minimum of 71°C, poultry to 82°C, and fish to 60°C.
7. Immediately, get rid of dented cans and any expired canned or packaged food and do not use them.
8. If any unused food will not be eaten within four hours, immediately refrigerate it.
9. Avoid leftover foods that have been left out of the refrigerator for a long period in restaurants or at social gatherings.

Self-Assessment Questions

1. Symptoms of food poisoning include
   a. Fever
   b. Abdominal pain
   c. Loss of appetite
   d. All of the above

2. Which of the following is not true about food poisoning?
   a. It can be caused by bacteria or its toxins
   b. It can affect people to the same extent
   c. Travelers have a greater risk
   d. Symptoms can begin after hours to days

Nosebleed

Usually occurs due to nose hit, picking the nose, blowing or sneezing hardy (causing rupture of the blood vessels in the nostrils). It can be also caused by the usage of anticoagulant drugs or increased blood pressure. In children and young adults, it usually originates from the septum. In older adults, it can also start from the septum but it can also begin in the nose interior (might be due to arteries hardening).

First Aid Steps

1. Encourage the casualty to sit down upright. This posture reduces blood pressure in the veins and decreases bleeding.
2. Tilt the causality's head forwards to help the blood drain from his nostrils. Never put the casualty's head back as this will only make the blood run down his throat and can make him feel sick.
3. Ask the casualty to breathe through his mouth. This will help him calm down.
4. Apply pressure by pinching his nostrils together for up to 10 minutes. Ask him not to speak or sniff during this time as this can dislodge blood clots that have started forming in the casualty's nose. Repeat for more than 10 minutes if necessary.
5. Once bleeding has stopped, ask the casualty not to pick or blow his nose or bend down until several hours to avoid rebleeding.
6. If rebleeding occurs, ask him to sniff in forcefully to clear your nose of blood clots, and use a decongestant nasal spray containing oxymetazoline. Pinch the nose again and arrange to take him to see a doctor.

> To avoid frequent nosebleeds, your doctor may advise you to have your blood vessel cauterized.
>
> *Cautery* means burning the blood vessel with electric current, silver nitrate, or a laser.
>
> Use a water-based lubricant on your nostrils to avoid nose bleeding if you are using supplemental oxygen using the nasal tube.

Self-Assessment Questions

1. What steps would you take to control bleeding from nosebleeds?
   a. Sit the victim down, lean forward, and pinch the soft part of the nose
   b. Sit the victim down, lean backward, and pinch the soft part of the nose
   c. Lie victim down and pinch the soft part of the nose
   d. Lie victim down and pinch the top of the nose

2. In children and young adults, nose bleeds:
   a. Starts from the septum
   b. Caused by hardening of arteries
   c. Very difficult to be controlled
   d. All of the above

3. If rebleeding occurs in a nose bleed, you should:
   a. Spray the nostrils with oxymetazoline
   b. Not pinch your nose
   c. Not sniff
   d. All of the above

Severe Bleeding

Severe bleeding from an artery is dark red, usually spurting and it is very serious. It can lead to death within six minutes. However, bleeding from a vein is bright red and flowing and it is not that serious. If applicable, to avoid infection, wash your hands with soap and water and use synthetic gloves first. Never try to reposition any displaced organs or push them back to their places. Only, cover the wound with a dressing.

First Aid Steps

1. Firstly, wear synthetic disposable gloves and get rid of any clothing, dirt, or debris on the wound. Never, remove large or deeply embedded objects. In such a case, your main target is to stop bleeding.
2. To stop bleeding, put a sterile bandage or clean cloth on the wound. Press it firmly using your palm. Press constantly until the bleeding stops. You may maintain pressure by binding the wound tightly with a thick bandage or a piece of clean cloth.
3. Help the injured person lie down. If possible, cover the victim with a blanket to avoid hypothermia. Slightly, elevate his legs to increase blood flow to the brain to reduce the risk of fainting
4. If the bleeding seeps through the bandage or the cloth, do not try to remove it, just put another bandage on the top and press firmly.
5. If the bleeding doesn't stop, squeeze the main artery. In the arms, pressure points are on the inside of the arm just above the elbow and just below the armpit. Pressure points of the leg are just behind the knee and in the groin.
6. If the bleeding has stopped, immobilize the injured part. Leave the bandages in place and get the injured person to the emergency room.
7. Seek immediate help if there are any signs of internal bleeding (bleeding from body cavities, bruising on the neck, chest, and abdomen, vomiting or coughing up blood, wounds penetrating the skull, chest, or abdomen, abdominal tenderness, fractures, shock).

Self-Assessment Questions

1. A victim of a train crash has bleeding from the nose and tender abdomen. His pulse is weak and fast. What is most likely wrong?
   a. The victim is having angina
   b. The victim anaphylaxis
   c. The victim has internal bleeding
   d. The victim is having a heart attack

2. One of your friends has cut his arm and is bleeding severely. How do you treat this injury?
   a. Put the injured limb in some cold water
   b. Apply direct pressure over the wound
   c. Give him an aspirin
   d. All of the above

Cuts and Scrapes

In general, minor cuts and scrapes do not need calling the EMS or going to the emergency room. However, it is very essential to properly take care of the wound to avoid any infections.

First Aid Guidelines

1. Stop bleeding by applying gentle pressure using a clean cloth or bandage continuously for 20 to 30 minutes. To avoid dislodging or damage of the fresh clot, do not keep checking to see if the bleeding has stopped or not.
2. Clean the wound with clear water only. do not use soap as it may irritate the wound. Debris or dirt remaining after washing is removed using alcohol-sanitized tweezers. The area around the wound can be cleaned using soap and water only (hydrogen peroxide and iodine-containing cleanser can irritate living cells).
3. Use bandages to cover the wound. This will help the wound to remain clean and away from any infection. Once it healed enough remove the bandage and expose the wound to air as this can speed up healing.
4. Change the dressing daily or if it becomes wet or dirty.
5. If the wound cuts deeply through the skin, it might require stitches. A strip of surgical tape can be used for minor cuts; otherwise, larger wounds require a visit to a doctor for proper closure of the wound as soon as possible.
6. If you notice any signs of infection such as redness, swelling, drainage, or warmth, immediately seek medical attention.

Self-Assessment Question

1. Which of the followings is contraindicated in the first aid of cuts and scrapes?
   a. Applying gentle pressure with a clean cloth for 20 – 30 min.
   b. Clean the wound with soap and water.
   c. Remove the bandage from time to time to make sure the bleeding had stopped
   d. a and b.

Spinal Injury

A person might have a spinal injury if there is evidence of a head injury or an injury that has excerpted a substantial force on the head, the neck or the back is twisted oddly, the victim suffers from severe pain in the neck or back and can not move his neck, the victim complains of weakness, numbness or paralysis or loss of control of his limbs, bladder or bowels.

As a rule, never move a victim if you suspect a back or neck injury to avoid any complications such as permanent paralysis.

If you presume that the victim has a spinal injury:

1. Call EMS immediately.
2. Keep the victim still.
3. Add heavy towels on both sides of the neck or hold the head and neck to prevent movement.

First-Aid Measures

N.B. The main and very important goal of first aid for a spinal injury is to keep the victim still in the same position he was found.

1. If there are no signs of circulation, begin CPR, without tilting the head back. Use your fingers to gently grasp the jaw and lift it forward.
2. If there is no pulse, start chest compressions.
3. If the victim is vomiting or choking and you must roll him, you need at least one other person to help you. One of you holding the head and the other sitting along the side of the victim and then working together to keep the person's head, neck, and back aligned while rolling the person onto one side.

Self-Assessment Questions

1. You find a person at the bottom of the stairs. He appears to have fallen and seems badly hurt you should
   a. Roll the victim on his stomach keeping the head and back in a straight line
   b. Roll the victim onto one side
   c. Attempt to keep the victim from moving
   d. None of the above

2. In spinal injury:
   a. To begin CPR, you have to tilt the head back
   b. If the person is wearing a helmet, do not remove it
   c. You can put the victim in the recovery position with the help of another person
   d. All of the above

3. The victim has spinal injury if:
   a. The person complains of severe pain in his or her neck or back
   b. The person won't move his or her neck
   c. An injury has exerted substantial force on the back or head
   d. All of the above

Corneal Abrasions

It is one of the most common types of eye injury that involves the cornea. It occurs due to direct contact with dust, dirt, sand, wood shavings, metal particles, or even an edge of a piece of paper. If the corneal abrasion becomes infected it can lead to a corneal ulcer. Abrasions by plant matter (such as a pine needle) may lead to delayed iritis. Symptoms include tears, redness, blurred vision, feeling like you have sand in your eye, and pain.

First-Aid Measures

1. Flush your eyes with water or saline solution if available. Use an eye cup if available with its rim resting on the bone at the base of your eye socket.
2. Blink several times as this may remove small particles such as dust or sand.
3. Pull the upper eyelid over the lower eyelid as the lashes of your lower eyelid can brush foreign objects from the undersurface of your upper eyelid.
4. Never try to remove an object embedded in your eyeball and do not touch your eyeball with cotton swabs, tweezers
5. Avoid rubbing your eye as this can worsen and increases the abrasion.

Self-Assessment Questions

1. If a boy has a piece of wood in his eye, you should:
   a. Rub the eye several times
   b. Attempt to remove the wood with a tweezers
   c. Flush the eye with water or saline
   d. All of the above

2. Which of the following most commonly cause iritis after corneal abrasions?
   a. Dust
   b. Pine needle
   c. Edge of a piece of paper
   d. a and b

Black Eye

Black eye results from bleeding under the skin around the eye. Even though black eye injuries aren't serious, they may denote further extensive injury such as fractures in the skull. Hyphema occurs if the bleeding reaches within the eye. It leads to the accumulation of blood in the space between the cornea and the iris, causing eye pain, blurred vision, sensitivity to light, and later damage to the cornea.

First Aid Steps

1. During the first 48 hours and to minimize swelling, apply cold compresses (20 minutes on and 20 minutes off).
2. After two days, use warm compresses as they can help open blood vessels and fluid drainage.
3. Always, keep your head up at least for the first 48 hours (reduces swelling).
4. Immediately, seek medical help if you suffer from blurred vision, double vision, severe pain, or bleeding from the eye or the nose.

Self-Assessment Question

Black eye:

a. Is caused by bleeding beneath the skin around the eye
b. It can indicate a skull fracture
c. Bleeding within the eye is called a Hyphema
d. All of the above

Chemical Splash in the Eye

First Aid Steps

1. Rinse your eye using clean warm tap water for a minimum of 20 minutes. Use one of the following techniques:
   a. Go into the shower and apply a gentle stream of water to your forehead over the affected eye.
   b. If both eyes are affected directly the stream on the bridge of your nose. Keep your eyes always open then, hold your affected eye open under a gently running tap.
   c. In the case of young children, let them lie down in the bathtub and pour a gentle stream of water on the forehead over the affected eye or on the bridge of the nose for both eyes.
2. To make sure that there is no chemical in your hand carefully; rinse them with soap and water.
3. Take off your contact lenses if they didn't come out during washing.

4. Never rub the eye as this can cause additional damage.
5. Never use eye drops unless directed by your doctors.

After applying the previous steps, seek emergency care. It is very important to take the chemical container or to know at least its name. Wear sunglasses as your eyes will be sensitive to light.

Self-Assessment Question

In chemical splash:

a. Wash the affected eye for at least 20 minutes
b. Rub your eye to remove the chemical
c. Put any medical eye drop on it
d. All of the above

Foreign Object in the Ear

A foreign object in the ear can be anything that enters the ear canal such as a small earring or cotton swab. Symptoms include uncomfortable feelings and pain if the ear canal or the eardrum is injured. Hearing might be affected. If an insect enters the ear canal, the casualty can hear buzzing or feel tickling sensations and the insect may bite inside the ear canal.

First Aid Steps

1. Do not try to remove the object with any tool such as a cotton swab, or matchstick. This may increase the risk of pushing the object farther into the ear and destroying the fragile structures of the middle ear such as the ear drum.
2. If you see the object clearly from the outside, remove it using tweezers.
3. Small objects can fall out of the ear canal with the aid of gravity/ if the ear is turned toward the ground. Gently shake the head in the direction of the ground.
4. If there is an insect inside the ear canal, do not push your finger into the ear as the insect may sting. Turn the head so the affected ear faces up. The insect may crawl out on its own. If it doesn't, try to float the object by adding a few drops of warm mineral oil or olive oil into the ear. The insect will suffocate and float.
5. Never use oil in case of perforation in the eardrum, bleeding, discharge from the ear, or removing any object other than an insect.
6. If all the above-mentioned methods fail or the casualty still suffers from pain in the ear experiences pain or a sensation of something lodged in the ear, seek medical assistance.

Self-Assessment Question

If an object becomes lodged in the ear which of the following steps is true?

a. Try to remove the foreign object with a cotton swab
b. Try using gravity and striking the person's head hardly
c. If the object is visible, remove it with a tweezers
d. Use oil in case of insects even if the eardrum is perforated.

Foreign Object on the Skin

There are many types of foreign objects that commonly get under the skin such as splinters, fish hooks, glass, and others. Symptoms include pain and the sensation of something under the skin.

First Aid Steps

1. When the foreign object is protruding from your skin, flush your hand and sanitize the affected area, then use tweezers to remove the foreign object.
2. In case of an object completely embedded in the skin
   a. Wash your hands and sanitize the affected area or wash it with soap and water.
   b. Rub a clean sharp needle with alcohol to sterilize it.
   c. With the aid of the needle, break the skin that lies over the object.
   d. Remove the embedded object using tweezers. You can use a magnifying glass to see the object better.
   e. Wash and dry the area.
   f. If the object doesn't come out easily or there are any signs of infection, immediately seek medical attention.

Self-Assessment Question

If a foreign object in the skin:
a. Wash your hands and clean the area with soap and water
b. Use a sterilized needle to break the skin over the object
c. Remove the embedded object with tweezers
d. All of the above

Frostbite

It happens when the skin and its underneath tissues start to freeze. Exposure to cold weather is the most prevailing cause of frostbite. It usually starts with very cold skin then numbness and after that skin becomes hard and pale. Generally, frostbite usually affects smaller and exposed areas of the body such as cheeks, chin, nose, fingers, toes, and ears.

Main conditions that can cause frostbite include: wearing light clothes in cold, wet, or windy weather, uncovered skin in very cold weather, spending a long time out in the cold, and direct contact and touching freezing materials such as frozen metals or ice packs. Frostbite occurs due to losing body heat (hypothermia). As the body temperature lowers, circulation decreases and this can threaten vital organs. This actuates a "life over limb" action. The body starts to protect vital organs at the expense of the extremities. Skin and underneath tissues start to freeze. Additionally, it can occur due to direct exposure to very cold objects. Heat will be conducted away from the body. This lowers skin temperature and leads to tissue freezing. Symptoms of frostbite include: painful, itchy, and burning sensation, red then white pale waxy skin, numbness, muscle stiffness, and blisters (in severe cases).

Stages of Frost Bite

1 - Frostnip	The first stage of frostbite. It is a mild form of frostbite. Skin is red and very cold. When the skin is warm pain and tingling sensation may occur. In this stage, there is no permanent damage to the skin.
2 - Superficial frostbite:	This stage follows frostnip. Skin becomes very pale and white with the appearance of some ice crystals. At this stage after rewarming, skin appears blue or purple and mottled. Blisters may appear 24-36 hours after rewarming and there is a burning sensation.
3 - Severe frostbite:	In this stage, frostbite affects all layers of the skin. Numbness occurs in the tissues that lie below. There is numbness, pain, and discomfort. Large blisters appear 24 to 48 hours after rewarming. The affected area becomes hard and black due to tissue death.

Complications of frostbite include:

1. Sensitivity to cold is raised and there is an increased risk of getting frostbite again.
2. Permanent nerve numbness at the site of frostbite.
3. Development of frost bit arthritis (damage of cartilage between joints.
4. If the growth plate is affected in children, growth defects may develop.
5. Infection.
6. Gangrene due to interruption o blood flow.

> Immediately seek medical attention if there is pale skin, severe blisters and loss of sensation in the affected area, severe increasing pain associated with fever, swelling, redness or discharges, and dizziness.

First-Aid Steps

The main aim of first aid here is gradually rewarming the affected area of the skin, main steps include:

1. Avoid further exposure and protect the skin. If you remain outside, tuck your frostbitten hands into your armpits outside
2. Try to cover your face, nose, or ears with dry or gloved hands.

3. Once possible, move to an indoor place and take off wet clothes.
4. Gently and gradually rewarm the frostbitten areas (arms and feet) by putting them in warm water (40- 42° C) for 15-30 minutes.
5. Other areas are covered using a warm blanket. Direct heat, such as a stove, heat lamp, fireplace, or heating pad is forbidden as they may cause burns
6. To avoid further damage to the tissue, never walk on the frost-bitten toes or feet.

Medical Treatment

1. The doctor will wrap the affected areas using thick bandages or dressings. If a bone or a muscle is affected use a splint and additionally, elevate the limb to avoid swelling.
2. For proper healing, the damaged tissue needs to be removed (debridement). This is usually done after 1-3 months.
3. Whirlpool (quickly rotating water) baths help in rapid and proper healing of the skin as it keeps the skin clean and aids in removing dead tissue.
4. In severe cases, amputation might be required to remove dead tissues.

Self-Assessment Questions

1. When caring for someone who is suffering from frostbite, you should not:
   a. Soak the affected part in warm water (40 – 42 °C)
   b. Rub vigorously until the skin appears red
   c. Wrap the area with a thick dressing
   d. Avoid walking on a frostbitten foot

2. In which stage does skin appear blue or purple when it is warmed after frostbite?
   a. Frostnip
   b. Superficial frost bite.
   c. Severe frostbite
   d. b and c

Fainting

Fainting is usually provoked by a transient decline in blood flow or glucose supply to the brain leading to a loss of responsiveness. When a casualty faints, he usually doesn't remember the fall, and it is hard to rouse or move by himself. Normally it is caused by a reaction to pain, exhaustion, and emotional stress. Additionally, it can occur when the casualty was drinking a lot of alcohol or stayed in hot humid weather for a long time. Fainting might also occur due to some medical conditions such as hypoglycemia, anemia, hemorrhage, heart attack, head injury, and stroke.

First Aid Management

1. Help the casualty lie on the floor with his ankles raised to increase blood flow to the brain.
2. Open the windows to assure that the casualty gets fresh air.
3. Assess ABCs and if the casualty is breathing and there is no need for CPR, roll him into the recovery position.
4. Keep monitoring the casualty and if at any time breathing or circulation has stopped roll the person back and begin CPR.

Self-Assessment Question

If someone faints, the first thing you should do is:

a. Give the casualty something to drink
b. Raise the casualty's feet
c. Have casualty lie on his face
d. Place cool water on his face

Heart Attack

A heart attack appears when there is an obstruction in the blood supply reaching the heart. Loss of blood flow can destroy a part of the heart muscle. Warning symptoms of heart attack usually appear hours, days, or weeks preceding. Symptoms include chest pain (tightness, shortness of breath, burning feeling in the chest), pain in the arm, stomach, jaw, and back, sweating, nausea, and vomiting.

First Aid Steps

1. Call an ambulance or drive the casualty to the nearest hospital if you can get fast to the hospital.
2. Help the casualty into a half-sitting position to alleviate the strain. You can put some cushions behind him to support his head and shoulders.
3. Raise his knees.
4. Help the casualty to chew or take an aspirin tablet (300mg) unless he is allergic or not allowed to take aspirin.
5. Check ABCs and start CPR if the victim is not breathing.

Self-Assessment Questions

1. Your colleague is complaining of breathlessness and tight pain in the chest. You suspect a heart attack. What should you do?

a. Get him to lay down flat
b. Encourage him to stand and move around
c. Lay him down with legs up
d. None of the above

2. Which is not a symptom of a Heart attack?
   a. Squeezing chest pain
   b. Red hot dry skin
   c. Shortness of breath
   d. Sweating and nausea

First Aid Kit

A first aid kit is one of the basic requirements that should be available at home and stored in a place to be easily retrieved. You can make your first aid kit by yourself or purchase a readymade first aid it is commercially available. You can purchase first-aid kits at many drugstores or assemble your own. In case of traveling for a few days or more carry on, in addition, your medications and your detailed medical information.

Basic Supplies Included in the First Aid Kit

- First aid manual
- Adhesive plaster in assorted sizes.
- Medium and large sterile dressings.
- Sterile eye pad
- Triangular and roller bandage
- Safety pins in different sizes
- Alcohol gel
- Tweezers
- Disposable gloves
- Wound cleaning wipes (Alcohol–free)
- Adhesive tape
- Plastic face shield or a face mask
- Notepad and a pencil
- Antibiotic cream
- Instant cold packs
- Cotton balls
- Thermometer
- Syringe, medical cup, or spoon

If you are traveling by car, carry on in addition

- Cellular phone and a recharger that can be plugged into your car or a power bank.
- Emergency phone numbers such as your family doctor, local emergency services, emergency road service, and the regional poison control center.
- Small waterproof torch with extra batteries.
- Candles and matches
- Blanket
- Fire extinguisher

First aid kit to be checked at least every 3 months to revise the expiry date and replace any expired item.

Self-Assessment Questions

1. Basic supplies in the first aid kit include:
   a. Instant cold packs
   b. Cotton balls and cotton-tipped swabs .
   c. Disposable latex or synthetic gloves, a least two pair
   d. All of the above

2. Medication in the first aid kit includes all the following EXCEPT:
   a. Acetaminophen
   b. Oral antibiotic
   c. Antihistaminic
   d. Calamine lotion

References

[1] American Heart Association. *AHA information*. 2020. May 25, [2020-05-25]. Https://www.heart.org/.

[2] Carta, T. (2019). gawaziuk jp, diaz-abele j, liu s, jeschke m, logsetty s. Properties of an ideal burn dressing: a survey of burn survivors and front-line healthcare providers. *Burns;*45(2):364–68.

[3] *First aid kit list of contents, essentials, and types* (emedicinehealth.com).

[4] Furst, J. (2018). *The complete first aid pocket guide: step-by-step treatment for all of your medical emergencies.* Massachusetts. Adams Media.

[5] Gary a. Smith, G. (2010). Policy statement—prevention of choking among children. *I Am acad Pediatr.* 125(3):601–7.

[6] George E. Dvorchak, G. E. (2010). *Skyhorse Pocket Guides: The Pocket First-Aid Field Guide.* New York, NY: Skyhorse Publishing.

[7] Greif, R. (2021). *European resuscitation council guidelines 2021: education for resuscitation.* Elsevier, resuscitation; 161:38 8– 4 0 7.

[8] Hammett, E. A. (2017). *Burns falls and emergency calls: The ultimate guide to the prevention and treatment of childhood accidents.* New York, NY.

[9] kit contents - Canadian red cross.

[10] Le, T., Mendoza, M., Coffa, D., Saint-Hilaire, L. (2017). *First Aid for the Family Medicine Boards*, 3rd Edition. New York, NY: McGraw Hill.

[11] The British Red Cross society. *British Red Cross first aid resources*. [2020-05-20]. Https://www.Redcross.org.uk/first-aid/

Chapter 3

Clinical Pharmacokinetics

Hoda Rabea[1,*]
Mohammed Almeziny[2]
Haitham Saeed[1]
Salah M. Seif[1]
Yassmin Madaney[1]
Amira B. Kassem[3]
Ramy Ibrahim Elwaraky[4]
Sherok Okda[3]
and Mohamed Emam Abdelmobdy Abdelrahim[1]
[1]Clinical Pharmacy Department, Faculty of Pharmacy, Beni-Suef University, Beni Suef, Egypt
[2]Prince Sultan Military Medical City (PSMMC), Riyadh, Saudi Arabia
[3]Clinical Pharmacy and Pharmacy Practice Department, Faculty of Pharmacy Damanhour University, Abadiyyat Damanhur, Egypt
[4]Kidney and Urology Center, Alexandria, Egypt

Learning Objectives

After completing this chapter, the reader would be able to:

- Understand the basic concepts of pharmacokinestics and clinical phramacokinetics.
- Understand the pharmacokinetic alterations in patients with kidney disease.
- Recommend the appropriate methods for assessment of kidney function for different patient categories and understand the limitations of each method.
- Design a personalized dosing regimen for patients with kidney disease.
- Understand the absorption, metabolism, elimination alterations in patients with liver disease.

* Corresponding Author's Email: Hoda.ahmed@pharm.bsu.edu.eg.

In: Clinical Pharmacist Tools to Deliver Rational Medication Use
Editor: Mohamed Emam Abdelmobdy Abdelrahim
ISBN: 979-8-88697-857-5

- Recommend the appropriate methods for assessment of liver function
- Design a personalized dosing regimen for patients with liver disease.
- Understand the different kinetics of selected medications and the manner of solving kinetics related issues.

Overview to Clinical Pharmacokinetics

Pharmacokinetics could be defined as the branch of pharmaceutical science that focuses on what happens to the drug in the body starting from the rate and extent of absorption, then distribution inside the body fluids and tissues, followed by metabolism and clearance. While, the application of pharmacokinetic principles to the administration of medications in a manner that is both safe and effective for the treatment of a specific patient is known as clinical pharmacokinetics.

There are four phases for drug pharmacokinetics

1) *Absorption;* Absorption is the process through which medication molecules move from the site of drug delivery (Gastrointestinal tract, intramuscular and skin) to enter the bloodstream. The method of delivery affects the rate of drug absorption and its extent. The lipid solubility of the drug, its formulation, and the mode of administration all influence drug absorption. To pass through membranes, a medicine must be lipid-soluble unless it has an active transport system or is so tiny that it can pass through the aqueous channels.
   Bioavailability is the proportion of a medicine that is absorbed into the systemic circulation following extravascular delivery.
2) *Distribution;* medication distribution is the movement of an unmetabolized drug through the blood and tissues. The distribution of a drug in specific tissues determines its efficacy or toxicity, which partially explains the lack of correlation between plasma levels and observed effects.
   The volume of distribution (Vd) is defined as the volume of plasma that would be necessary to account for the total amount of drug in the patient's body, if drug concentration were present throughout the body at the same concentration as found in the plasma.
   Several factors pertaining to the drug and the body influence drug distribution. pH, blood and tissue-binding proteins, and perfusion are some of the drug-related variables. The body-related components consist of fat composition, body water content, and disease prevalence such as burns, volume depletion, and edema.
3) *Metabolism;* the metabolic process is the chemical transformation of pharmaceuticals from a lipid-soluble state suited for absorption and distribution into a water-soluble form suitable for excretion. The method eliminates the parent substance completely.
   Metabolism of a drug has two phases, in phase I, drug molecules are chemically changed through hydrolysis, oxidation, or reduction to prepare them for Phase II reactions or excretion. Oxidation is the most prevalent type of Phase 1 reaction and includes mostly membrane-bound cytochrome P450 enzymes in the smooth endoplasmic reticulum of liver cells. The majority of products of Phase 1 metabolism

are pharmacologically inert, however, some retain action to a greater or lesser degree, and some possess activity not present in the parent drug (prodrug). Prodrug is defined as a pharmacologically inactive drug that is transformed in the body into a pharmacologically active drug. Following phase I, Phase II starts, in which molecules of the Phase I metabolite interact with an endogenous substrate to generate an inactive conjugate that is far more water-soluble than the Phase I metabolite. Synthesis of glucuronide or sulphate products, acetylation or methylation, and conjugation with glutathione are Phase II processes.

The medicine's lipid solubility, formulation, and route of administration all affect drug absorption. A drug must be lipid-soluble to pass across membranes unless it has an active transport system or is so small that it may pass through aqueous channels.

4) *Excretion;* it is the process through which medicines and their metabolites are eliminated from the body. They may be eliminated in fluids such as urine and bile, solids (faeces), or gases during expiration.

   Low-molecular-weight medicines that are not metabolized and are sufficiently water-soluble to evade renal tubular reabsorption are often eliminated via urinary excretion. Small water-soluble compounds that enter the bloodstream as a result of liver or other organ metabolism are also eliminated via this route. Small molecules that are not attached to plasma proteins are filtered by the glomeruli and enter the tubules, where they may be reabsorbed if they are still lipid-soluble, but not if they are water-soluble. Larger molecular-weight medications, particularly those conjugated with glucuronide in the liver, and any pharmaceuticals that are not absorbed and are preferentially eliminated via faeces. Molecules of drug or metabolite that enter the bile following liver metabolism are transported into the intestinal lumen, transit through the digestive tract, and are removed in the faeces. Some molecules of unmodified medication or metabolite may be reabsorbed and re-enter the portal vein if they are sufficiently lipid-soluble. This recycling between the liver, bile, intestine, and portal vein is referred to as entero-hepatic circulation. After absorption and distribution are complete, the half-life is the time necessary for blood concentrations to decline by half. It determines the time necessary to reach steady state and the dosing interval. The half-life is a dependent kinetic variable since its value is dependent on the clearance and Vd.

   Membrane transporters are protein molecules that actively transport medicines across cell membranes. The role of transport proteins in the bioavailability, excretion, and distribution of drugs continues to develop. P-glycoprotein is a major transport protein involved in the transfer of medicines across biological membranes. Numerous organs contain P-glycoprotein, including the gastrointestinal tract, liver, and kidney. Organic cation transporters, organic anion transporters, and organic anion-carrying polypeptides are further transport protein families.

Dose Adjustment of Drugs in Patients with Liver Disease

Introduction

There is no naturally occurring material that can be used to estimate the hepatic clearance of medications, even though measurements of the creatinine clearance level can be utilized for dose modifications in cases of compromised renal function. The Child-Pugh score, which is made up of a number of clinical factors, is frequently used to evaluate the prognosis in patients with liver cirrhosis [1].

Liver Function Assessment

In clinical practice, the Child-Turcotte classification as modified by Pugh has been widely used to classify patients according to the severity of liver function impairment. The Pugh modification of the Child- Turcotte's scale was initially intended to stratify the risk of portocaval shunt surgery in cirrhotic patients, but it has since been demonstrated that it also correlates with survival and the development of cirrhosis complications. Included in the Child-Pugh classification (Table 1) are five variables to assess the severity of liver disease: serum bilirubin, serum albumin, prothrombin time, the presence of encephalopathy, and the presence of ascites [2].

Disease severity is then classified as mild (class A), moderate (class B), or severe (class C). This categorization system is helpful in assessing the progression of a patient's condition individually and in comparing patient populations. It may also provide the clinician with some dose adjustment advice. Another classification scheme, the model for end-stage liver disease (MELD), is based on serum bilirubin concentration, serum creatinine, the international normalized ratio (INR) of prothrombin time, and the underlying cause of liver disease [2].

The MELD score has been adopted to use for allocating priority in patients awaiting liver transplants because it correctly predicts 3-month mortality among patients on a liver-transplant waiting list. These classification schemes lack the sensitivity to quantify the specific capacity of the liver to metabolize particular drugs, in contrast to renal patients where estimates of glomerular filtration rate (creatinine clearance, inulin clearance) correlate with kinetic parameters of drug elimination like renal clearance [2].

In an effort to more accurately predict how each patient would handle a particular medicine, dynamic liver function tests have been created in addition to the Child-Pugh and MELD classification systems. These tests include giving an exogenous drug, which is primarily or entirely removed by the liver, either orally or intravenously. The test is based on the identification of a metabolite in plasma, urine, or even expired air in the event of a breath test, or the assessment of the probe's plasma disappearance (i.e., clearance). Exogenous chemicals that are used as model substrates to assess a person's ability to remove drugs can be broadly divided into two categories: substances with a high extraction ratio and those with a low extraction ratio [2].

As with the creatinine clearance test used for drug dose adjustment in renal patients, the challenge is to design a dynamic liver function test that assesses the remaining liver elimination capacity in a patient with hepatic failure and serves as the cornerstone for dosage adjustment. Clinical professionals currently rely more on the Child-Pugh score, which may not be better but is more easily accessible for liver patients, than on these dynamic liver function tests for dosage modification purposes in patients with hepatic dysfunction [2].

Table 1. Child-Pugh classification and scoring of the severity of liver disease

Clinical/biochemical indicator	1 point	2 points	3 points
Serum bilirubin(mg/dl)	<2	2-3	>3
Serum albumin (g/dl)	>3.5	2.8-3.5	<2.8
Prothrombin time (s>control)	<4	4-6	>6
INR (more accurate than Prothrombin time	<1.7	1.7-2.2	>2.2
Encephalopathy(grade)	None	1 or 2	3 or 4
Ascites	Absent	Slight	Moderate

Points are summed, and the total score is classified according to severity as follows: 5–6 points = group A (mild), 7–9 points = group B (moderate), 10–15 points = group C (severe) [2]

Effect of liver dysfunction on pharmacokinetic processes.

Hepatic Blood Flow and Intrinsic Clearance and Hepatic Extraction Ratio

Hepatic drug clearance (CLH), defined as the volume of blood from which drug removed completely by the liver per unit time, is a function of hepatic blood flow (QH) and the hepatic extraction ratio (EH) of the drug.

CLH = QH x EH [2]

Since EH depends on liver blood flow, the intrinsic clearance of unbound drug (CLint), and the fraction of unbound drug in blood (fu), the following fundamental equation for CLH has been derived [2]

CLH= QH x fu x Clint
QH+fu x Clint [2]

This equation is based on the "well-stirred" or "venous equilibration" model, a kinetic model that is frequently used to describe the relationship between hepatic drug clearance and the three main factors that affect hepatic drug elimination, namely blood flow, drug binding in blood, and intrinsic clearance (the activity of enzymes and transporters involved in the hepatic elimination of drugs by metabolism and biliary excretion). According to this model, the liver is a single, thoroughly mixed compartment, and drugs present in arterial blood that enters the liver instantly equilibrate with those present in venous blood. The model sheds light on how changes in liver blood flow and intrinsic clearance affect hepatic medication clearance and dosage.

Drugs can be categorized according to the efficiency of the liver in removing the substance from the circulation as having a high (EH>0.7), low (EH<0.3) or intermediate (0.3<EH<0.7) hepatic extraction ratio. The hepatic clearance of highly extracted drugs approaches and becomes limited by liver blood flow, The hepatic clearance of these drugs is said to be blood flow limited and is relatively insensitive to changes in binding of drug to blood components or enzyme/transporter activity, i.e., CLint. Hepatic clearance of these medications approaches and becomes limited by liver blood flow. Cirrhosis and other conditions that affect liver blood flow and portosystemic shunting will significantly affect the hepatic clearance of these medications, especially when taken orally. However, the intrinsic hepatic clearance and variations in blood/plasma binding are the key factors affecting the hepatic clearance of poorly extracted drugs, which is why it is thought to be enzyme/transporter-capacity limited.

Last but not least, some medications have intermediate hepatic extraction efficiency, in which case modifications to any one of its three main determinants, i.e., QH, CLint and fu.

Example of high extraction ratio drugs include antipsychotics, opioids, beta blockers, statins, tricyclic antidepressants, Selective Serotonin Reuptake Inhibitor (SSRI) and nitrates [1].

Example of low extraction ratio drugs include Anticonvulsants most Sulphonylureas, Spironolactone, Theophylline, Paracetamol, Warfarin, Nonsteroidal Anti-Inflammatory Drug (NSAIDs) and Steroids [1].

Absorption

Patients with liver disease have been reported to experience gastrointestinal dysfunction, which may be a factor in the complications of cirrhosis. However, decreased presystemic hepatic metabolism is the main cause of chronic liver disease's impact on the bioavailability of medications taken orally. All medications absorbed from the gastrointestinal tract—aside from those inhaled through the mouth and the lower part of the rectum—are exposed to the liver's metabolizing enzymes and bile excretory transport systems before entering the systemic circulation as a result of the liver's special position in the circulatory system. Drugs with an intermediate to high hepatic extraction ratio will undergo an important presystemic elimination or 'first-pass effect' [1].

The fraction of an absorbed oral dose that escapes first-pass hepatic clearance, can be described by the following equation: (1)

$$FH = 1- fH*EH = QH + fu * CLint(1-fH)/ QH + fu * Clint \qquad (1)$$

Where, fH is the fraction of the mesenteric blood flow passing through the functioning liver [1].

Plasma Protein Binding and Distribution

The distribution of a drug inside the body depends on its reversible binding to blood cells, plasma proteins, and tissue macromolecules since only the unbound drug is capable of entering and exiting the tissue compartments. In patients with chronic liver illness, several medications that are strongly bound to albumin or 1-acid glycoprotein have a noticeably greater unbound fraction.

Mechanisms for decreased binding of certain drugs to plasma proteins include

1) Decreased production of albumin and 1-acid glycoprotein, resulting in low levels of these crucial binding proteins in the plasma of chronic liver disease patients,

2) Buildup of endogenous substances, such as bilirubin, which prevents some drugs from binding to plasma proteins, and (1)

Potential Qualitative Changes in Albumin and 1-Acid Glycoprotein

The Vd of some medications may be higher in these patients due to the decreased plasma binding. Additionally, patients with ascites will have a marked rise in the Vd of water-soluble medications, which may call for higher loading doses. For instance, it was discovered that patients with cirrhosis had three times the apparent Vd of the the lactam antibiotic cefodizime compared to healthy individuals.

Metabolism

The primary organ involved in drug metabolism is the liver. When there are no flow limitations, the liver can remove unbound drugs from the blood according to its intrinsic clearance (CLint). The function of sinusoidal and canalicular transporters, as well as the activity of metabolic enzymes, all affect CLint. The relationship between poor drug metabolism and chronic liver disease in general has long been understood.

In fact, decreased drug metabolism may result from a decrease in the absolute mass of liver cells or a decrease in enzyme activity as a result of changes in the function of surviving cells in chronic liver disease. Additionally, sinusoidal capillarization may impair the uptake of some medications and oxygen across the capillarized endothelium, which may result in a reduction in the hepatic drug metabolism in chronic liver disease.

Phase I oxidative metabolism is carried out by the microsomal mixed function oxidase system, which is found in the smooth endoplasmic reticulum of hepatocytes. Cytochrome P450 (CYP450) and nicotinamide adenine dinucleotide phosphate (NADPH)-dependent cytochrome P450 reductase are the two enzymes that make up this system. For these enzymes to work, NADPH and molecular oxygen are also necessary. Due to the shortage of oxygen brought on by shunting, sinusoidal capillarization, and decreased hepatic perfusion, CYP450 enzymes are typically more sensitive than phase II conjugating enzymes.

Studies have assessed the amount of protein or the activity of key drug-metabolizing enzymes in the livers of cirrhotic patients have revealed that, generally, enzyme activities and protein content decrease with increasing disease severity. These investigations also appear to show that patients with chronic liver illness have a selective regulation of the different drug metabolising enzymes. In fact, CYP450 activity reductions in chronic liver disorders are diverse and non-uniform and do not relate to decreased hepatic blood flow.

Biliary Excretion

Bile flow obstruction and extrahepatic cholestasis can be caused by common bile duct stones, sclerosing cholangitis, or pancreatic malignancy. Some medications, including erythromycin, phenol-thiazines, and anabolic steroids, can cause intrahepatic cholestasis as a result of functional disturbance of the hepato-canalicular bile secretory system. Reduced bile production or secretion into the duodenum will affect the amount of chemicals that are cleared by biliary excretion, both endogenous and exogenous.

The biliary excretion of antibiotics such ampicillin, piperacillin, certain cephalosporins, clindamycin, and ciprofloxacin was significantly hindered in individuals with obstructed biliary tract, according to studies in patients having surgery for obstruction of the common bile duct.

Drugs and drug metabolites that are typically eliminated mostly through the bile may therefore accumulate in patients with common bile duct obstruction. Furthermore, biliary blockage may cause hepatocellular damage and hinder the metabolic clearance of drugs. In fact, it has been demonstrated that the activity of several CYPs, including CYP2C and CYP2E1, is impaired in livers removed during transplantation for patients with end-stage cirrhosis, both with and without cholestasis. However, the protein of CYP3A was significantly reduced only in the cirrhotic livers without cholestasis. As a result, dosage adjustments may be necessary for medications whose clearance depends heavily on hepatic metabolism in cholestasis patients [1].

Guidelines of dosage adjustment in patients with hepatic dysfunction:

Both the Food and Drug Administration (FDA) and the European Medicines Agency (EMEA) have published a guidance for industry on the evaluation of the pharmacokinetics of medicinal products in patients with impaired hepatic function.

These recommendations recommend performing a pharmacokinetic study while a medicinal product is being developed if it will likely be used by patients with impaired hepatic function and if the pharmacokinetics of the drug substance or its active metabolite will likely be significantly affected by hepatic impairment (s). Such a study's main goals are to identify individuals who are at risk and determine if patients with decreased liver function need to have their dosage adjusted. These recommendations advise using the Child-Pugh classification to group individuals based on the severity of their liver impairment. Additionally, they promote the use of exogenous markers to evaluate the patients' potential for elimination via various methods.

A recent study revealed that there are currently relatively few drugs that have specific recommendations for dosage adjustment based on hepatic function as assessed by the Child-Pugh score. More often than not, patients with a Child-Pugh classification C, or severe liver illness, are not included if the pharmacokinetics of a medicinal product are evaluated during development. However, the ethical and practical issues surrounding the administration of investigational drugs to patients with advanced liver disease who have no chance of benefiting from them warrant proper consideration. In any case, in addition to clinical evaluation by a semi-quantitative Child-Pugh score, characterization of the status of hepatic function would benefit from being quantified on the basis of an independent measure of the metabolism of a marker known to be altered by liver disease.

The following general considerations will be useful if there are no recommendations for dosage adjustment in patients with hepatic dysfunction based on their Child-Pugh score. The medication is assumed to be primarily removed by hepatic mechanisms (metabolism, biliary excretion).

1) Drugs with a relatively high hepatic extraction ratio: In patients with chronic liver illness, the oral bioavailability of these drugs might dramatically rise; as a result, the dosage should be adjusted. If hepatic blood flow is decreased after systemic injection (IV, IM, SC, etc.), the plasma clearance may be reduced.
2) Low hepatic extraction medications with high plasma protein binding (> 90%) include: The intrinsic capacity of the hepatic elimination pathways and the unbound drug fraction in blood or plasma determine the oral and intravenous clearance of these medicines. The liver's functional capacity and the specific metabolic pathway(s) used for drug removal will both influence how much the intrinsic clearance is diminished. Because the unbound fraction of the drug in blood or plasma may be much higher in patients with chronic liver disease, the dosage may need to be adjusted even though total blood or plasma concentrations are within the normal range for pharmacokinetic evaluation.
3) Drugs with low plasma protein binding (90%) and low hepatic extraction ratio include: The intrinsic capacity of the hepatic elimination pathways and the unbound drug fraction in blood or plasma determine the oral and intravenous clearance of these drugs. The liver's functional capacity and the specific metabolic pathway(s) used for drug removal will both influence how much the intrinsic clearance is diminished. Fluctuations in the unbound drug fraction in blood or plasma are relatively minor and won't have a big impact on the medication' clearance. The goal of dosage adjustment should be to maintain normal total plasma concentrations (bound plus unbound).
4) In patients with hepato-renal syndrome, the clearance of medications that are partially excreted by the kidneys in unchanged form will be impaired. It should be noted that in these patients, glomerular filtration rate is greatly overestimated by creatinine clearance.
5) In individuals with chronic liver disease who have edema or ascites, the Vd of hydrophilic drug may be increased. Therefore, if a rapid and complete medication effect is needed in these patients, the loading dose might need to be increased. Renal function should be considered as many hydrophilic medicines are largely removed by the kidneys in unaltered form.
6) Extreme caution should be taken when prescribing any medication to individuals with severe liver failure and when using medications with a narrow therapeutic index in those with liver disease (Child-Pugh class C).

Carmen C. Franz et al. performed a cross sectional retrospective study to assess the dose adequacy of drug treatment of 400 cirrhotic patients at hospital admission based on the authors' own previous studies and standard literature to assess drug-related problems in patients with liver cirrhosis by investigating the prevalence of inadequately dosed drugs and their association with adverse drug reactions (ADRs) and hospitalizations and the following algorithm, as shown in figure 1, was designed to guide dosage recommendations of drugs in patients with liver cirrhosis [3].

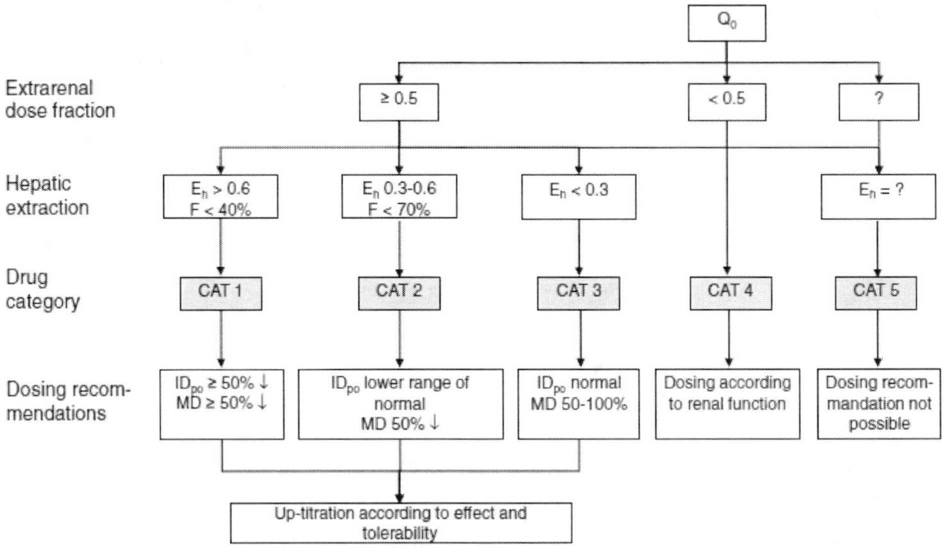

Figure 1. Classification and dosage recommendations of drugs in patients with liver cirrhosis. Drugs were classified into 5 categories (CAT) according to their pharmacokinetic parameters Q0 (extrarenal dose fraction) and Eh (hepatic extraction). If published data for Eh were not available, Eh was estimated. If bioavailability after oral administration (F) was available, intestinal absorption was also taken into account to estimate Eh. CAT 1 High hepatic extraction drugs, CAT 2 intermediate hepatic extraction drugs, CAT 3 low hepatic extraction drugs, CAT 4 renal elimination drugs, CAT 5 drugs with unknown elimination pathway, IDpo initial dose administered orally, MD maintenance dose [3].

Deepak N. Amarapurkar et al. designed an algorithm (Figure 2) for drug dosing in liver failure and advised of Possibly avoiding drugs which are metabolized by liver and/or have potential hepatotoxicity. Deepak N. Amarapurkar et al. concluded that Most medications, in the opinion of experts, can be used in cirrhotic patients safely, but cirrhotic patients may not tolerate drug-induced hepatotoxicity well; as a result, potential hepatotoxins should be avoided in cirrhotic patients. In individuals with liver cirrhosis, potentially hepatotoxic medications may be given depending on clinical needs and when no other options are available [4].

When giving drugs to individuals with cirrhosis, drug dosage should be tailored to each patient's needs and take into account things like adherence, renal function, nutritional status, and drug interactions. It is strongly recommended to often monitor liver function despite these recommendations, both patients and doctors do not adhere to the need for alanine transaminase monitoring of drug-induced liver injury. As clinicians, it is our responsibility to inform patients about the warning symptoms of drug-induced liver impairment, such as nausea, jaundice, and stomach discomfort, so they can stop taking their medications and seek medical attention [4].

Fabiola Delcò et al. concluded that Agents can be categorized based on their hepatic extraction in order to predict the kinetic behavior of medications in cirrhotic patients. In cirrhotic individuals, bioavailability rises, and hepatic clearance falls for medicines with a high hepatic extraction (poor bioavailability in healthy persons) [5].

When giving such medications orally to cirrhotic patients, the initial dose must be lowered in accordance with hepatic extraction. Kinetic studies in cirrhotic individuals also suggest that their maintenance dose should be adjusted, regardless of the route of administration, if possible liver disease has little effect on the bioavailability of medications with poor hepatic extraction, but it may have an impact on hepatic clearance According to the projected decrease in hepatic drug metabolism, only the maintenance dose needs to be decreased for such medications.

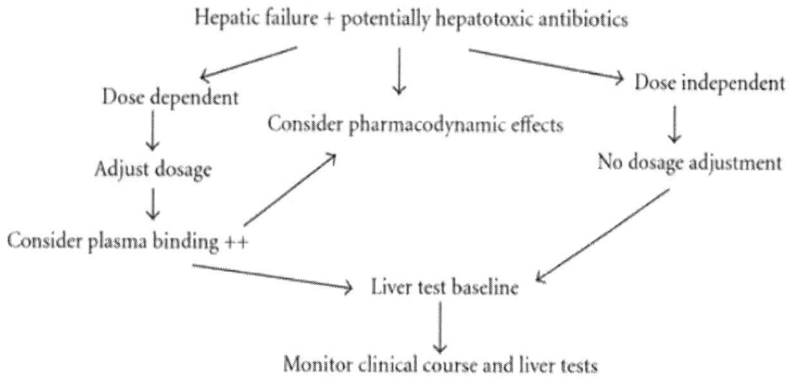

Figure 2. Algorithm for drug dosing in liver failure [4].

Initial oral dosages for medications with an intermediate hepatic extraction should be selected in the low range of normal in cirrhotic patients, and maintenance doses should be decreased as for medications with a high extraction.

The clearance of medications with a predominance in biliary elimination may be reduced in cholestatic individuals. Many antineoplastic treatments include guidelines for dose reduction in cholestasis, but other medications with biliary elimination typically don't. Therefore, dose adaptation of such medications in cholestatic patients is challenging and must be done in accordance with pharmacological impact and/or toxicity.

Importantly, in patients with liver illness, the dose of medications with a predominance in renal elimination may also need to be adjusted. Despite having a normal serum creatinine level, cirrhotic patients may have decreased renal function. Therefore, creatinine clearance should be evaluated or calculated in cirrhotic patients to provide recommendations for the dosage of medications with a predominance of renal elimination.

Case

A 62-year-old, 65-kg male with hepatic cirrhosis (total bilirubin = 2.6 mg/dL, serum albumin = 2.5 mg/dL, prothrombin time prolonged over normal by 8 seconds, slight amount of ascitic fluid, no hepatic encephalopathy) and severe chronic obstructive pulmonary disease. The patient is not a tobacco smoker and does not have heart failure., patient medical history includes cystic fibrosis for which he takes ivacaftor.

1) Compute the patient's Child-Pugh score
2) What is your recommendation for dose adjustment of ivacaftor considering patient's hepatic impairment? Knowing that standard dose is morning dose of ivafactor of 100 mg PO and evening dose of 100 mg PO.

Clinical Pharmacokinetics in Kidney Diseases

Introduction

Kidney disease affect the pharmacokinetics (PK) and pharmacodynamics (PD) of many drugs by various degrees that depend on both the drug and the clinical setting. Drugs eliminated by the kidneys would require dosage adjustment in kidney disease. However, prescribing to patients with kidney disease is complicated, as estimating kidney function in acute and chronic kidney disease is challenging. Moreover, renal replacement therapies (RRT) influence the disposition of various drugs. Clinicians must assess kidney function accurately and understand the impact of changes associated with kidney disease on multiple organ systems and on drugs and their active or toxic metabolites to optimize treatment regimen of individual patients.

Table 2. Staging of kidney function based on GFR [1]

GFR category	GFR range (mL/min/1.73 m^2)	Description
G1	≥90	Normal or high
G2	60 to 89	Mildly decreased
G3a	45 to 59	Mildly to moderately decreased
G3b	30 to 44	Moderately to severely decreased
G4	15 to 29	Severely decreased
G5	<15	Kidney failure

Assessment of Kidney Function

The kidneys play a major role in the elimination of many drugs. When kidney functions deteriorate, there would be a compelling need for dosage adjustment of renally eliminated drugs, particularly for drugs with narrow-therapeutic range. Glomerular filtration rate (GFR) has been considered for decades as the principal measure of kidney function (Table 2). Theoretically, the GFR measures the volume of plasma filtered across the glomeruli per unit of time. The measurement of GFR can be determined by using exogenous or endogenous substances.

Exogenous Substances

There are many exogenous compounds that has been utilized in the assessment of GFR, of them, the urinary clearance of inulin is considered the gold standard, however, it is rarely performed except for research purposes due to limited availability, cost, and complexity of the procedure. Other exogenous agents such as iothalamate, iohexol, and the radioactive Technetium-99m-labeled diethylenetriaminepentaacetic acid (^{99m}Tc DTPA) also have limitations. Iothalamate and iohexol are not completely eliminated by glomerular filtration and are also secreted by the tubules. Both previous agents cannot be used in patients with allergies to Iodine. The use of non-radioactive iothalamate requires an expensive assay, whereas the use of Iodine-125 tracer with iothalamate or Technetium-99m-labeled tracer with DTPA requires an equipped laboratory for storage, administration, and disposal of radioactive substances [2]. Due to these limitations, the determination of GFR utilizing administration of exogenous substances is currently considered not practical for routine use.

Endogenous Substances

Estimation of GFR utilizing an endogenous substance is therefore the most common used method in clinical practice (Figure 3). Serum creatinine (S_{cr}) has been widely used to estimate GFR. Creatine is a product of protein metabolism synthesized primarily in the liver, pancreas, and kidneys, then it is stored into muscle tissue. Creatinine is produced as a breakdown product of creatine in muscle tissue at an approximately constant rate depending on muscle mass, then released into the circulation. Creatinine then undergoes passive glomerular filtration, with partial active tubular secretion. Urinary clearance of creatinine derived from a 24-hour urine collection is a method for determination of GFR. However, this method is cumbersome, prone to errors even with shorter urine collection periods, and associated with delay in reporting of results, limiting its clinical value. Hence, GFR is estimated in clinical practice from the measurement of an endogenous substance, such as serum creatinine, combined with patient factors such as age, weight, gender, and race. Due to availability, ease, reliability, and low cost, serum creatinine is one of the most used measures in clinical laboratories worldwide.

Limitations of Serum Creatinine

As creatinine generation is related to muscle mass and diet, people with extremes of muscle mass (for example, people with malnutrition, muscle wasting, amputees, or contrarywise obesity or body builders) or those on a vegan or vegetarian diet will have different values than expected, that could misinterpret the result of the equation and either overestimate or underestimate GFR, regardless of which equation is used, predisposing patients to treatment failure or adverse drug events [3]. Also, there are age and gender differences in creatinine generation, as S_{cr} was found to increase with age, equal for boys and girls, up to 14 years and with a much steeper slope for boys than for girls between 14 and 20 years. Serum creatinine then remains constant for the average healthy subject between 20 and 70 years of age, with a mean of 0.90 mg/dL for Caucasian men and with a mean of 0.70 mg/dL for Caucasian women. Above the age of 70 years, serum creatinine starts to slowly increase again in both genders [4]. Serum creatinine must be at steady state to be incorporated into an equation, otherwise, it would either overestimate or underestimate GFR.

Another limitation is that creatinine is not only cleared by glomerular filtration, as some creatinine also undergoes tubular secretion. Thus, creatinine clearance (CLcr) equations, such as Cockcroft and Gault, overestimates GFR [5]. Drugs can also interfere with this tubular secretion and famous examples are trimethoprim and cimetidine. This can lead to an increase in serum creatinine values while GFR remains unchanged [6, 7].

Historically, there have been variations in S_{cr} assays among laboratories, made by either enzymatic methods or alkaline picric acid (Jaffe) method, with the resulting bias primarily associated with instrument manufacturer, not with type of method used [8]. In 2005, the Laboratory Working Group of the National Kidney Disease Education Program in collaboration with the International Federation of Clinical Chemistry and Laboratory Medicine and the European Communities Confederation of Clinical Chemistry created the Creatinine Standardization Program, to reduce interlaboratory variation in creatinine assay calibration and to enable more accurate estimates of GFR. The standardization of creatinine calibration was traceable to an isotope dilution mass spectrometry (IDMS) reference measurement procedure [9]. Comparing the old Jaffe methods with the new IDMS-standardized S_{cr} values showed that the Jaffe techniques overestimated S_{cr} by values between 10 to 21% [10].

However, although the old method yielded higher S_{cr}, this used to compensate the error of GFR overestimate caused by tubular secretion of creatinine, and the IDMS-standardized S_{cr} reintroduced the problem, necessitating modifying the used equations to account for standardization. Also, this variation between the old and standardized assay does affect the reported results from the old PK and PD studies, and their interpretation in dosing adjustments in the product labeling. As it is not possible or practical to repeat all the PK studies with the standardized S_{cr}, it is still reasonable to use the old drug dosing adjustments in the product labeling [11]. However, while these differences may not influence dosing of drugs with a wide therapeutic range, they may have significant clinical effects with safety and effectiveness of drugs with a narrow therapeutic range.

Some substances may interfere with the assay of S_{cr} measurement. The alkaline picrate colorimetric assay is affected by chromogens, such as acetoacetate in diabetic ketoacidosis [12].

Moreover, as creatine is synthesized in the liver before being stored in muscles where it is phosphorylated as creatinine, serum creatinine should be interpreted with caution in patients with liver cirrhosis due to potential overestimation of renal function [13].

Cystatin C

Cystatin C is a low-molecular-weight protein, produced by all nucleated cells, that is freely filtered by the glomerulus, then metabolized by tubular epithelial cells, with small amount excreted in urine, that limit its use to directly measure urinary clearance. The rate of generation of cystatin C has been thought to be less variable than creatinine. However, cystatin C levels was found to be influenced by older age, male gender, greater weight, greater height, race/ethnicity, uric acid, thyroid dysfunction, diabetes, higher C-reactive protein, and use of corticosteroids in a dose-dependent manner [14–17]. Another limitation of cystatin C is the variation in reported results due to inaccuracy of measurement procedures. In 2010, the International Federation for Clinical Chemists Working Group for the Standardization of serum cystatin C and the Institute for Reference Materials and Measurements produced a certified reference material to reduce bias [18]. However, later studies showed that the bias persisted, and more efforts are needed to improve traceability to the reference material [19, 20]. Compared with S_{cr}, cystatin C was more sensitive, but less specific for the estimation of GFR in patients with CKD or kidney transplant patients [21, 22]. Cystatin C might be a promising marker to accurately assess kidney function in patients with liver cirrhosis [23]. The combination of both S_{cr} and cystatin C in the same equation is proposed to provide more accurate estimate of GFR [24].

> You are reviewing the medications of a 70-year-old female with a longstanding history of hypertension and diabetes. She was diagnosed with CKD 2 years ago, with a stable Scr of 2 mg/dL. She is currently on valsartan/hydrochlorothiazide, felodipine, metformin, vildagliptin, aspirin, and rosuvastatin. On a follow-up visit, her HbA1c was 7%, and her urinary albumin/creatinine ratio was 450 mg/g. Her weight is 55 kg and her height is 150 cm. She is on a vegetarian diet. Her doctor is considering prescribing a sodium/glucose cotransporter 2 (SGLT2) inhibitor.

Question 1: How would you assess her GFR? And what is the impact of GFR assessment of medications?

a) 24-Hour urine for creatinine clearance (CLcr)
b) eGFRcr by CKD-EPI equation
c) eGFRcr by MDRD equation
d) estimated CLcr by CG equation
e) eGFRcys by CKD-EPI equation
f) Measured GFR by plasma clearance of iohexol

Equations Used for Estimation of CLcr and GFR

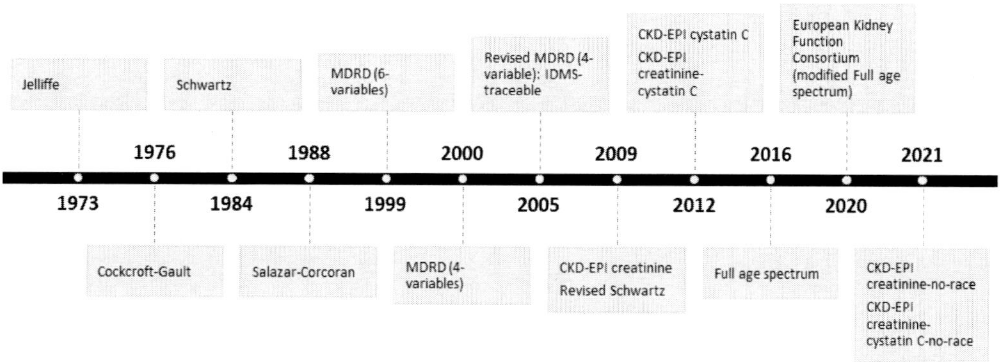

Figure 3. Timeline of equations used for estimation of CLcr and GFR.

Cockcroft-Gault Equation

$$\text{eCLcr}_{\text{(males)}}\ (\text{mL/min}) = \frac{(140 - Age) \times (W)}{(72) \times (Scr)}$$

$$\text{eCLcr}_{\text{(females)}}\ (\text{mL/min}) = \frac{(140 - Age) \times (W)}{(72) \times (Scr)} \times 0.85$$

Where age is in years, (W) is weight in kilograms, and S_{cr} in mg/dL.

Historically, most of the research work and clinical practice have been using the Cockcroft and Gault (CG) equation to estimate GFR [25]. The CG equation was developed to estimate CLcr (eCLcr) in adults using serum creatinine measured with a kinetic Jaffe assay, but has been used as a surrogate of GFR as well, regardless of that creatinine also undergoes tubular secretion. The CG equation has been shown to overestimate GFR with the use of standardized creatinine assays [26].

The CG equation report eCLcr in mL/min, and muscle mass is incorporated by using body weight, though not including height to represent accurate body surface area (BSA). For females, the authors of the equation made a hypothetical assumption of a modification factor of 0.85 to be multiplied by the resulting estimate to account for smaller muscle mass. There has been a debate since the introduction of Cockcroft-Gault equation, about which type of weight to be used in the equation. The original study developed the equation using actual body weight

(ABW). However, Cockcroft and Gault stated that S_{cr} may be falsely low and give an artificially high predicted eCLcr when muscle wasting has occurred, as well as patients with marked obesity who also excreted less creatinine per kilogram than expected. They suggested a correction to lean or ideal body weight when these abnormalities are pronounced (Table 3) [25].

Table 3. Equations used for estimation of weight parameters

Ideal body weight (Devine 1974) [36] Where (H) is height (cm)	*IBW (males) (kg) = 50 + [0.9 (H – 152)]* *IBW (females) (kg) = 45.5 + [0.9 (H – 152)]* *OR* *IBW (males) (kg) = 50 kg + 2.3 kg per inch over 5 feet* *IBW (females) (kg) = 45.5 kg + 2.3 kg per inch over 5 feet*
Adjusted body weight	$BW_{adj} = IBW + 0.4\ (ABW - IBW)$
Body mass index (1967) [37]	$BMI\ (Kg/m^2) = weight\ (kg) / [height\ (m)]^2$
Body surface area (Du Bois method) [38]	$BSA = 0.007184 \times Height\ [cm]^{0.725} \times Weight\ [kg]^{0.425}$
Lean body weight (2005) [39] Where ABW is in kg, and body mass index (BMI) is in kg per meter^2	$LBW_{(males)}\ (kg) = (9270 \times ABW) / [6680 + (216 \times BMI)]$ $LBW_{(females)}\ (kg) = (9270 \times ABW) / [8780 + (244 \times BMI)]$

ABW, actual body weight; BMI, body mass index; BSA, body surface area; BW_{adj}, adjusted body weight; IBW, ideal body weight; LBW, lean body weight.

Some authors proposed the use of ABW in underweight patients and ideal body weight (IBW) in patients of normal weight, while using an adjusted body weight (BW_{adj}) by multiplying ABW by a factor of 0.4 (ABW × (0.4)) for overweight, obese, and morbidly obese patients [27, 28]. The use of lean body weight (LBW) in CG equation have been proposed for estimating CLcr in obese and morbidly obese patients [29–31]. Other authors proposed using a range for drug dosing purposes, with the lower boundary defined by using IBW in the and the upper boundary by using TBW, and applying result as precisely as possible to the benefit versus risk analysis for a specific patient [32]. However, these proposals have not been validated on a large scale [30, 33, 34].

There has been a debate about rounding up S_{cr} in patients with low concentrations to account for the tendency of CG equation to overestimate GFR, however, there is no substantial evidence to support these suggestions, and it may lead to medication dosing errors [28, 35].

MDRD Study Equations

MDRD (Six-variable) Equation

$$eGFR\ (mL/minute/1.73\ m^2) = 170 \times (S_{cr}^{-0.999} \times age^{-0.176}) \times [1.180\ if\ black] \times [0.762\ if\ female] \times [SUN^{-0.170}] \times [Albumin^{0.318}]$$

MDRD (Four-variable) Equation

$$eGFR\ (mL/minute/1.73\ m^2) = 186 \times (S_{cr}^{-1.154} \times age^{-0.203}) \times [1.212\ if\ black] \times [0.742\ if\ female]$$

MDRD (Four-variable) Equation for IDMS Traceable S_{cr}

eGFR (mL/minute/1.73 m²) = 175.6 × (S_{cr} $^{−1.154}$ × Age $^{−0.203}$) × [1.212 if black] × [0.742 if female]

$$eGFR\ (mL/minute/1.73\ m^2) = 175.6 \times (S_{cr}^{-1.154} \times Age^{-0.203}) \times [1.212\ if\ black] \times [0.742\ if\ female]$$

Where:

Age is in years; S_{cr} in mg/dL; serum albumin concentration in g/dL; and SUN is serum urea nitrogen concentration in mg/dL.

The resulting eGFR values are 'normalized', as expressed for a BSA of 1.73 m^2. When using the equation for individuals with a different BSA, especially in extremes of BSA, the result should be readjusted, by converting it into units of mL/min. This is done by multiplying the result by individual's BSA divided by 1.73 m^2. For example, for a patient with eGFR of 40 mL/minute/1.73 m^2, and an actual BSA of 1.4 m^2, the adjusted eGFR = 40 ×1.4/1.73 = 32.4 mL/min.

The original Modification of Diet in Renal Disease (MDRD) Study equation was developed from a large cross-sectional study on predominantly nondiabetic patients with CKD, and a measured GFR (mGFR) using renal clearance of ^{125}I-iothalamate was also obtained for comparison. It had shown to be more accurate than measured creatinine clearance from 24-hour urine collections or estimated by the CG equation [40]. First, MDRD equation required six-variables, then, a simpler equation with four-variables was developed, and later, the equation was re-expressed for the standardized IDMS traceable S_{cr} assay. The MDRD Study equation has been validated in Caucasian and African American CKD patients between the ages of 18 and 70 with eGFR < 60 mL/min/1.73 m^2 [41, 42]. However, the equation has been shown to be less accurate in GFR > 60 ml/min per 1.73 m^2. The MDRD study equation was once recommended by the National Kidney Disease Education Program (NDKEP) in the United States to estimate GFR in adults along with the CLcr estimated by the CG equation.

CKD-EPI Equations

The original CKD-EPI equation was developed in 2009 to provide more precise estimates of GFR at higher values (i.e., eGFR > 60 mL/min/1.73 m^2). Authors used pooled data sets that included 8254 participants in 10 studies and validated their results against 3896 participants in another 16 studies, in which GFR was measured by exogenous markers (iothalamate in the development data set; iothalamate and other markers in the validation data set). The CKD-EPI creatinine equation was more accurate than the MDRD study equation at higher GFR and was as accurate as the MDRD study equation among individuals with eGFR less than 60 mL/min per 1.73 m^2 [43].

Later in 2012, other equations that included cystatin C were developed. The combined creatinine-cystatin C equation performed better than equations based on either of these markers alone, and can be useful as a confirmatory test for the diagnosis of CKD in patients with a decreased GFR as estimated from creatinine alone [44]. This can also be useful in obtaining a more accurate estimation of GFR in patients with differences in diet, extremes of muscle mass (such as body builders or patients with muscle wasting), or chronic illness.

As with the MDRD study equation, the CKD-EPI 2009 and 2012 equations included a factor for race, to account for the hypothetical increased muscle mass in black individuals. However, there have been several debates, as many advocates that race is rather a social construct that ignore the relative biological differences between individuals that we assume to be from the same race. This have been supported by studies that undermined the importance of race in improving accuracy of eGFR as the black coefficient did not predict well in non-American European and African black patients, and studies that showed variations among black individuals in the non-GFR determinants of serum creatinine [45–47]. Less data is available for other ethnicities. Using a four-level race variable (Black, Asian, Native American and Hispanic, and White and other) instead of the two-level variable for race (Black and White and other) did not improve performance, as the two-level race equation had minimal bias in Black, Native American and Hispanic, and White and other cohorts, while the four-level ethnicity equation significantly improved bias in Asians of the validation data set and in Chinese, and both equations had a large bias in Japanese and South African patients [48]. Estimating GFR in Asian populations is another controversial topic. In 2010, authors proposed the Japanese coefficient–modified CKD-EPI equation, with a coefficient of 0.813, resulting in a decrease in eGFR and a lower estimated prevalence of CKD in Japan [49]. While another study created a calibrated CKD-EPI ($eGFR_{cr\text{-}PK}$) equation for the general Pakistan population, an example of a south Asian population. The proposed equation is: ($eGFR_{CKD\text{-}EPI(PK)} = 0.686 \times eGFR_{CKD\text{-}EPI}^{1.059}$) [50]. When compared later with the 2012 Cystatin C-based CKD-EPI equations ($eGFR_{cys}$ and $eGFR_{cr\text{-}cys}$), the $eGFR_{cys}$ underestimated mGFR in South Asians and $eGFR_{cr\text{-}cys}$ did not offer substantial advantage compared with $eGFR_{cr\text{-}PK}$ [51]. However, although these proposed modifications reduced bias in studied cohorts, they are based on small size, cross-sectional trials with a temporal relationship of non-GFR determinants, and future studies are warranted to validate their accuracy.

On the other hand, other authors advocate that eliminating Race from GFR estimates may lead to systematic errors and underestimation of eGFR in black individuals even when height and weight are included [52].

Thus, accounting for race when estimating GFR continue to be controversial. Although it may be inaccurate and doesn't reflect variation in non-GFR determinants of serum creatinine, it may remain of importance in many cases in the absence of suitable surrogates for these physiologic variables, and inaccuracy from eliminating race could disadvantage blacks [53, 54].

The CKD-EPI group developed the 2021 CKD-EPI equation for estimating GFR from serum creatinine without a factor for race (Table 4). The new equation used the same dataset of the 2009 CKD-EPI creatinine equation and was validated in a new dataset of 4050 participants in 12 studies. The 2021 equation is slightly less accurate than the 2009 equation, but the overall accuracy is acceptable, as it underestimates mGFR in Black individuals (median, 3.6 ml per minute per 1.73 m^2; 95% CI, 1.8 to 5.5) but overestimates mGFR in non-Blacks by approximately same amount (median, 3.9 ml per minute per 1.73 m^2; 95% CI, 3.4 to 4.4) [55]. The American Society of Nephrology (ASN) and National Kidney Foundation (NKF) task force recommended the adoption of the 2021 CKD-EPI creatinine equation, and facilitating increased, routine, and timely use of cystatin C, especially to confirm estimated GFR in adults who are at risk for or have CKD, as combining creatinine and cystatin C is more accurate and would support better clinical decisions than either marker alone. The task force also recommended encouraging and funding research on GFR estimation with new endogenous filtration markers and on interventions to eliminate race and ethnic disparities [56].

Table 4. CKD-EPI equations

CKD-EPI Creatinine (2009) [43] Where: α is −0.329 for females and −0.411 for males	$eGFR_{cr}$ *(mL/minute/1.73 m²) =* $141 \times min (S_{cr}/\kappa, 1)^{\alpha} \times max (S_{cr}/\kappa, 1)^{-1.209} \times 0.993^{Age} \times 1.018$ *[if female]* $\times 1.159$ *[if black]*
CKD-EPI Cystatin C (2012) [44]	$eGFR_{cys}$ *(mL/minute/1.73 m²) =* $133 \times min (S_{cys}/0.8, 1)^{-0.499} \times max (S_{cys}/0.8, 1)^{-1.328} \times 0.996^{Age} \times 0.932$ *[if female]*
CKD-EPI Creatinine–Cystatin C (2012) [44] Where: α is −0.248 for females and −0.207 for males	$eGFR_{cr\text{-}cys}$ *(mL/minute/1.73 m²) =* $135 \times min (S_{cr}/\kappa, 1)^{\alpha} \times max (S_{cr}/\kappa, 1)^{-0.601} \times (min (S_{cys}/0.8, 1)^{-0.375} \times max (S_{Cys}/0.8, 1)^{-0.711} \times 0.995^{Age} \times 0.969$ *[if female]* $\times$ *[1.08 if black]*
CKD-EPI Creatinine (2021) [55] Where: α is −0.241 (female) or −0.302 (male)	*eGFR (mL/minute/1.73 m²) =* $142 \times min (S_{cr}/\kappa, 1)^{\alpha} \times max (S_{cr}/\kappa, 1)^{-1.200} \times 0.9938^{Age} \times 1.012$ *[if female]*
CKD-EPI Creatinine-Cystatin Equation (2021) [55] Where: α is −0.219 for females and −0.144 for males	$eGFR_{cr\text{-}cys}$ *(mL/minute/1.73 m²) =* $135 \times min (S_{cr}/\kappa, 1)^{\alpha} \times max (S_{cr}/\kappa, 1)^{-1.200} \times (min (S_{cys}/0.8, 1)^{-0.323} \times max (S_{Cys}/0.8, 1)^{-0.778} \times 0.9961^{Age} \times 0.963$ *[if female]*

Age in years; κ is 0.7 for females and 0.9 for males; S_{cr} is serum creatinine in mg/dL; S_{cys} is serum cystatin C in mg/L; min (Scr/κ, 1) is the minimum of S_{cr}/κ and 1.0; max (S_{cr}/κ, 1) is the maximum of Scr/κ and 1.0; min (S_{cys}/0.8, 1) indicates the minimum of S_{cys}/0.8 or 1; and max (S_{cys}/0.8, 1) indicates the maximum of S_{cys}/0.8 or 1.

The 2021 CKD-EPI equation showed similar performance to the prior CKD-EPI equations in a study on 415 kidney transplant recipients, with same day measurements of creatinine, cystatin C, and mGFR (^{99m}Tc-DTPA). No significant difference in performance was observed between the 2021 CKD-EPI$_{Cr}$ and 2021 CKD-EPI$_{cr\text{-}cys}$ equations in the kidney transplant population [57]. However, the study had limitations that include the small overall sample size, with only 11% of the validation set with eGFR <30 mL/min/1.73 m², and the racial representativeness, with 87% of the recipients self-identified as White, 3% Black, and the remaining as other races.

Answer to *Question 1*: The patient eGFR using CKD-EPI$_{cr}$ 2021 equation is 26 mL/min/1.73 m². As her BSA is 1.49 m², the adjusted eGFR would be 26 x 1.49/1.73 = 22.39 mL/min. Her estimated CLcr by CG equation is 22.73 mL/min. For this patient, the estimation of GFR would affect management, as whether to start an SGLT2 inhibitor. The precise estimation would prevent potential adverse events and would assure that she would not be denied from beneficial treatment. She would probably stop metformin. Extremes of muscles mass and vegetarian diet are known to affect Scr. As eGFR$_{cr}$ may be less accurate, confirmation test with eGFRcr-cys would be beneficial, assuming that the patient does not have other conditions that would affect eGFRcys, such as obesity, thyroid dysfunction, smoking, steroids use, or edema, then a measured GFR would be appropriate. The current KDIGO recommendation is to initiate SGLT2 inhibitors in patients with eGFR > 25 mL/min, and to continue until initiation of RRT.

Full Age Spectrum Equations

$$FAS\text{-}eGFR\ (for\ 2 \leq age \leq 40\ years) = \frac{107.3}{(Scr)/(Q)}$$

$$FAS\text{-}eGFR\ (for\ age > 40\ years) = \frac{107.3}{(Scr)/(Q)} \times 0.988^{(Age-40)}$$

The Full age spectrum (FAS) equation was developed on 2016, based on normalized serum creatinine (S_{cr}/Q), where Q is the median S_{cr} from healthy populations to account for age and sex. Coefficients for the equation were mathematically obtained by requiring continuity during the pediatric-adult and adult-elderly transition. The study was validated with mGFR (inulin, iohexol and iothalamate clearance) and IDMS traceable S_{cr}. The FAS equation was less biased and more accurate than the Schwartz equation for children and adolescents; less biased and as accurate as the CKD-EPI 2012 equation for young and middle-age adults; and less biased and more accurate than CKD-EPI 2012 for older adults. However, as the study used the Belgian growth curves to be representative for European children, matching other national growth curves to Q-values may be needed. Also, cystatin C equations were not considered in the comparison, and the study was validated for Caucasians only [58].

Later, a modified FAS equation was developed and validated on 2020, combining design features of the FAS and CKD-EPI equations. The new European Kidney Function Consortium (EKFC) equation is a FAS equation that showed less bias in children and adults) across the FAS (2 to 90 years) and S_{cr} range (0.45 to 5.54 mg/dL) and with fewer estimation errors exceeding 30% (6.5% [CI, 3.8% to 9.1%] in children and 3.1% [CI, 2.5% to 3.6%] in adults) compared with the Chronic Kidney Disease in Children Study (CKiD) equation for children and CKD-EPI equations (Table 5). However, the EKFC equation was not validated in black patients [59].

Table 5. The new EKFC equation [59]

Age	S_{cr}/Q	Equation
2-40 y	< 1	$107.3 \times (S_{cr}/Q)^{-0.322}$
	≥ 1	$107.3 \times (S_{cr}/Q)^{-1.132}$
> 40 y	< 1	$107.3 \times (S_{cr}/Q)^{-0.322} \times 0.990^{(Age-40)}$
	≥ 1	$107.3 \times (S_{cr}/Q)^{-1.132} \times 0.990^{(Age-40)}$
Q Values		
For ages 2–25 y	Males	$ln(Q) = 3.200 + 0.259 \times Age - 0.543 \times ln(Age) - 0.00763 \times Age^2 + 0.0000790 \times Age^3$
	Females	$ln(Q) = 3.080 + 0.177 \times Age - 0.223 \times ln(Age) - 0.00596 \times Age^2 + 0.0000686 \times Age^3$
For ages >25 y	Males	$Q = 80\ \mu mol/L\ (0.90\ mg/dL)$
	Females	$Q = 62\ \mu mol/L\ (0.70\ mg/dL)$

Q values (in µmol/L or mg/dL) correspond to the median S_{cr} values for the age- and sex-specific populations. EKFC = European Kidney Function Consortium. To convert µmol/L to mg/dL, divide by 88.4.

Schwartz Equations

The Schwartz formula was developed in 1976 to estimate GFR in children from S_{cr} and body length [60]. Since then, several modifications to the original equation had been published. In 2009, the formula was revised to avoid overestimation of eGFR after standardization of the IDMS traceable S_{cr} methods [61]. The revised "Bedside Schwartz" formula was developed using data from the CKiD study, and was later validated in a sample of pediatric patients with less impaired renal function [62]. The bedside Schwartz formula is validated for use in children 1-18 years old. The equation uses a constant "k" that is directly proportional to the muscle component of body and varies with age. The eGFR also depends on the laboratory assay used to measure serum creatinine (i.e., Jaffe or enzymatic method for creatinine) [63]. Later in 2012, equations utilizing cystatin-C were developed [64]. These equations may be useful as a confirmatory test in specific circumstances when eGFR based on S_{cr} is less accurate, or when the clinical scenario warrants a secondary test. However, back in 2012, the cystatin C values were not yet standardized to the International Federation of Clinical Chemistry (IFCC standards). In 2021, newer age and sex dependent CKiD Under 25 (U25) GFR estimating equations based on enzymatic method for creatinine and IFCC-standardized cystatin C have been developed by the CKiD study for children and young adults with CKD up to age 25 years old [65]. The eGFR derived from the average of the two single-marker eGFR values is less biased, more accurate, and more precise than either of the two single-marker estimates [66] (See Table 6).

Table 6. Equations for eGFR in children and young adults

Revised Schwartz (2009) [61]	$eGFR\ (mL/min/1.73\ m^2) = "k" \times height\ in\ cm / S_{cr}$
Where values of "k":	
Method for creatinine	*k*
- Jaffe method	
Premature infants through the first year of life	*0.33*
Term infants through the first year of life	*0.45*
Children and adolescent girls	*0.55*
Adolescent boys	*0.7*
- Enzymatic method	
All children with CKD between ages 1 and 16 years	*0.413*
Cystatin C-based equation (2012) [64]	$eGFR_{cys}\ (mL/min/1.73\ m^2) = 70.69 \times (S_{Cys})^{-0.931}$
Creatinine-cystatin C-based CKiD equation (2012) [64]	$eGFR_{cr\text{-}cys}\ (mL/min/1.73\ m^2) = 39.8 \times [ht/S_{cr}]^{0.456} \times [1.8/S_{Cys}]^{0.418} \times [30/BUN]^{0.079} \times [1.076\ if\ male] \times [ht\ in\ meters/1.4]^{0.179}$
CKiD Under 25 (U25) equation [65]	Online calculator: https://ckid-gfrcalculator.shinyapps.io/eGFR/

BUN (blood urea nitrogen) = mg/dL; SCys (cystatin C) = mg/L; Scr (standardized serum creatinine) = mg/dL.

Drug Dosing Considerations

Historically, most drug dosing recommendations have been developed using the CG equation to guide dose adjustment in renal impairment. But as mentioned before, the standardization of creatinine assay introduced another limitation of using the CG equation, as most pharmacokinetic studies for drug dosing in kidney disease were done before the era of standardization. In 2011, The Kidney Disease Improving Global Outcomes (KDIGO) published a clinical update on drug dosing in patients with AKI and CKD [11]. In this report, KDIGO recommended that clinicians should use the most accurate method/tool to assess kidney function for the individual patient (i.e., eCLcr or eGFR or mGFR) and that clinical laboratories should report eGFR in ml/min as well as ml/min per $1.73m^2$. As noted, if the reported eGFR is in units of ml/min per $1.73m^2$, then it should be multiplied by BSA and divided by 1.73 to convert it to units of mL/min. Equations for estimating GFR require stable renal function, as a steady-state concentration of S_{cr} is mandator. Other considerations would affect drug dosing in patients with AKI and patients requiring RRT.

Patients with CKD

Chronic kidney disease alters many PK and PD parameters. Volume overload increase the V_d of many drugs (hydrophilic drugs) and hypoalbuminemia increase the free fraction of protein bound drugs. Nonrenal clearance is also affected. Accumulated uremic toxins and inflammatory cytokines may affect uptake and efflux transporters and hepatic drug metabolism cytochrome P450 enzymes [67]. Drug metabolites and parent compounds may accumulate in patients with CKD, and the effects of accumulated parent compounds and metabolites in CKD may be markedly different than in normal renal functions.

The current staging of kidney function based on eGFR (Table 2) may differ from many drug dosing recommendations that classified renal impairment according to arbitrary terms of mild, moderate and severe, which may not express the exact definitions among dosing recommendations and the related PK studies. Moreover, many dosing recommendations use broad adjustment ranges of eGFR, putting different classes of CKD in the same range, which may not be optimal for drugs with narrow-therapeutic index. Avoiding nephrotoxic drugs is recommended in all stages as possible. To achieve therapeutic goals, KDIGO recommended a stepwise approach that ensure individualization (Figure 4).

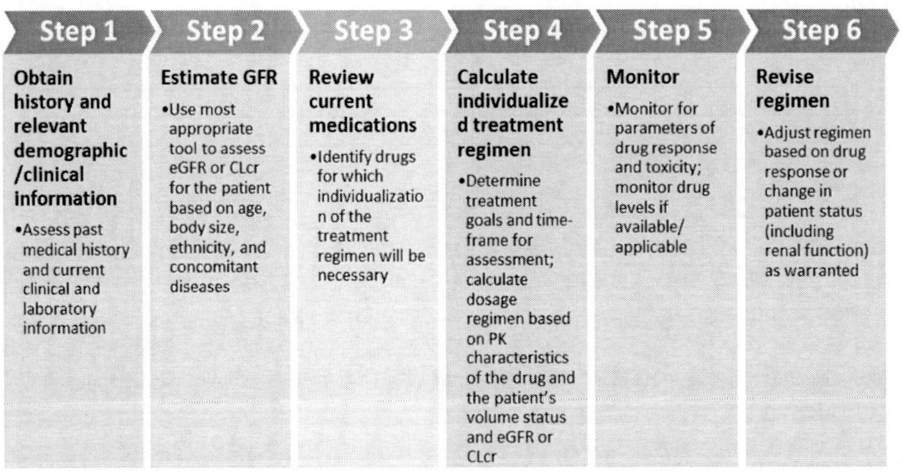

AKI, acute kidney injury; CKD, chronic kidney disease; CLcr, creatinine clearance; eGFR, estimated GFR; GFR, glomerular filtration rate.

Data from: Matzke et al. 2011 (*Kidney Int*. https://doi.org/10.1038/ki.2011.322).

Figure 4. Stepwise approach to adjust drug dosage regimens for patients with CKD and AKI.

Loading Dose

Generally, loading doses are required when there is a need to rapidly achieve steady-state concentration with a drug that has a long half-life. When the V_d of a drug is significantly increased due to volume overload or hypoalbuminemia, a loading dose will likely be needed even if not routinely recommended for patients with normal renal function, as the loading dose is proportional to the V_d. Fluid overload is more likely to affect the V_d of hydrophilic drugs (for example, aminoglycoside and β-lactams). The modified loading dose could be calculated according to the degree of change in the V_d as follows:

Patient's loading dose = Usual loading dose × Patient's V_d/Normal V_d

Maintenance Dose

Subsequent doses require careful consideration of drug PK and PD, along with monitoring of response and side-effects, as the maintenance dose depends on clearance. Prolonging dosing interval, dose adjustment, or both, can be choices to attain similar steady-state concentrations similar to those in patients with normal renal functions.

> The previous patient in *Question 1* suffered from gastroenteritis with persistent vomiting and diarrhea. She presented to the hospital with hypotension, dehydration, and oliguria. Her serum creatinine raised to 2.8 mg/dL.
>
> *Question 2*: How would you assess her GFR at hospitalization?

Patients with AKI

AKI commonly occurs in critically ill patients, often in the context of multiple organ dysfunction syndrome, where a dynamic change occurs in affected organs and fluid status that ultimately affect several PK parameters. These changes markedly affect drug concentrations if not properly adjusted. The challenge is that serum creatinine would not be at steady state, limiting the use of equations for estimating GFR, as if the serum creatinine is falling, the eGFR would underestimate the actual GFR, and vice versa. Instead, the change in trend in serum creatinine and urine output should be utilized to judge the decline or recovery in kidney function. If the patient is anuric, then GFR should be presumed to be 0 mL/min. Dose adjustment may be required on a daily basis accordingly during the course of AKI to limit the risk of adverse effects without compromising efficacy. For medications with a directly measurable physiologic response (e.g., antihypertensives or vasopressors), the dose should be titrated to the desired clinical endpoint.

The V_d of many drugs could increase significantly during sepsis and AKI. This could be caused by large volume of fluids used for resuscitation, increased capillary permeability, third space compartments (e.g., pleural effusion or ascites), as well as changes in protein binding. This change in V_d will influence hydrophilic antimicrobial dosing strategies, whereas for lipophilic drugs, the V_d would remain unchanged [68].

Loading Dose

Clinicians should carefully review the PK and PD characteristics of medications. As the V_d of hydrophilic drugs is significantly increased during AKI, especially antibiotics, including b-lactams, cephalosporins, and carbapenems, administration of aggressive loading doses (25–50% greater than normal) are highly recommended, even if a loading dose is not routinely recommended for patients with normal renal function [11].

Maintenance Dose

Clinicians should carefully monitor the degree and rate of change in kidney function and fluid volume status. The dosing regimen for many drugs, especially antimicrobial agents, should be initiated at normal or near normal, especially if AKI is likely reversible (e.g., prerenal due to decreased perfusion), and the drugs have a wide therapeutic index, such as antibiotics for septic shock. The exception is when the drug accumulation would be associated with adverse events, such as neurotoxicity with cefepime. Close daily monitoring for the change in trend in serum creatinine and urine output is recommended to adjust further doses.

Use of Equations to Estimate GFR during AKI

Several equations for estimating unstable renal function based on two non-steady-state serum creatinine values have been proposed, including the Jelliffe (1972), Chiou (1975), Brater (1983), and Jelliffe (2002) methods [69–72]. All these equations lack the robust evidence of the equations for stable renal function and are poorly validated in a large group of patients.

An alternative method is to measure CLcr based on urine measurements, either a 24-hour collection, or a shorter duration. The amount of creatinine excreted in urine (concentration × volume × time) is divided by the mean S_{cr} concentration (average of the S_{cr} at the beginning and the end of the 24-hour urine collection) and converted into mL/min.

In 2013, a kinetic eGFR (KeGFR) equation was proposed [73]. This method has not yet been validated in comparison with a measured GFR. In a small retrospective study, the KeGFR equation predicted the AKI and the need for RRT more accurately than MDRD [74]. The utility of KeGFR equation requires validation in larger prospective studies.

$$KeGFR = SSP_{Cr} \times CLcr / Mean\ P_{Cr} \times [1 - (24 \times \Delta P_{Cr} / \Delta Time\ (h) \times Max\ \Delta P_{Cr}/Day)]$$

Where:

SSP_{Cr} is a previous baseline steady-state plasma creatinine; CLcr is the creatinine clearance based on the previous steady-state plasma creatinine; the Mean P_{Cr} is arithmetic mean of the starting and the ending values of two creatinine endpoints, ΔP_{Cr} refers to the change in plasma creatinine. It is defined as the ending creatinine minus the starting creatinine or P_{Cr} (end) – P_{Cr} (start); ΔTime (h) is the interval in hours between the two consecutive creatinine measures; Max ΔP_{Cr}/Day refers to the maximal change (increase) in the plasma creatinine that can occur per day if renal function is completely lost. In anuric AKI, the customary teaching is that the plasma creatinine can rise at most by 1.0–1.5 mg/dl per day.

Therapeutic Drug Monitoring (TDM)

Measurement of drug concentrations should be used whenever possible, especially for drugs with a narrow therapeutic range. However, this could be limited by unavailability of assay, delayed results, and high cost. When TDM is not possible, patients should be carefully monitored for therapeutic effects and toxicities and use them as a surrogate for need for dosage adjustment.

Answer to *Question 2*: The patient presented with AKI, probably due to hypovolemia after vomiting and diarrhea. Estimation of GFR using equations requires a stable Scr at steady state. Equations like KeGFR would offer some help, however it is not validated till now, and may either over-estimate or underestimate actual GFR. Monitoring trend in Scr and urine output is recommended. Understanding the drug specific PK and PD is essential. The patient would probably require fluid resuscitation, that would cause an increase in the V_d of hydrophilic drugs.

RRT

The impact of RRT on drugs is dependent on several factors, including the drug physiochemical and pharmacokinetic characteristics, the dialysis prescription, and the clinical condition. Drug characteristics include the V_d, water solubility, molecular weight, and degree of protein binding. The mechanical properties of the dialyzer affect drug clearance, as the dialyzability would increase with the larger surface area of the dialyzer and the higher porosity of the dialysis membrane. High-flux membranes have larger pore sizes allowing the passage of most solutes. The higher dialysate and blood flow rates also increase dialyzability. The dialysis prescription and frequency affect drug clearance by varying degrees. There are two main types of dialysis: hemodialysis (HD) and peritoneal dialysis (PD). Different HD modalities exist, including conventional intermittent HD, continuous renal replacement therapy (CRRT), and prolonged intermittent renal replacement therapy (PIRRT). The indication for RRT differs according to clinical condition, including fluid overload and removal of uremic toxins in patients with AKI or in end-stage kidney disease (ESKD) patients. CRRT and hybrid modalities like PIRRT are usually utilized in hemodynamically unstable patients, and intermittent HD is usually utilized in ESKD patients on maintenance RRT. The patient's residual kidney function is an added factor in drug clearance and should be accounted for. Also, the non-renal clearance of some drugs was found to be changed during RRT, this could be related to the removal of uremic toxins that inhibit CYP450 and drug transporters [75, 76]. Although some drugs have an observable clinical effect that can be titrated to the desired clinical response (e.g., analgesics, sedatives, and vasopressors), others cannot be evaluated by the same methods, and subtherapeutic concentration or toxicities could occur. Optimizing antimicrobials is of great concern especially in critically ill patients with sepsis, and though TDM is recommended for medications with a narrow therapeutic index (e.g., vancomycin, phenytoin, and gentamicin), the serum concentrations of most antimicrobials cannot be measured in the clinical setting.

You are reviewing the condition of a 45-year-old male who was admitted to the ICU with sepsis. He is an ESKD patient on maintenance hemodialysis thrice weekly through a right internal jugular long-term hemodialysis catheter. He is suspected to have a catheter-related blood stream infection. Blood cultures were withdrawn, and the catheter was removed. Empirical antibiotics are to be initiated with meropenem and vancomycin. His weight is 75 kg and his height is 170 cm. The patient has a residual renal clearance of 8 mL/min.

Question 3: What would you recommend to optimize vancomycin dosing in this patient?

Conventional intermittent HD utilize rapid solute clearance and ultrafiltration over a brief duration (usually 3-5 hours) performed thrice weekly in outpatient regimens. The common approach is to administer drugs with high dialyzability after the end of the session. A supplemental dose could be administered after session for partly dialyzed drugs. However, for some drugs, predialysis dosing could be beneficial. An example is gentamicin, where a larger predialysis dose is proposed to optimize the concentration–time profile [77, 78]. Clinicians should maintain a simple consistent schedule on dialysis and non-dialysis days to avoid errors and wasting of resources. It is important to note that drug dosing regimens for intermittent HD are mostly based on thrice weekly sessions, and for patients receiving more or less sessions, an individualized therapeutic plan would be needed.

Continuous and hybrid modalities provide more gradual solute clearance and ultrafiltration over prolonged duration. CRRT can be useful to manage hemodynamically unstable AKI patients, with sessions optimally reaching 24 hours per day. Several factors affect drug removal, including modes (convective, diffusive, or both), filters used, and effluent flow rates. Modalities include continuous veno-venous hemofiltration (CVVH), continuous veno-venous hemodialysis (CVVHD), and continuous veno-venous hemodiafiltration (CVVHDF). The challenge in optimizing drug dosing regimens for patients receiving CRRT or PIRRT is the interaction between many factors, including those related to RRT, along with nonrenal clearance, residual kidney function, and changes in Vd and protein binding [79, 80]. Only few drugs have clear recommendations for dosing adjustment during CRRT, and guidance is not often provided in a product labeling.

Hybrid PIRRT modalities utilize higher dialysate flow rates than those used in CRRT, but shorter treatment periods (6–12 hours), and lower blood and dialysate flow rates with longer periods compared with intermittent HD. PIRRT is becoming an increasingly popular alternative to CRRT in critically ill patients due to cost-effectiveness [81]. Modalities include slow low-efficiency dialysis (SLED), extended daily dialysis, continuous SLED, slow low-efficiency daily dialysis (SLEDD), and slow low-efficiency daily hemodiafiltration (SLEDD-f). The main challenge in drug dosing in patients receiving PIRRT is its inconsistent nature that complicates drug dosing, as patients would require different regimens for dialyzable drugs during PIRRT (intradialytic) and different regimens during days without PIRRT (interdialytic). Another challenge is whether drugs should be administered before, during, or after PIRRT. There are only few data regarding drug dosing adjustment during PIRRT due to scarcity of PK studies. [82-88]

Conclusion

Clinicians should understand the varying PK and PD effects of AKI and CKD and be vigilant with the dynamic changes that can occur during the treatment course, especially in critical illness, and can predispose patients to therapeutic failure or significant adverse events. TDM can be useful in optimizing a tailored patient-centered regimen for drugs with a narrow therapeutic index, however, this requires availability of standardized assays, a fast turnaround time, and a reasonable cost.

Carbamazepine

Carbamazepine (CBZ) is used for treatment of various types of seizures where its chemical structure resembles the tricyclic antidepressant agent. Many dosage forms are available in the market containing carbamazepine as oral tablets, chewable tablets, extended-release tablets or even oral suspension [89-95]. The intended therapeutic concentration of carbamazepine, which is preferred by many clinicians, should be in the range of 4 to 8 mg/L instead of 4 to 12 mg/L, as shown in Table 6. Carbamazepine toxicity symptoms may occur in patients if the drug concentration exceeds 9 mg/L. 10,11 epoxide, a carbamazepine metabolite can elevate carbamazepine concentration to some extent due to cross reactivity especially with the concomitant administration of valproic acid which increases its formation [96, 97].

Absorption of carbamazepine from the gastrointestinal tract is slow and variable despite being a lipid soluble compound. Therefore, carbamazepine administration with high fat meal can increase the rate not the extent of drug absorption (AUC). Following the administration of rapid or immediate release preparations, the peak concentration (C_{max}) is attended after 6 h (2 to 24 h). This drug undergoes first pass metabolism so giving the drug with grapefruit juice can inhibit CYP 3A4 in the liver and the gut so increases the drug bioavailability. Being a neutral compound, carbamazepine binds to both albumin and alpha1-acid glycoprotein where its free fraction is estimated to be in the range of 20 to 30% of total drug and this fraction significantly increases in uremic patient. Carbamazepine has a mean Vd of 1.4 L/kg (0.8 to 1.9 L/kg) [98].

Loading doses of carbamazepine are not recommended due to auto-induction where it is preferred to use maintenance doses of the drug to allow gradual increase in concentration until reaching steady state. In addition, patients should be started on a fraction of calculated maintenance dose which should be then increased in an interval of 1 to 2 weeks until reaching the full calculated dose. CBZ auto-induction refers to the induction of its own metabolism by CYP 3A4, which is thought to subside after 5 to 7 days after use. CBZ is mainly metabolized by the liver via CYP 3A4 isoenzyme where only a small fraction (<2%) is excreted in the urine. CBZ is considered a liver microsomal enzyme inducer where it induces the metabolism (cross induction) of other drugs through induction of CYP 1A2, CYP 3A4, CYP 2C9 and CYP2C19 [92, 108].

The mean clearance of the drug when given chronically will differ from that if it is given as monotherapy (~0.064 L/kg/h) or with other enzyme inducing antiepileptics (~0.1 L/kg/h). Consequently, additional monitoring of plasma carbamazepine concentration is needed when it is concomitantly used with other anticonvulsants to assure the desired drug response. The average elimination half-life of the drug is about 10 h when administered with other enzyme-inducing antiepileptics as phenytoin, phenobarbital, primidone and about 15 h when given alone [91].

Table 7. Therapeutic drug monitoring medications for carbamazepine

Drug	Therapeutic Serum Conc.	When to Sample
Carbamazepine	4 to 12 mg/L Recommended 4 to 8 mg/L SI units 17-51 (μmol/L) Converting factor 1 mg/L= 4.23 μmol/L	Trough: Immediately prior to the next dose, 5 days after start or change in dose. If toxicity suspected, sample peak 3-4 hours post dose.
Interventions/Comments		
Low Level	No Adverse Events/ Seizures not Controlled: Titrate upward by 200-400mg /day until seizure control. Maximum maintenance dose: 1600mg/day	
High Level	Adverse Events/ With Seizure Control: Reduce dose by slow tapering down of 200 mg/day. Adverse Events/Seizure not Controlled: Consider other drug therapy	

Inhibitors of carbamazepine metabolism include erythromycin, clarithromycin, azole antifungals, protease inhibitors,cimetidine, diltiazem, verapamil and grapefruit juice. Since children are rapid drug metabolizers, the elimination half-life will be in a range of 4 to 12 hours. Although plasma sampling of carbamazepine during the first weeks of administration is not useful for long term monitoring, it can serve as a guidance of the relation between therapeutic response and drug concentration. Trough concentration (prior to the next dose) or obtaining a sample in the morning prior to the first dose of the drug (Table 7) is usually preferred for plasma monitoring once the drug reaches the steady state [92, 109].

Self-Assessment Questions

1. Loading doses of carbamazepine are not recommended as the drug is subjected to
   a. First pass metabolism
   b. Auto-induction
   c. Elevated absorption

2. _______ decreases plasma drug concentration of carbamazepine
   a. Erythromycin
   b. Diltiazem
   c. Grapefruit juice
   d. Phenobarbital

3. Which of the following sentences best describes carbamazepine?
   a. It is a lipophilic drug and rapidly absorbed from GIT
   b. It is an acidic drug and highly bound to plasma albumin
   c. It undergoes first pass metabolism in the gut and liver
   d. Its free fraction is less than 10% of total drug

Cyclosporine

Cyclosporine is an immunosuppressant used to prevent the rejection of transplanted organs but not for treatment where it is usually administered with other immunosuppressive drugs. Also, it has an important role in treatment of autoimmune diseases as psoriasis and rheumatoid arthritis. Various preparations are available in the market in the form of capsules or liquid solutions.

Generally, cyclosporine is found in two forms: original formulation (cyclosporine prepared in olive oil Sandimmune®) and cyclosporine modified solution (Sandimmune® Neoral®). The main difference between these two forms is the need for bile salts for emulsification and subsequently absorption from the gastrointestinal tract. Absorption of original preparation definitely depends on the presence of bile while cyclosporine modified solution is prepared as a micro-emulsion with no need for the presence of bile to be absorbed [99,100]. From that, disorders as cholestasis, diarrhea and external biliary drainage will decrease the absorption of original formulations not modified solutions.

Also, modified formulations offer the advantages of rapid rate and great extent of absorption (higher C_{max} and AUC) and that explains the current preference of their use over original formulations. Side effects associated with cyclosporine use include neurotoxicity, reversible renal dysfunction, hirsutism, gingival hyperplasia, malignancies and opportunistic infections. Sandimmune® and Neoral® are not bioequivalent and cannot be used interchangeably.

To prevent rejection of transplanted organs, cyclosporine is usually initiated in an approximate dose of 2.5 to 5 mg/kg twice daily. The intended therapeutic range may differ based on transplant organ and exact time of administration after transplantation, as shown in table 8. Cyclosporine is lipophilic and highly bound to blood cells (red and white blood cells) and lipoproteins where only less than 10% of total drug is found free in plasma. The binding affinity of cyclosporine to blood components depends on temperature. So, it is preferred to use whole blood sample for concentration monitoring or keeping the temperature at 37°C during assay of other blood samples (serum or plasma) to guarantee accurate results [100, 101].

Various assay techniques can be used for monitoring drug concentration as high performance liquid chromatography (HPLC), monoclonal and polyclonal radioimmunoassay and fluorescence polarization immunoassay. Therapeutic ranges determined by any type of polyclonal assays are usually higher than that of monoclonal ones where this returned to lower specificity of polyclonal assays. Both the drug and its metabolites can be determined by polyclonal assay. HPLC is the preferred assay method due to its lower cost, its ability to detect drug metabolite or any interference.

Despite the high lipophilicity of cyclosporine, its bioavailability is limited where that of conventional formulations is about 30%. For oil based formulations, cyclosporine reaches its peak concentration 4 to 6 hours post dose administration where modified formulations only require 1 to 2 hours to reach C_{max}. Cyclosporine is affected by first pass metabolism by CYP3A4 in the gut and is transported by P-glycoprotein which is a drug efflux pump. Vd of cyclosporine is relatively large (~4 to 5 L/kg) which indicates its significant binding to blood elements and extensive distribution into extravascular tissues and only less than 10% of drug is found free in plasma. Cyclosporine is extensively metabolized in the liver and gut by CYP3A4 into less active metabolites than parent drug.

The total drug clearance from plasma is considered low (~ 5 to 10 mL/kg/min) and this is returned to the low free fraction of drug which is susceptible to elimination. The elimination half-life of the drug ranges from 6 to 12 h [92, 102].

Measuring trough concentration is the most common method used for monitoring cyclosporine therapy. This concentration monitoring is essential after dosage adjustment and when starting or stopping a drug which is liver microsomal enzyme (CYP3A4) inducer or inhibitor or when patient experiences any seizures. Determination of area under the concentration-time curve (AUC_{0-12}) through collecting several blood samples over a period of 12 h post dose administration can be used as alternative method for monitoring cyclosporine therapy as it is strongly related to clinical outcomes. Despite being an accurate reflection of exposure to the drug, AUC method has a major drawback due to its high cost and impracticality. For that, a new method called sparse sample method or abbreviated AUC can replace AUC_{0-12} which depends on measuring drug concentration at 2 or 3 hourly points to predict AUC [99-101].

Table 8. Therapeutic drug monitoring medications for cyclosporine

Drug	Therapeutic Serum Conc.	When to Sample
Cyclosporine*	50-300 ng/mL SI units 42-250 (nmol/L) Converting factor 1 ng/mL = 0.832 nmol/L	12-hour trough (C0) concentrations **Two-hour post-dose (C2) Level checked two to three days after starting cyclosporine and after any dose change
Interventions / Comments		
Low	Increase by 25 -50 mg/ dose	
high	Decrease by 25 -50 mg/ dose	
Supra therapeutics	>400 ng/mL: Check if it is true level Hold until the concentration returns to the therapeutic range Resume with lower dose	

Notes:
*Immunosuppressant Target concentrations Vary depends on:

- Organ transplanted (Kidney, liver, pancreas, lung or heart)
- Time after transplant (early vs. late)
- Patient specific factor (infection, drug-drug, or drug-food interaction)

** C2 monitoring may be more accurate but is often more difficult (not practical) and less convenient for the patient. In rare circumstances, assessing both may be beneficial in a patient with absorption issues.

Self-Assessment Questions

1. _______ method reflects drug exposure during cyclosporine monitoring and is considered impractical
   a. Trough Conc
   b. AUC0-12
   c. Sparse sample

2. Which of the following is true about cyclosporine modified formulations?
   a. They are absorbed only in the presence of bile
   b. Their absorption is decreased by external biliary drainage
   c. They result in higher C_{max} and greater AUC
   d. They are less used than original formulations

3. Volume of distribution of cyclosporine is relatively large due to
   a. Its high binding affinity to blood elements
   b. Its low distribution into extravasular space
   c. Its high free fraction

Lithium

Lithium is an alkali metal that is delivered to the human body as monovalent (Li^+). Its psychiatric uses were discovered in 1940s, but its mechanism of action is still mainly unknown. It is prescribed for the primary management of bipolar disorders, the acute and mixed episodes of mania in patients having bipolar 1 or 2 disorders, and the maintenance therapy of bipolar disorders to avoid or reduce the severity of subsequent manic episodes. It is also used for the management of tardive dyskinesia, cluster headaches, and alcoholism,. Lithium is available in orally administered citrate and carbonate salts. Electrolytes levels are measured in the body in mmol/L or mEq/L. Lithium is available as 300 mg lithium carbonate in the market that equalizes 8.12 mEq of lithium salt [89], as shown in table 9.

Although, Lithium has small therapeutic range, its plasma therapeutic concentration is clearly established. The usual serum level of lithium for acute mania is 0.8-1.2 mEq/L (Table 9), and levels of 1.2-1.5 mEq/L are rarely required. The majority of clinicians use various treatment concentration in the light of medical circumstances of the patient. Once the therapeutic level is controlled, the long-term maintenance level can be 0.6-1 mEq/L and may rarely reach 1.2 mEq/L. Such target serum levels adopt a frequent daily dosing model. Lithium concentration after oral delivery exhibits complicated concentration/time curve that is explained by multi-compartment models [90].

Gastrointestinal (GI) and central nervous system (CNS) related- side effects are two of the most well-known lithium-related adverse effects. About 30% of patients may show GI adverse effects that may include diarrhea, nausea, bloating, and vomiting. However, about 40%-50% of patients have CNS adverse effects that may involve lethargy, confusion, headache, mild loss of memory, and tremors especially hand tremors. These CNS adverse effects may be related to great peak concentration. That is why delivering immediate-release lithium preparations with food is favorable to minimize such effects. All patients on lithium therapy have their thyroid gland monitored for any signs or symptoms of hypothyroidism such as hypotension, fatigue, and cold intolerance. Thyroid-stimulating hormone (TSH) should be examined at baseline and every 6-12 months. Lithium is sorted as pregnancy category D, as it is teratogen. Lithium toxicity can be predicted from its serum levels [91].

It is available as oral liquid, tablet, and capsule preparation. It is rapidly absorbed and attains the peak serum level 30-60 min with liquid syrup and 1-3 hr with immediate-release capsules and tablets. The absorption of immediate-release preparations form GIT is approximately complete (95-100%), the oral bioavailability (f) therefore, is 1.

Lithium is not bound to plasma proteins, is widely distributed throughout the body equal to that of water. Its distribution is governed by two-compartment open model of pharmacokinetics. The central compartment is where lithium rapidly distributes in organs with a good blood supply, while the peripheral compartment, such as skin, muscle, and bone, is where lithium less quickly distributes. Blood samples should, therefore, be taken after complete distribution. The final Vd is 0.7 L/kg after the distribution is terminated, but it is reduced in the elderly.

Lithium is monovalent cation, so it is not metabolized. In patients with normal sodium balance, lithium clearance is equal to 25% of creatinine clearance (CrCl). Its clearance is directly correlated to glomerular filtration rate. The clearance for adults is 0.024 L/hr/kg, while it is reduced in the elderly.

Lithium has two half-lives, the first is called alpha half-life and specific to distribution (6 hr), and the second is called beta half-life and specific to elimination (20-24 hr). It takes 3-5 days to attain lithium steady state (Css). However, Health care providers should be attentive that full therapeutic outcomes may take 14-21 days [91, 92].

The optimum time to take a lithium blood sample is either just prior to the morning dose (trough concentration) or 8-12 hr after the evening dose so that a full distribution and equilibrium can be attained. Any factor that can change GFR or sodium balance will influence lithium clearance and therefore its serum level. Concomitant use of certain medications such as thiazide diuretics, NSAIDs, and angiotensin-converting enzyme inhibitor (ACEs) can achieve lithium toxicity. In contrary, methylxanzines (theophylline-caffeine) may achieve sub-therapeutic level of lithium [91].

Table 9. Therapeutic drug monitoring for Lithium medication

Drug	Therapeutic Serum Conc.	When to Sample
Lithium	Usually: 0.4-1.0 mmol/L Elderly: 0.4-0.8 mmol/L Acute bipolar disorder: up to 1.2 mmol/L Lithium is a monovalent cation; the conversion factor is 1 from mEq to mmol.	Ideally, 12 hours after last dose
Interventions/Comments		
300 mg of Lithium Carbonate is equivalent to 8 mEq of Lithium. During the first 6-10 hours after a dose, serum lithium concentrations fluctuate due to circadian variation in elimination. Renal disease and dehydration increase levels. • Acute bipolar disorder may require concentrations up to 1.2 mmol/L • 0.8 mmol/L preferred upper end of target range • Relapses more likely below approximately 0.5 mmol/L		

Case Study

M.S is a 43-year-old white female to be placed on lithium carbonate for refractory acute mania. Her serum creatinine = 1.1 mg/dl. What is the maintenance dose to attain a steady-state lithium serum level of 1.5 mEq/L?

The salt factor (S) equals 1. Bioavailability (F) =1. Height: 5′6″, Weight: 70 kg

Step 1: We should work out the patient's lithium clearance:

She is female so a factor of 0.85 is used for a creatinine clearance calculation.

Crcl = $0.85\frac{(140-\text{age})*\text{IBW}}{72*\text{Srcr}} = 0.85\frac{(140-43)*70\ kg}{72*1.1\ mg/dl}$=72.8 ml/min * 60 min/1000 ml =4.37 l/hr.

whilst sodium level is normally balanced, lithium clearance equalizes 25% of creatinine clearance.

Licl= 0.25* Crcl

Licl= 0.25*4.37=1.09 l/hr

Step 2: We should work out the maintenance dose (MD) using the following equation:

$$MD = \frac{Cssav*CL*\tau}{S*F}$$

MD= maintenance dose required, Cssav= steady state needed to achieve, τ = daily dosing interval, S= salt factor, F= bioavailability.

$$MD = \frac{1.5\frac{mEq}{L}*1.09\ L/hr*24hr}{1*1}$$

$$MD = 39.24\ mEq/day$$

Note that daily dosing interval (τ) may be 24 hr or 1 day depending on the units of data in the equation such that all units should be of the same type.

Step 3: We should convert lithium carbonate milliequivalents into the equivalent lithium carbonate dose in milligrams using the following formula:

$$\text{Lithium carbonate (mg)} = \frac{Lithium\ dose\ mEq * 300\ mg}{8.12\ mEq}$$

$$\text{Lithium carbonate (mg)} = \frac{39.24\ mEq * 300\ mg}{8.12\ mEq}$$

$$\text{Lithium carbonate (mg)} = 1449\ mg \approx 1500\ mg/\text{day}$$

If 300-mg capsule is available, this patient may be placed on any of the following regimens:

1) Lithium carbonate 300 mg: 1 capsule 5x/day.
2) Lithium carbonate 300 mg: 2 capsules in the morning, 1 capsule in the afternoon, 2 capsules in the evening.

If M.S has an acute episode of asthma, and theophylline is currently added to her medical regimen, lithium therapy then needs dosing adjustment. If theophylline affects LiCl by 20%, LiCl will increase to 120% and maintenance dose should be then increased to 120%, so as to keep the desired steady state. The maintenance dose of lithium will be 1500 *1.2 = 1800 mg (600 mg three times daily).

Self-Assessment Questions

1. The concurrent use of _______ may produce lithium therapy failure.
   a. lisinopril
   b. aminophylline
   c. naproxen
   d. hydrochlorothiazide

2. Which of the following best describes lithium therapy.
   a. It has a wide therapeutic range.
   b. It is distributed into two compartments.
   c. It is extensively metabolized by the liver.
   d. Its serum level is not afflicted by sodium or any electrolyte levels.

Phenytoin

Phenytoin, barbiturates-related compound, is indicated for the treatment of seizures. It is approved by FDA for long-term controlling the partial, generalized seizures (tonic-clonic), and for acute management of generalized status epilepticus. It is used for other multiple conditions such as arrhythmia.

Oral suspensions, chewable tablets, sustained-release capsules, and intravenous (IV) formulations are all various dosage forms of phenytoin that are accessible in the market. Phenytoin should not be delivered Intra-muscularly (IM) owing to unpredictable absorption and painful injection. Only fosphenytoin (phosphate ester of phenytoin) can be safely delivered by IM route. Owing to the potential for hypotension, the rate of IV delivery should not be more than 50 mg/min in adults and not exceed 20 mg/min in case of the elderly and patients with preexisting cardiovascular issues. However, when oral dosage form is provided, no greater than 400 mg should be given at one time with 2 hr dosing interval in an attempt to minimize GI side effects and guarantee full absorption [91, 94].

The therapeutic serum level of total phenytoin for the management of seizures ranges from 10-20 mg/L, as shown in table 10. Based on the usual fraction of unbound (free) phenytoin (10%) in patients with normal phenytoin plasma binding, the suggested therapeutic serum concentration of free phenytoin is 1-2 mg/L. If a patient on phenytoin exhibits diplopia and nystagmus (concentration-related toxicity), it means that serum level is above 20 mg/L. However, if serum level exceeds 30 mg/L, these clinical manifestations fade and others such as nausea, vomiting, and ataxia appear. Owing to phenytoin-associated cardiotoxicity, all patients on IV phenytoin should have their heart monitored. Phenytoin crosses the placenta and may cause congenital malformations, that is why it is sorted as pregnancy category D.

The bioavailability of phenytoin significantly differs based on the type of dosage form. It barely dissolves in water. It quickly distributes to the brain where the equilibrium between the brain and blood levels occurs within 20 min. The Vd ranges between 0.6 and 0.7 L/kg in children and adults and higher in neonates and infants (1.2 L/kg). About 92% of phenytoin is bound to plasma proteins and the other portion remains free in the body. This free portion which can be equilibrated and then produces either efficacy or toxicity. The reported phenytoin levels from clinical labs represent the total phenytoin (bound and unbound level), and referred to as phenytoin observed.

Hence, any condition can influence the affinity of phenytoin to plasma protein binding will cause a change in the free fraction. Toxicity can, therefore, appear even though the total observed phenytoin appears normal as a result of increased free portion responsible for activity and toxicity. As a result, the observed phenytoin becomes a poor index of the true level of phenytoin in such patients [91, 93].

Phenytoin is highly protein bound 90%. In addition, it is an acidic drug. In patients with renal failure, the accumulation of uremic toxins may also modify protein binding for many drugs including phenytoin moreover, hypoalbuminemia is a common in renal failure. Decreased plasma protein binding will result in lower measured total phenytoin concentrations, and the calculated apparent Vd may increase. The free fraction (active form) of phenytoin is increased in renal failure up to 20% to 25%. A number of mechanisms have been suggested to explain the decreased binding, including (a) reduced albumin concentration, (b) accumulation of uremic byproducts that displace phenytoin from its binding sites, and (c) alteration in the structure of albumin in renal patients, resulting in a decreased number of binding sites or reduced affinity for phenytoin.

The following equation (2) was suggested to correct for altered binding in renal dysfunction and hypoalbuminemia [103].

$$Cp_{\text{Normal Binding}} = \frac{Cp'}{(0.48)(1-\alpha)\left(\frac{P'}{P_{NL}}\right)+\alpha} \quad (2)$$

Where Cp' is the measured plasma concentration. CpNormal Binding is the corrected plasma concentration that would be seen if the patient had normal renal function and normal albumin. Alpha (α) is the normal free fraction (0.1), P' is the patient's serum albumin, and PNL is normal albumin (4.4 g/dL). Decreased affinity of phenytoin for albumin. The factor 0.48 should be used only to estimate changes in protein binding for patients with ESRD receiving hemodialysis.

Loading dose of phenytoin is needed to attain desired serum level rapidly in case of recently-diagnosed patients who will start on phenytoin therapy or those who are sub-therapeutic and their seizures are not controlled. The serum phenytoin level is supposed to be observed and the desired level is needed to be set to work out a loading dose.

Phenytoin is mainly metabolized by the liver. It has a limited capacity of metabolism. In other words, the greater the dosing, the higher the metabolism rate will be, but in a certain point the metabolism become saturated. As a result, any small elevation in dose can produce toxic serum levels due to stopping the liver to metabolize any more. Phenytoin, therefore, follows Michaelis-Menten kinetics and produces nonlinear kinetics (zero-order kinetics). The dose at which phenytoin metabolism is saturated is not known.

In case of limited capacity of metabolism, half-life is not relevant to the metabolism, but it depends on the medication's serum level. The more the phenytoin serum level, the higher the half-life will be, and vice versa. Hence, phenytoin doses not have a constant half-life. The use of half-life to determine when phenytoin reaches the steady state and when to eliminate from the body is very challenging. The exact half-life is very variable and cannot be predicted. It ranges from 10 and 95 hr in adults [104].

Case Study

(1) RS is a 65-year-old female (70 kg) recently diagnosed with seizure disorder. She has normal albumin level and renal function. She needs to be loaded with phenytoin to attain peak serum level of 20 mg/L. Calculate a loading dose using phenytoin intravenously and in suspension and describe the appropriate dosing delivery for both. Phenytoin's average Vd = 0.65 L/kg, f = 1, S_{iv} = 0.92, and $S_{suspension}$

Solution

$LD = ((C_{desired}-C_{observed})*Vd)/(s*f)$

Because she is recently diagnosed with phenytoin (phenytoin-naïve), the $C_{observed}$ is equal to zero

$LD_{iv} = ((20-0)*0.65*70)/(0.92*1) = 989 \approx 1000$ mg, IV route is employed when more quick peak serum phenytoin level must be provided. IV phenytoin formulation contains propylene glycol as a diluent, which accounts for cardiotoxicity when delivered quickly. So, the rate of IV administration shouldn't overtake 50 mg/min, but it is favorable to apply an infusion rate no more than 20 mg/min, in case of the elderly and those with a history of heart disease to further minimize the incidence of cardiotoxicity.

RS is 65 years old, so IV phenytoin shouldn't exceed 20 mg/min (1000/20). In other words, it should be given no faster than 50 min.

$$LD_{suspension} = ((20\text{-}0)*0.65*70)/(1*1) = 910 \text{ mg} \approx 900 \text{ mg}.$$

Owing to the limited gastrointestinal absorption of phenytoin, it is advisable to deliver small, frequent doses rather than all the dose at one time. Hence, no more than 400 mg can be delivered at one time with dosing interval 2 hr. Therefore, for RS, 400 mg of oral phenytoin suspension is administered at time 0 hr, 400 mg at time 2 hr, and finally 100 mg at time 4 hr of delivery. Another option is to give 400 mg at time 0 hr, 300 mg at time 2 hr, and 200 mg at time 4 hr of oral administration.

(2) If RS has been started on phenytoin suspension 300 mg daily as a maintenance dose. After three weeks, a blood sample was taken to determine her observed phenytoin level which was 14 mg/L. Is this reported level likely to be at steady-state?

As previously mentioned, owing to the capacity-limited metabolism, phenytoin's half-life is variable and dependent on the serum drug level so that it can't be employed to determine the steady-state plasma concentration. Hence, another solution ($t_{90\%}$ formula) should be looked for. $t_{90\%}$ formula determines the time needed for phenytoin to achieve 90% of its steady state value. However, it should be noted that this formula is based on a 70 kg patient

$$\mathbf{90\%t = (115+(35)(C))\,(C) / (S)(F)(Dose/day)}$$

Step 1: Adjust the dose based on a 70 kg patient. However, if you looked back at the problem, you would find that RS is a 70 kg female, so it isn't needed to convert the existing dose into an equivalent 70 kg based-dose.

Table 10. Therapeutic drug monitoring for phenytoin medication

<table>
<tr><td>Drug</td><td colspan="2">Therapeutic Serum Conc.</td><td>When to Sample</td></tr>
<tr><td>Phenytoin</td><td colspan="2">Adult: Total Phenytoin: 10-20 mg/L
Si Unit 40-80 μmol/L
Converting factor 1mg/L= 3.96 μmol/L
Free Phenytoin: 1-2 mg/L
Si Unit 4-8 μmol/L</td><td><u>After Loading Dose:</u>
2-4 hr after an IV load
24 hrs after an oral load
<u>After Initiating MD or adjusting:</u>
Trough Level (before dose) 5 – 7 days</td></tr>
<tr><td colspan="4"><u>Interventions / Comments</u></td></tr>
<tr><td rowspan="5">Low Level</td><td>Measured Level</td><td>Current dose</td><td>Max. Dose Increase</td></tr>
<tr><td>< 20 μmol/L</td><td><4.5mg/kg/day
Increase to 4.5-6mg/kg/day</td><td>100 mg/day</td></tr>
<tr><td>20 -40 μmol/L</td><td>4.5 -6 mg/kg/day</td><td>50 mg/day</td></tr>
<tr><td>50 μmol/L</td><td>>6mg/kg/day</td><td>30 mg/day</td></tr>
<tr><td>>50 μmol/L</td><td colspan="2">Any change may result in a significant increase in serum level and should be done very carefully</td></tr>
<tr><td>High Level
>80μmol/L</td><td colspan="3">Withhold dose and check level daily until target concentration achieved (40 – 80 μmol/L).
New Maintenance dose should be recalculated.</td></tr>
</table>

Step 2: Calculate $t_{90\%}$ based on a 70 kg patient.

$$t_{90\%} = (115+35*(14 \text{ mg/L}))*(14 \text{ mg/L})/(1*1*300 \text{ mg/day})$$
$$t_{90\%} = 28.23 \approx 28 \text{ days}$$

Based on the estimated $t_{90\%}$, the determined time to attain a steady state is about 28 days. The blood sample was drawn on day 21, so this serum level observed doesn't represent a steady state.

Self-Assessment Questions

1. Phenytoin _______.
   a. is liver microsomal enzymes inducer.
   b. is liver microsomal enzymes inhibitor.
   c. has no effect on liver microsomal enzymes.
   d. can elevate other drug's concentration.

2. All of the following is correct for phenytoin except _______.
   a. It follows zero kinetic order.
   b. It has capacity-limited metabolism.
   c. It follows first kinetic order.
   d. It has non-linear kinetics.

3. IV phenytoin formulation can not be given as bolus because
   a. It can produce phlebitis and pain.
   b. It has a limited- gastrointestinal absorption.
   c. It can cause cardiovascular events.
   d. It may produce much high plasma drug level.

Ethosuximide

For the management of petit mal (absence) seizures, ethosuximide is very effective. The recommended therapeutic range for ethosuximide is 40-100 mg/L and may be as great as 150 mg/L as suggested by some specialists with adequate follow-up of serum level and potential side effects. The most common ethosuximide-related side effects are nausea, vomiting, and gastric upset. The delivery of small doses with more frequency can cause these effects to subside. Some adverse-effects such as drowsiness, ataxia, fatigue, and headache can appear owing to the rise in serum concentration above 70mg/L, and referred to as concentration-associated adverse effects. Patients should be watched for these adverse effects [91].

Table 11. Therapeutic drug monitoring for Ethosuximide medication

Drug	Therapeutic Serum Conc.	When to Sample
Ethosuximide	40–100 mg/L (283–708 mmole/L) Si Unit 283–708 mmole/L Converting factor 1mg/L= 7.07 mmol/L	At steady state, the fluctuation in serum drug concentration during a dosing interval is negligible, therefore, samples can be collected at any time
Interventions / Comments		
Steady state will generally be attained in 7 to 10 days after the maintenance dose has been established. Many patients with absence seizures respond at a concentration in the 125 to 150 mg/L range.		

The aim of any anticonvulsant is to minimize the frequency of seizures and boost the life's quality with no or a few adverse effects of the medication. Patients will have better compliance, then. The importance of routinely measuring the medication's serum concentration is to assure that the concentration is in the therapeutic range and avoid the adverse effects.

Ethosuximide is mainly eliminated by the liver (70-80%) and the rest is excreted unchanged in the urine. In case of acute hepatitis or liver cirrhosis, decreased ethosuximide clearance is observed. The clearance rate of oral ethosuximide is 0.288 L/kg/day for adults and children above 12 years old, but, for the young children under 12 years, the clearance rate is 0.384 L/kg/day. Hence, its half-life average is 60 hr for adults and 30 hr for the young children, its half-life is relatively long such that it is required a loading dose to accomplish the target steady state quickly. Ethosuximide doesn't induce or inhibit hepatic enzymes like other anti-epileptics do [91, 92, 95].

The Vd is supposed to be 0.7 L/kg for both children and adults, and the affinity of Ethosuximide to plasma proteins is scanty (<10%). Ethosuximide is therefore extensively eliminated by hemodialysis (≈50%). Hence, additional dose is required to be delivered following each dialysis session. In order to individualize the medication's dose for each patient, the pharmacokinetic parameters for each patient are calculated employing the average parameters form other patients with similar medical conditions (pharmacokinetic dosing method). If the true clearance and Vd values are reported for a patient, elimination-rate constant (K) and half-life ($t_{½}$) can then be calculated form the following equation: $t_{½}$ = (0.693*Vd)/Cl, K = 0.693/$t_{½}$ = Cl/Vd [91, 92].

Case Study

N.S. is a girl with 30 kg in weight (11 years old). She experiences 3 absence seizures daily. Her physician prescribed an oral ethosuximide syrup (250 mg/5 ml) to control her seizures. The prescribed dose provided a steady state concentration 70 mg/L. Her creatinine clearance is below 30 ml/min/1.73 m^2, so she is on dialysis three times weekly. After dialysis, serum drug level falls to 35 mg/L. What is the maintenance dose and post-dialysis replacement doses in mls (milliliters) to recover the steady state average dropped down after dialysis and how to propose the patient will take them. Knowing that the average population Cl = 0.39L/kg/day, ethosuximide's distribution volume, = 0.7 L/kg, s =1, f=1.

MD = (Cssave*Cl*τ)/(s*f)
MD = (70*0.39*30*1)/(1*1)

MD = 819 mg/day, which can be converted into mls by the following formula using the given strength (250 mg/5ml), MD = (819/250)*5= 16.38 ≈16 ml/day. The daily dose should be divided to minimize the most common ethosuximide-related gastric upset. Hence, the dose will often be 8 ml/12 hr.

Post dialysis replacement dose = Cssave*Vd*(fraction lost during dialysis)

For ethosuximide, the serum drug level usually falls to half following dialysis. However, if mathematical equation is needed to calculate the fraction lost during dialysis for any another drug with significant removal, the following formula can be applied.

Fraction lost during dialysis = 1-(post-dialysis serum drug level/predialysis serum drug level) = 1- (35/70) = 1-0.5 =0.5

Post dialysis replacement dose = 70*0.7*30*0.5 = 735 mg /dialysis session = (735/250)*5 = 14.7 ≈ 15 ml /dialysis session

The dose should be divided into two halves, the first is delivered before the dialysis session to minimize the incidence of seizures during the session due to the significant drop in serum drug level to sub-therapeutic level, and the second is administered after the session. Hence, 7.5 ml of ethosuximide is delivered prior the dialysis session and 7.5 ml thereafter.

Self-Assessment Questions

1. Which is of the following is correct about Ethosuximide?
   a. It is liver microsomal enzymes inducer.
   b. It is liver microsomal enzymes inhibitor.
   c. None of the above

2. Which is of the following best describes Ethosuximide?
   a. The prescribed dose can be given at one time.
   b. In order to limit GI-associated adverse effect, the total daily dose is needed to be split with more frequent dosing.
   c. The daily dose is not liable to any change in case of liver cirrhosis or renal failure.

Methotrexate

Methotrexate is an antimetabolite-class antineoplastic Its function is to reversibly inhibit dihydrofolate reductase, the enzyme that reduces folic acid into tetrahydrofolic acid thereby interfering with DNA synthesis, repair and cellular replication. Methotrexate is most commonly used in chemotherapy to treat leukemia and certain types of cancer of the breast, skin, head and neck, lung, or uterus and immunosuppressant in auto-immune diseases severe psoriasis and rheumatoid arthritis.

Methotrexate is administered orally or parenterally while the parenteral route is preferred when doses exceed 30 mg/m^2 because oral absorption is limited. Current dosing regimens range from as low as 2.5mg to as high as 12 g/m^2 or more. High-dose methotrexate is administered over a period as short as 3 to 6 hours to as long as 40 hours. The MTX therapeutic levels are not usually seriously toxic as long as good renal function and adequate hydration are maintained and also when the methotrexate concentration normally falls below 1×10^{-7} molar (0.1 micromolar) within 48 hours following the initiation of therapy [91, 105].

Approximately 50% of methotrexate is bound to plasma proteins. Methotrexate is mainly cleared by the kidneys. At low pH, the drug has limited solubility and may precipitate in the urine, causing nephrotoxicity. Therefore, a patient receiving high-dose methotrexate should receive hydration, and the urine pH should be maintained above 7. Methotrexate is metabolized in liver into 7-hydroxy-methotrexate. The concentration of this metabolite may become significant with high doses of methotrexate. It may precipitate in the renal tubules causing acute nephrotoxicity due to poor solubility. This solubility problem is an additional reason why patients receiving high doses of methotrexate should be adequately hydrated and have their urine alkalinized.

The most common toxic effects of methotrexate include myelosuppression, oral and gastrointestinal mucositis, and acute hepatic dysfunction that may occur when plasma concentrations exceeding 1×10^{-7} molar for 48 hours or more. One of the primary goals of methotrexate plasma monitoring is to ensure that all patients receive adequate doses of rescue factor (Leucovorin Rescue) to prevent serious toxicity. Leucovorin is administered every 4 to 6 hours in doses that range from 10 to 100 mg/m^2 to prevent methotrexate toxicities in moderate and high-dose treatment regimens. Plasma concentration monitoring can be used to detect unusual methotrexate concentrations that require intervention either by increasing the dose of leucovorin or using carboxypeptidase. Carboxypeptidase is a recombinate enzyme that metabolizes circulating methotrexate to the inactive metabolite. Methotrexate is partially eliminated by dialysis (About 50%).

Methotrexate is a folate analog that, following administration, distributes primarily to the non-fatty tissues of the body. The distribution of methotrexate follows the multi-compartmental modeling. When loading doses are required, a Vd of 0.2 to 0.5 L/kg is usually employed. The presence of third-space fluids such as ascites, edema, or pleural effusions can influence the Vd of methotrexate. The high concentrations of methotrexate that accumulate in these spaces makes equilibration with plasma delayed. The initial elimination half-life appears to be normal; however, the second elimination phase is prolonged. In this case, additional doses and/or higher doses of leucovorin rescue factor may be required [92, 106].

The vast majority of methotrexate is eliminated by the renal route. Methotrexate clearance ranges from 1 to 2 times the creatinine clearance. Methotrexate clearance by an active transport mechanism that may be saturable results in a renal clearance value that varies with methotrexate plasma concentrations. Weak acids such as Probenecid, salicylates, proton pump inhibitors, sulfisoxazole have been associated with delays in methotrexate clearance and prolong methotrexate half-life.

Serious toxicity and death have been reported with doses as low as 10 mg of methotrexate when administered to a patient with inadequate renal function. Concomitant use of the prostaglandin inhibitors e.g., indomethacin and ketoprofen with methotrexate has been associated with an acute renal failure and methotrexate toxicity.

A relatively small percentage of methotrexate is metabolized into7-hydroxy-methotrexate that can be found in the urine when large doses are administered. This is especially true during the late phase of methotrexate elimination when the majority of the parent compound has been eliminated.

The initial α half-life of methotrexate is approximately 3 hours and the β or terminal half-life is 10 hours. The terminal half-life does not appear until plasma concentrations decline into the range of 5×10^{-7} molar (0.5×10^{-6} or 0.5 μmolar).

Methotrexate plasma concentrations can be used to evaluate the potential efficacy or toxicity of a given dosing regimen. There are two situations when monitoring methotrexate levels for efficacy is useful. The first is in patients receiving prolonged methotrexate infusions, the infusion rate may require adjustment. The second is in patients who are going to receive repeated methotrexate doses, in which case future doses can be adjusted to achieve the desired target concentration.

When using methotrexate levels to evaluate the leucovorin rescue dosage regimen, samples are obtained 24 to 48 hours following the initiation of therapy to determine whether additional leucovorin will be required. For example, plasma levels greater than 1×10^{-6} molar at 48 hours are usually associated with increased methotrexate toxicity unless leucovorin rescue doses are increased from 10 mg/m^2 every 6 hours to 50 to 100 mg/m^2 every 3 to 6 hours. For patients with plasma levels below 1×10^{-6} but above 1×10^{-7} molar, a leucovorin rescue dose of 10 mg/m^2 every 6 hours is generally adequate. All patients should have documented methotrexate concentrations below 1×10^{-7} molar or 0.5×10^{-7} molar before leucovorin rescue is discontinued.

Methotrexate can be administered intrathecally. The standard intrathecal dose of methotrexate is only 12 mg regardless of body size. The risk of systemic methotrexate toxicity is relatively low unless the patient develops renal dysfunction [91, 107].

Self-Assessment Questions

1. The vast majority of methotrexate is eliminated by _______ route
   a) Renal
   b) Hepatic
   c) Both renal and hepatic

2. _______ is a recombinant enzyme that metabolizes circulating methotrexate to the inactive metabolite
   a) Leucovorin
   b) Carboxypeptidase

3. The distribution of methotrexate follows _______ model
   a) One compartment
   b) Two compartment
   c) Multi-compartment

4. Indomethacin and ketoprofen may _______ the terminal half-life of methotrexate
   a) Prolong
   b) shorten

References

[1] Hossain R, Jannat RA, Chadni SA, Das C, Hassan H, Islam MT. *Dosage adjustment in hepatic patients: a literature-based review.* 2019 [cited 2022 Aug 12];2:113–37. Available from: http://pharmacologyonline.silae.i.

[2] Verbeeck RK. Pharmacokinetics and dosage adjustment in patients with hepatic dysfunction. *European journal of clinical pharmacology*. 2008 Dec;64(12):1147-61.

[3] Franz CC, Hildbrand C, Born C, Egger S, Rätz Bravo AE, Krähenbühl S. Dose adjustment in patients with liver cirrhosis: impact on adverse drug reactions and hospitalizations. *European journal of clinical pharmacology*. 2013 Aug;69[8]:1565-73.

[4] Amarapurkar DN. Prescribing medications in patients with decompensated liver cirrhosis. *International journal of hepatology*. 2011 Aug 22;2011.

[5] Delco F, Tchambaz L, Schlienger R, Drewe J, Krähenbühl S. Dose adjustment in patients with liver disease. *Drug safety*. 2005 Jun;28[6]:529-45.

[6] Kidney Disease: Improving Global Outcomes (KDIGO) CKD Work Group. KDIGO 2012 Clinical Practice Guideline for the Evaluation and Management of Chronic Kidney Disease. *Kidney Int Suppl* [Internet]. Elsevier; 2013;3:4. Available from: https://doi.org/10.1038/kisup.2012.76

[7] Stevens LA, Levey AS. Measured GFR as a confirmatory test for estimated GFR. *J Am Soc Nephrol*. 2009;20:2305–13.

[8] Delanaye P, Cavalier E, Pottel H. Serum Creatinine: Not so Simple! *Nephron*. 2017;136:302–8.

[9] Pottel H, Vrydags N, Mahieu B, Vandewynckele E, Croes K, Martens F. Establishing age/sex related serum creatinine reference intervals from hospital laboratory data based on different statistical methods. *Clin Chim Acta*. Netherlands; 2008;396:49–55.

[10] Stevens LA, Coresh J, Greene T, Levey AS. Assessing Kidney Function — Measured and Estimated Glomerular Filtration Rate. *N Engl J Med*. 2006;354:2473–83.

[11] van Acker BA, Koomen GC, Koopman MG, de Waart DR, Arisz L. Creatinine clearance during cimetidine administration for measurement of glomerular filtration rate. *Lancet* (London, England). England; 1992;340:1326–9.

[12] Delanaye P, Mariat C, Cavalier E, Maillard N, Krzesinski J-M, White CA. Trimethoprim, creatinine and creatinine-based equations. *Nephron Clin Pract*. Switzerland; 2011;119:c187-93; discussion c193-4.

[13] Greg Miller W, Myers GL, Ashwood ER, Killeen AA, Wang E, Thienpont LM, Siekmann L. Creatinine measurement: state of the art in accuracy and interlaboratory harmonization. *Archives of pathology & laboratory medicine*. 2005 Mar;129[3]:297-304.

[14] Myers GL, Miller WG, Coresh J, Fleming J, Greenberg N, Greene T, Hostetter T, Levey AS, Panteghini M, Welch M, Eckfeldt JH. Recommendations for improving serum creatinine measurement: a report from the Laboratory Working Group of the National Kidney Disease Education Program. *Clinical chemistry*. 2006 Jan 1;52[1]:5-18.

[15] Drion I, Cobbaert C, Groenier KH, Weykamp C, Bilo HJ, Wetzels JF, Kleefstra N. Clinical evaluation of analytical variations in serum creatinine measurements: why laboratories should abandon Jaffe techniques. *BMC nephrology*. 2012 Dec;13[1]:1-8.

[16] Matzke GR, Aronoff GR, Atkinson Jr AJ, Bennett WM, Decker BS, Eckardt KU, Golper T, Grabe DW, Kasiske B, Keller F, Kielstein JT. Drug dosing consideration in patients with acute and chronic kidney disease—a clinical update from Kidney Disease: Improving Global Outcomes (KDIGO). *Kidney international*. 2011 Dec 1;80(11):1122-37.

[17] Greenberg N, Roberts WL, Bachmann LM, Wright EC, Dalton RN, Zakowski JJ, Greg Miller W. Specificity characteristics of 7 commercial creatinine measurement procedures by enzymatic and Jaffe method principles. *Clinical chemistry*. 2012 Feb 1;58[2]:391-401..

[18] Francoz C, Glotz D, Moreau R, Durand F. The evaluation of renal function and disease in patients with cirrhosis. *J Hepatol* [Internet]. 2010;52:605–13. Available from: https://www.sciencedirect.com/science/article/pii/S0168827809008204

[19] Knight EL, Verhave JC, Spiegelman D, Hillege HL, De Zeeuw D, Curhan GC, De Jong PE. Factors influencing serum cystatin C levels other than renal function and the impact on renal function measurement. *Kidney international*. 2004 Apr 1;65[4]:1416-21.

[20] Manetti L, Pardini E, Genovesi M, Campomori A, Grasso L, Morselli LL, Lupi I, Pellegrini G, Bartalena L, Bogazzi F, Martino E. Thyroid function differently affects serum cystatin Cand creatinine concentrations. *Journal of endocrinological investigation*. 2005 Jun;28:346-9.

[21] Stevens LA, Schmid CH, Greene T, Li L, Beck GJ, Joffe MM, Froissart M, Kusek JW, Zhang YL, Coresh J, Levey AS. Factors other than glomerular filtration rate affect serum cystatin C levels. *Kidney international*. 2009 Mar 2;75[6]:652 60.

[22] Tsushita H, Tanaka R, Suzuki Y, Sato Y, Itoh H. Effects of dose and type of corticosteroids on the divergence between estimated glomerular filtration rates derived from cystatin C and creatinine. *J Clin Pharm Ther*. England; 2020;45:1390–7.

[23] Grubb A, Blirup-Jensen S, Lindström V, Schmidt C, Althaus H, Zegers I. First certified reference material for cystatin C in human serum ERM-DA471/IFCC. *Clin Chem Lab Med*. Germany;

2010;48:1619–21.

[24] Eckfeldt JH, Karger AB, Miller WG, Rynders GP, Inker LA. Performance in Measurement of Serum Cystatin C by Laboratories Participating in the College of American Pathologists 2014 CYS Survey. *Arch Pathol Lab Med*. United States; 2015;139:888–93.

[25] Bargnoux AS, Piéroni L, Cristol JP, Kuster N, Delanaye P, Carlier MC, Fellahi S, Boutten A, Lombard C, González-Antuña A, Delatour V. Multicenter evaluation of cystatin C measurement after assay standardization. *Clinical chemistry*. 2017 Apr 1;63[4]:833-41..

[26] Zhang M, Cao X, Cai G, Wu D, Wei R, Yuan X, Bai X, Liu S, Chen X. Clinical evaluation of serum cystatin C and creatinine in patients with chronic kidney disease: a meta-analysis. *Journal of international medical research*. 2013 Aug;41[4]:944-55..

[27] Pan Y, Hu B, Li M, Fan L, Ni Y, Zhou J, Shi X. A meta-analysis on diagnostic value of serum cystatin C and creatinine for the evaluation of glomerular filtration function in renal transplant patients. *African health sciences*. 2014;14[4]:1025-35..

[28] Yoo JJ, Kim SG, Kim YS, Lee B, Lee MH, Jeong SW, Jang JY, Lee SH, Kim HS, Kim YD, Cheon GJ. Estimation of renal function in patients with liver cirrhosis: Impact of muscle mass and sex. *Journal of Hepatology*. 2019 May 1;70[5]:847-54.

[29] Stevens LA, Coresh J, Schmid CH, Feldman HI, Froissart M, Kusek J, Rossert J, Van Lente F, Bruce III RD, Zhang YL, Greene T. Estimating GFR using serum cystatin C alone and in combination with serum creatinine: a pooled analysis of 3,418 individuals with CKD. *American journal of kidney diseases*. 2008 Mar 1;51[3]:395-406..

[30] Cockcroft DW, Gault MH. Prediction of creatinine clearance from serum creatinine. *Nephron*. Switzerland; 1976;16:31–41.

[31] Stevens LA, Coresh J, Schmid CH, Feldman HI, Froissart M, Kusek J, Rossert J, Van Lente F, Bruce III RD, Zhang YL, Greene T. Estimating GFR using serum cystatin C alone and in combination with serum creatinine: a pooled analysis of 3,418 individuals with CKD. *American journal of kidney diseases*. 2008 Mar 1;51[3]:395-406..

[32] Winter MA, Guhr KN, Berg GM. Impact of various body weights and serum creatinine concentrations on the bias and accuracy of the Cockcroft-Gault equation. *Pharmacotherapy*. United States; 2012;32:604–12.

[33] Wilhelm SM, Kale-Pradhan PB. Estimating creatinine clearance: a meta-analysis. *Pharmacotherapy*. United States; 2011;31:658–64.

[34] Demirovic JA, Pai AB, Pai MP. Estimation of creatinine clearance in morbidly obese patients. *Am J Heal Pharm AJHP Off J Am Soc Heal Pharm*. England; 2009;66:642–8.

[35] Pai MP. Estimating the glomerular filtration rate in obese adult patients for drug dosing. *Adv Chronic Kidney Dis*. United States; 2010;17:e53-62.

[36] Brunetti L, Back H, Yu S, Jalil U, Kagan L. Evaluation and enhancement of standard equations for renal function estimation in individuals with components of metabolic disease. *BMC Nephrol* [Internet]. 2021;22:389. Available from: https://doi.org/10.1186/s12882-021-02588-4

[37] Brown DL, Masselink AJ, Lalla CD. Functional range of creatinine clearance for renal drug dosing: a practical solution to the controversy of which weight to use in the Cockcroft-Gault equation. *Ann Pharmacother*. United States; 2013;47:1039–44.

[38] Erstad BL, Nix DE. Assessment of Kidney Function in Patients With Extreme Obesity: A Narrative Review. *Ann Pharmacother* [Internet]. SAGE Publications Inc; 2020;55:80–8. Available from: https://doi.org/10.1177/1060028020935580

[39] Brunetti L, Back H, Yu S, Jalil U, Kagan L. Evaluation and enhancement of standard equations for renal function estimation in individuals with components of metabolic disease. *BMC Nephrol*. 2021;22:389.

[40] Nguyen T, Foster Y, Cekaj S. Older Adult Kidney Function Assessment and Rounding Creatinine Led to Medication Dosing Error. *Am J Ther*. United States; 2018;25:e439–46.

[41] McCarron MM, Devine BJ. Clinical Pharmacy: Case Studies: Case Number 25 Gentamicin Therapy. *Drug Intell Clin Pharm* [Internet]. SAGE Publications; 1974;8:650–5. Available from: https://doi.org/10.1177/106002807400801104

[42] Khosla T, Lowe CR. Indices of obesity derived from body weight and height. *Br J Prev Soc Med*

[Internet]. 1967;21:122–8. Available from: https://pubmed.ncbi.nlm.nih.gov/6033482

[43] Du Bois D, Du Bois EF. Clinical calorimetry: tenth paper a formula to estimate the approximate surface area if height and weight be known. *Arch Intern Med* [Internet]. 1916;XVII:863–71. Available from: https://doi.org/10.1001/archinte.1916.00080130010002

[44] Janmahasatian S, Duffull SB, Ash S, Ward LC, Byrne NM, Green B. Quantification of lean bodyweight. *Clin Pharmacokinet.* Switzerland; 2005;44:1051–65.

[45] Levey AS, Bosch JP, Lewis JB, Greene T, Rogers N, Roth D. A more accurate method to estimate glomerular filtration rate from serum creatinine: a new prediction equation. Modification of Diet in Renal Disease Study Group. *Ann Intern Med.* United States; 1999;130:461–70.

[46] Levey AS, Greene T, Kusek JW, Beck GJ. A simplified equation to predict glomerular filtration rate from serum creatinine. *J Am Soc Nephrol*. 2000;11:155A.

[47] Levey AS, Coresh J, Greene T, Stevens LA, Zhang Y, Hendriksen S, Kusek JW, Van Lente F, Chronic Kidney Disease Epidemiology Collaboration*. Using standardized serum creatinine values in the modification of diet in renal disease study equation for estimating glomerular filtration rate. *Annals of internal medicine.* 2006 Aug 15;145[4]:247-54..

[48] Levey AS, Stevens LA, Schmid CH, Zhang Y, Castro III AF, Feldman HI, Kusek JW, Eggers P, Van Lente F, Greene T, Coresh J. A new equation to estimate glomerular filtration rate. *Annals of internal medicine*. 2009 May 5;150[9]:604-12.

[49] Inker LA, Schmid CH, Tighiouart H, Eckfeldt JH, Feldman HI, Greene T, Kusek JW, Manzi J, Van Lente F, Zhang YL, Coresh J. Estimating glomerular filtration rate from serum creatinine and cystatin C. *New England Journal of Medicine*. 2012 Jul 5;367[1]:20-9.

[50] Bukabau JB, Yayo E, Gnionsahé A, Monnet D, Pottel H, Cavalier E, Nkodila A, Makulo JR, Mokoli VM, Lepira FB, Nseka NM. Performance of creatinine-or cystatin C–based equations to estimate glomerular filtration rate in sub-Saharan African populations. *Kidney international.* 2019 May 1;95[5]:1181-9.

[51] Flamant M, Vidal-Petiot E, Metzger M, Haymann JP, Letavernier E, Delatour V, Karras A, Thervet E, Boffa JJ, Houillier P, Stengel B. Performance of GFR estimating equations in African Europeans: basis for a lower race-ethnicity factor than in African Americans. *American Journal of Kidney Diseases.* 2013 Jul 1;62[1]:182-4.

[52] Delanaye P, Mariat C, Maillard N, Krzesinski J-M, Cavalier E. Are the Creatinine-Based Equations Accurate to Estimate Glomerular Filtration Rate in African American Populations? *Clin J Am Soc* Nephrol [Internet]. 2011;6:906 LP – 912. Available from: http://cjasn.asnjournals.org/content/6/4/906.abstract

[53] Stevens LA, Claybon MA, Schmid CH, Chen J, Horio M, Imai E, Nelson RG, Van Deventer M, Wang HY, Zuo L, Zhang YL. Evaluation of the Chronic Kidney Disease Epidemiology Collaboration equation for estimating the glomerular filtration rate in multiple ethnicities. *Kidney international.* 2011 Mar 1;79[5]:555-62.

[54] Horio M, Imai E, Yasuda Y, Watanabe T, Matsuo S. Modification of the CKD Epidemiology Collaboration (CKD-EPI) Equation for Japanese: Accuracy and Use for Population Estimates. *Am J Kidney Dis* [Internet]. Elsevier; 2010;56:32–8. Available from: https://doi.org/10.1053/j.ajkd.2010.02.344

[55] Jessani S, Levey AS, Bux R, Inker LA, Islam M, Chaturvedi N, Mariat C, Schmid CH, Jafar TH. Estimation of GFR in South Asians: a study from the general population in Pakistan. *American journal of kidney diseases*. 2014 Jan 1;63[1]:49-58.

[56] Wang Y, Levey AS, Inker LA, Jessani S, Bux R, Samad Z, Khan AR, Karger AB, Allen JC, Jafar TH. Performance and determinants of serum creatinine and cystatin C–based GFR estimating equations in South Asians. *Kidney International Reports*. 2021 Apr 1;6[4]:962-75.

[57] Levey AS, Tighiouart H, Titan SM, Inker LA. Estimation of Glomerular Filtration Rate With vs Without Including Patient Race. *JAMA Intern Med*. 2020;180:793–5.

[58] Levey AS, Titan SM, Powe NR, Coresh J, Inker LA. Kidney Disease, Race, and GFR Estimation. *Clin J Am Soc Nephrol* [Internet]. 2020;15:1203 LP – 1212. Available from: http://cjasn.asnjournals.org/content/15/8/1203.abstract

[59] Eneanya ND, Yang W, Reese PP. Reconsidering the Consequences of Using Race to Estimate Kidney

Function. *JAMA* [Internet]. 2019;322:113–4. Available from: https://doi.org/10.1001/ jama.2019.5774

[60] Inker LA, Eneanya ND, Coresh J, Tighiouart H, Wang D, Sang Y, Crews DC, Doria A, Estrella MM, Froissart M, Grams ME. New creatinine-and cystatin C–based equations to estimate GFR without race. *New England Journal of Medicine*. 2021 Nov 4;385(19):1737-49.

[61] Delgado C, Baweja M, Crews DC, Eneanya ND, Gadegbeku CA, Inker LA, Mendu ML, Miller WG, Moxey-Mims MM, Roberts GV, Peter WL. A unifying approach for GFR estimation: recommendations of the NKF-ASN task force on reassessing the inclusion of race in diagnosing kidney disease. *American Journal of Kidney Diseases*. 2022 Feb 1;79[2]:268-88.

[62] Hundemer GL, White CA, Norman PA, Knoll GA, Tangri N, Sood MM, Hiremath S, Burns KD, McCudden C, Akbari A. Performance of the 2021 Race-Free CKD-EPI Creatinine-and Cystatin C–Based Estimated GFR Equations Among Kidney Transplant Recipients. *American Journal of Kidney Diseases*. 2022 May 16.

[63] Pottel H, Hoste L, Dubourg L, Ebert N, Schaeffner E, Eriksen BO, Melsom T, Lamb EJ, Rule AD, Turner ST, Glassock RJ. An estimated glomerular filtration rate equation for the full age spectrum. *Nephrology Dialysis Transplantation*. 2016 May 1;31[5]:798-806.

[64] Pottel H, Björk J, Courbebaisse M, Couzi L, Ebert N, Eriksen BO, Dalton RN, Dubourg L, Gaillard F, Garrouste C, Grubb A. Development and validation of a modified full age spectrum creatinine-based equation to estimate glomerular filtration rate: a cross-sectional analysis of pooled data. *Annals of internal medicine*. 2021 Feb;174[2]:183-91.

[65] Schwartz GJ, Haycock GB, Edelmann CMJ, Spitzer A. A simple estimate of glomerular filtration rate in children derived from body length and plasma creatinine. *Pediatrics*. United States; 1976;58: 259–63.

[66] Pottel, H., et al., Alternatives for the bedside Schwartz equation to estimate glomerular filtration rate in children. *Advances in Chronic Kidney Disease*, 2018. 25(1): p. 57-66.

[67] Staples A, LeBlond R, Watkins S, Wong C, Brandt J. Validation of the revised Schwartz estimating equation in a predominantly non-CKD population. *Pediatr Nephrol.* Germany; 2010;25:2321–6.

[68] Srivastava T, Alon US, Althahabi R, Garg U. Impact of standardization of creatinine methodology on the assessment of glomerular filtration rate in children. *Pediatr Res.* United States; 2009;65:113–6.

[69] Schwartz GJ, Schneider MF, Maier PS, Moxey-Mims M, Dharnidharka VR, Warady BA, Furth SL, Muñoz A. Improved equations estimating GFR in children with chronic kidney disease using an immunonephelometric determination of cystatin C. *Kidney international*. 2012 Aug 2;82[4]:445-53.

[70] Pierce CB, Muñoz A, Ng DK, Warady BA, Furth SL, Schwartz GJ. Age- and sex-dependent clinical equations to estimate glomerular filtration rates in children and young adults with chronic kidney disease. *Kidney Int*. 2021;99:948–56.

[71] Ng DK, Pierce CB. Kidney Disease Progression in Children and Young Adults With Pediatric CKD: Epidemiologic Perspectives and Clinical Applications. *Semin Nephrol*. 2021;41:405–15.

[72] Lalande L, Charpiat B, Leboucher G, Tod M. Consequences of Renal Failure on Non-Renal Clearance of Drugs. *Clin Pharmacokinet* [Internet]. 2014;53:521–32. Available from: https://doi.org/ 10.1007/s40262-014-0146-1

[73] Blot S, Lipman J, Roberts DM, Roberts JA. The influence of acute kidney injury on antimicrobial dosing in critically ill patients: are dose reductions always necessary? *Diagn Microbiol Infect Dis.* United States; 2014;79:77–84.

[74] Jelliffe RW, Jelliffe SM. A computer program for estimation of creatinine clearance from unstable serum creatinine levels, age, sex, and weight. *Bellman Prize Math Biosci.* 1972;14:17–24.

[75] Chiou WL, Hsu FH. A new simple and rapid method to monitor the renal function based on pharmacokinetic consideration of endogeneous creatinine=. *Res Commun Chem Pathol Pharmacol.* United States; 1975;10:315–30.

[76] Brater DC. *Drug use in renal disease.* ADIS Health Science Press; 1983.

[77] Jelliffe R. Estimation of creatinine clearance in patients with unstable renal function, without a urine specimen. *Am J Nephrol.* Switzerland; 2002;22:320–4.

[78] Chen S. Retooling the creatinine clearance equation to estimate kinetic GFR when the plasma creatinine is changing acutely. *J Am Soc Nephrol.* United States; 2013;24:877–88.

[79] O'Sullivan ED, Doyle A. The clinical utility of kinetic glomerular filtration rate. *Clin Kidney J.* 2017;10:202–8.

[80] Michaud J, Nolin TD, Naud J, Dani M, Lafrance JP, Leblond FA, Himmelfarb J, Pichette V. Effect of hemodialysis on hepatic cytochrome P450 functional expression. *Journal of pharmacological sciences.* 2008 Jan 1;108[2]:157-63..

[81] Egeland EJ, Witczak BJ, Zaré HK, Christensen H, Åsberg A, Robertsen I. Chronic Inhibition of CYP3A is Temporarily Reduced by Each Hemodialysis Session in Patients With End-Stage Renal Disease. *Clin Pharmacol Ther.* United States; 2020;108:866–73.

[82] Sowinski KM, Magner SJ, Lucksiri A, Scott MK, Hamburger RJ, Mueller BA. Influence of hemodialysis on gentamicin pharmacokinetics, removal during hemodialysis, and recommended dosing. *Clin J Am Soc Nephrol.* 2008;3:355–61.

[83] Veinstein A, Venisse N, Badin J, Pinsard M, Robert R, Dupuis A. Gentamicin in hemodialyzed critical care patients: early dialysis after administration of a high dose should be considered. *Antimicrob Agents Chemother.* 2013;57:977–82.

[84] Pea F, Viale P, Pavan F, Furlanut M. Pharmacokinetic considerations for antimicrobial therapy in patients receiving renal replacement therapy. *Clin Pharmacokinet.* Switzerland; 2007;46:997–1038.

[85] Jang SM, Infante S, Abdi Pour A. Drug Dosing Considerations in Critically Ill Patients Receiving Continuous Renal Replacement Therapy. *Pharm* (Basel, Switzerland). 2020;8.

[86] Edrees F, Li T, Vijayan A. Prolonged Intermittent Renal Replacement Therapy. *Adv Chronic Kidney Dis.* United States; 2016;23:195–202.

[87] Rybak, M.J., Le, J., Lodise, T.P., Levine, D.P., Bradley, J.S., Liu, C., Mueller, B.A., Pai, M.P., Wong-Beringer, A., Rotschafer, J.C. and Rodvold, K.A., 2020. Therapeutic monitoring of vancomycin for serious methicillin-resistant Staphylococcus aureus infections: a revised consensus guideline and review by the American Society of Health-System Pharmacists, the Infectious Diseases Society of America, the Pediatric Infectious Diseases Society, and the Society of Infectious Diseases Pharmacists. *Clinical Infectious Diseases*, *71*[6], pp.1361-1364. Available from: https://doi.org/10.1093/ajhp/zxaa036.

[88] Rodríguez N, Gómez M, Rico N, María Campistol J, Maduell F. Vancomycin hemodialysis: Clearance differences between high-flux hemodialysis and on-line hemodiafiltration. *Artif Organs.* United States; 2019;43:261–9.

[89] Imaz ML, Soy D, Torra M, García-Esteve L, Soler C, Martin-Santos R. Case Report: Clinical and Pharmacokinetic Profile of Lithium Monotherapy in Exclusive Breastfeeding. A Follow-Up Case Series. *Frontiers in Pharmacology*. 2021 Jun 24;12:965.

[90] Sproule BA, Hardy BG, Shulman KI. Differential pharmacokinetics of lithium in elderly patients. *Drugs & aging*. 2000 Mar;16[3]:165-77.

[91] Cohen H. *Casebook in clinical pharmacokinetics and drug dosing*. 2015: McGraw-Hill Medical Publishing. 913.

[92] Bauer, L., *Applied Clinical Pharmacokinetics*. 2008: McGraw-Hill Medical. 842.

[93] Atkinson Jr AJ. Clinical pharmacokinetics. *Atkinson's Principles of Clinical Pharmacology*. 2022 Jan 1:11-26.

[94] Fischer JH, Patel TV, Fischer PA. Fosphenytoin. *Clinical pharmacokinetics*. 2003 Jan;42[1]:33-58.

[95] Glauser TA, Perucca E. Ethosuximide. *The treatment of epilepsy*. 2015 Oct 2:460-71.

[96] Kudriakova TB, Sirota LA, Rozova GI, Gorkov VA. Autoinduction and steady-state pharmacokinetics of carbamazepine and its major metabolites. *British journal of clinical pharmacology*. 1992 Jun;33[6]:611-5.

[97] Ding JJ, Zhang YJ, Jiao Z, Wang Y. The effect of poor compliance on the pharmacokinetics of carbamazepine and its epoxide metabolite using Monte Carlo simulation. *Acta Pharmacologica Sinica*. 2012 Nov;33(11):1431 40.

[98] Strandjord RE, Johannessen SI. A preliminary study of serum carbamazepine levels in healthy subjects and in patients with epilepsy. *Clinical pharmacology of antiepileptic drugs*. Schneider, H., Janz, D., Gardner-Thorpe, C., Meinardi, H., Sherwin, AL (ed.). 2012 Dec 6:181-8.

[99] Kahan BD. Individualization of cyclosporine therapy using pharmacokinetic and pharmacodynamic parameters. *Transplantation*. 1985 Nov 1;40[5]:457-76.

[100] Patel D, Wairkar S. Recent advances in cyclosporine drug delivery: Challenges and opportunities. *Drug delivery and translational research*. 2019 Dec;9[6]:1067-81.

[101] Kahan BD, Grevel J. Optimization of cyclosporine therapy in renal transplantation by a pharmacokinetic strategy. *Transplantation*. 1988 Nov 1;46[5]:631-44.

[102] Kahan BD, Welsh M, Rutzky LP. Challenges in cyclosporine therapy: the role of therapeutic monitoring by area under the curve monitoring. *Therapeutic drug monitoring*. 1995 Dec 1;17[6]:621-4.

[103] Wilfred PM, Mathew S, Chacko B, Prabha R, Mathew BS. Estimation of Free Phenytoin Concentration in Critically Ill Patients with Hypoalbuminemia: Direct-measurement vs Traditional Equations. *Indian Journal of Critical Care Medicine*: Peer-reviewed, *Official Publication of Indian Society of Critical Care Medicine*. 2022 Jun;26[6]:682.

[104] Valodia PN, Seymour MA, McFadyen ML, Miller R, Folb PI. Validation of population pharmacokinetic parameters of phenytoin using the parallel Michaelis-Menten and first-order elimination model. *Therapeutic Drug Monitoring*. 2000 Jun 1;22[3]:313-9.

[105] Pesenti G, Foppoli M, Manca D. A minimal physiologically based pharmacokinetic model for high-dose methotrexate. *Cancer chemotherapy and pharmacology*. 2021 Oct;88:595-606.

[106] Zhang Y, Sun L, Chen X, Zhao L, Wang X, Zhao Z, Mei S. A systematic review of population pharmacokinetic models of methotrexate. *European Journal of Drug Metabolism and Pharmacokinetics*. 2022 Mar;47[2]:143-64.

[107] Kawakatsu S, Nikanjam M, Lin M, Le S, Saunders I, Kuo DJ, Capparelli EV. Population pharmacokinetic analysis of high-dose methotrexate in pediatric and adult oncology patients. *Cancer chemotherapy and pharmacology*. 2019 Dec;84:1339-48.

[108] Djordjevic N, Jankovic SM, Milovanovic JR. Pharmacokinetics and pharmacogenetics of carbamazepine in children. *European Journal of Drug Metabolism and Pharmacokinetics*. 2017 Oct;42:729-44.

[109] Milovanovic JR, Jankovic SM. Factors influencing carbamazepine pharmacokinetics in children and adults: population pharmacokinetic analysis. *International Journal of Clinical Pharmacology and Therapeutics*. 2011 Jul 1;49[7]:428.

Chapter 4

Clinical Nutrition Management

Al Shaimaa Ibrahim Rabie[1,2,*]
and Sohailah Alzahrani[3]
[1]Clinical Pharmacy Department, Fayium Oncology Center, Fayium, Egypt
[2]Clinical Nutrition Department, Health Insurance Authority, Fayium, Egypt
[3]Department of Pharmacy, Prince Sultan Military Medical City, Riyadh, Saudi Arabia

Learning Objectives

After completing this chapter, the reader would be able to:

- Describe the Malnutrition screening and assessment as part of the Nutrition Care Process
- Enteral nutrition indications, types of formula and complication
- Different types of Drug nutrients interaction
- Total parenteral nutrition indication, formulation, complications and monitoring
- Overview of the Nutrition Care Process.

Introduction

Recognition of the importance of adequate and appropriate nutrition is paramount to the maintenance of optimal health. A nutritional issue can develop when there is an equilibrium between both the supply and demand for the body's sources of nutrients and energy.

Nutrient imbalance driven by insufficient protein and energy intake, absorption, or imbalance consumption leads to malnutrition. Changes in subcellular, cellular, or organ function driven on by undernutrition might raise a person's risk of morbidity and mortality.

The relationship between malnutrition and nutrition assessment is critical. Any elements that influence the development of malnutrition and the manifestations that result should both comprise the steps of assessment and provide reliable identifiers for nutrition screening. In theory, malnutrition will occur when intake falls below (or exceeds) what is required. In

* Corresponding Author's Email: alshaimaa.ph@gmail.com.

In: Clinical Pharmacist Tools to Deliver Rational Medication Use
Editor: Mohamed Emam Abdelmobdy Abdelrahim
ISBN: 979-8-88697-857-5

practice, this process is significantly more complex. Metabolic irregularities, physiologic alterations, decreased organ and tissue function, and the loss of vital body mass are the accompanying symptoms. For these reasons, Malnutrition is defined as any variation in physiology, components, or function linked to a diet or a condition that has an impact on nutritional outcomes. Malnutrition for the purposes of nutrition assessment in the clinical setting refers to a disease-related malnutrition that differs dramatically from that associated with natural disaster, conflict, or deprivation in the public health.

Malnutrition Syndromes

- Starvation-associated malnutrition, Anorexia nervosa, inadequate dietary intake when serious depression is present
- Chronic disease–associated malnutrition, Organ failure, pancreatic cancer, rheumatoid arthritis, sarcopenic obesity
- Acute disease– or injury-associated malnutrition, Major infection burns, trauma, or closed head injury.

Identification of malnutrition and the entire purpose of the nutrition assessment process require a general understanding of its risk factors and manifestations. Because it is estimated that malnutrition affects between 30% and 55% of hospitalized patients, many of whom are malnourished at baseline, nutrition assessment is fundamental to the evaluation of the acutely ill adult. A.S.P.E.N. stated unique diagnostic criteria that can be identified within the aforementioned domains:

- Unintentional weight loss over a certain period of time
- Insufficient energy intake, as determined by calculating the percentage of needs met
- Signs of muscle mass loss and/or subcutaneous fat loss discovered during a physical examination; or fluid accumulation (generalized or localized) that could conceal any recent weight loss.
- Decrease in functional status as detected by handgrip strength.

Screening

A Method of determining whether a person is malnourished or at risk of becoming one (immediate, minimum data). Hospitals are mandated by The Joint Commission on Accreditation of Healthcare Organizations (JCAHO) to perform nutrition checks within 24 hours of patient admission. In order to establish whether a patient is malnourished or at risk for malnutrition, nutrition screening determines whether a nutritional assessment is necessary.

Although some screening tools have been endorsed by international nutrition societies, there is no universal or empirical agreement on a single best tool. The four most well-known and widely used examples include Nutritional Risk Screening (NRS-2002), Malnutrition Universal Screening Tool (MUST), Short Nutritional Assessment Questionnaire (SNAQ), and Malnutrition Screening Tool (MST). Please note that while some of these tools were developed by professional groups outside of the United States, they are used widely across clinical practice.

Assessment

Nutrition assessment is the first step in developing a nutrition care plan and is a more comprehensive evaluation to make a diagnosis of malnutrition syndrome and to guide intervention and expected outcomes. A major assessment of both nutritional status and the degree of illness because of there is a correlation between the two. Diagnoses related with severe morbidity, such as Traumatic injuries, septic shock, and malignant tumors. This assessment should include a nutrition-focused history, Weight history, medication history, a physical exam including anthropometrics, and laboratory measurements.

Clinical Evaluation

Nutrition History

For a nutritional assessment to be successful, a nutrition history is essential. Malnutrition can be caused by a number of conditions, including those that the patient already has, their past medical history, and their socioeconomic situation. *Dietary data a* modified diet history and/or a 24-hour recall can be used to acquire dietary information in a practical way.

Weight History

Weight loss is an indication of an unbalanced protein and energy intake and is frequently linked to a bad prognosis for hospitalized patients. A reference for ideal body weight is frequently used to compare a patient's present weight to (IBW). Equation describes how to determine the percentage of IBW.

% Ideal Body Weight = [current Weight/ IBW] X 100

Involuntary weight loss is considered severe if loss exceeds 5% of usual weight within 1 month, or 10% of usual weight within 6 months. A nonvolitional weight loss of more than 10% is considered significant for malnutrition. A more patient specific method of evaluating weight is to compare current weight with the patient's usual weight. This can be determined using Equation:

% Usual body weight = [current Weight/ usual body weight] X 100

Anthropometric Data

Malnutrition can be detected by weight loss and an underweight condition. Measurements of body composition, height, weight, skin folds, circumferences, and others are useful.

Anthropometry is the science of body composition based on measurement of weight, stature, body circumferences, and subcutaneous fat thickness. These are physical measurements of the size, weight, and proportions of the human body used to compare an individual with normative population standards.

Body mass index (BMI) is another index of weight-for-height that is highly correlated with body fat.

Interpretation of BMI should include consideration of gender, frame size, and age. BMI values greater than 25 kg/m2 are indicative of overweight, and values less than 18.5 kg/m2 are indicative of undernutrition BMI <18.5 kg/m^2 possible initial identification for malnutrition, BMI <15 kg/m2 or less is correlated with mortality (see Table 1). BMI is calculated as follows: Body weight (kg)/[height (m)]^2

The most common measurements are weight, stature, head circumference (for children younger than 3 years of age) waist circumference, and measurements of limb size (e.g., skinfold thickness and midarm muscle and wrist circumferences), along with bioelectrical impedance analysis (BIA).

Bioelectrical Impedance Analysis (BIA)

Based on the theory that lean body mass has a higher electrical conductivity and lower impedance in comparison to fat due to its higher electrolyte content.

Estimates of total body water and fat-free mass are made using measurements of resistance and reactance (to a weak electrical current). BIA is a simple, noninvasive, and relatively inexpensive way to measure Lean Body mass (LBM).

Table 1. Analysis of body mass index (BMI)

BMI	
18.5	Underweight
18.5 -24.9	Normal
25-29.9	Overweight
30 – 34.9	Class 1 Obesity
35 – 39.9	Class 2 Obesity
Over 40	Class 3 Extreme Obesity

Skin Folds and Circumferences

Although they have had some success, but they have had limited practical application in patient care settings because appropriate training is required, developed from non-hospitalized populations may have a poor correlation with measurements made on hospitalized patients.

Physical Examination

Physical examination should focus on assessment of lean body mass (LBM) and physical findings of vitamin, trace element, and essential fatty acid deficiencies. A physical examination can identify specific nutrient deficits, weight increase or loss, and edema (Table 2, 3) [1].

Table 2. Physical examination parameters

Parameters	
Body mass index	BMI weight (kg)/(height (m))2 BMI <18.5 kg/m2 possible initial identification for malnutrition BMI <15 kg/m2 or less is correlated with mortality
Weight loss	Monitor for signs of muscle loss and subcutaneous fat accumulation.
Weakness/loss of strength	Lower extremity weakness may be seen with thiamin deprivation, which has been linked to loss of muscle mass and decreased hand-grip and leg extensor strength.
Peripheral Edema	Weight measures may be distorted by peripheral edema. Additionally, edema may be seen in thiamin deficient cases.
Hair exam	Some vitamin deficits are indicated by hair abnormalities. eg Brittle: biotin, Coiled, corkscrew: vitamins A and C
Skin exam	Skin conditions can indicate vitamin deficits Riboflavin deficit causes a desquamation vitamins A and C deficit cause Petechiae vitamin C deficit causes Perifollicular hemorrhage vitamins C and K cause Ecchymosis Xerosis, bran-like desquamation may related to essential fatty acid deficiency Pigmentation, cracking, crusting may be due to Niacin deficiency Acneiform lesions, follicular keratosis, xerosis may be due to vitamin A deficiency. Acro-orificial dermatitis, erythematous, vesiculobullous, and pustular related to zinc deficiency
Perioral exam	The presence of Perioral signs may indicate nutritional deficits. Angular stomatitis and cheilosis: B complex, iron, and protein Glossitis may be related to niacin, folate, and vitamin B12 deficiency, Magenta tongue may due to Riboflavin deficiency Bleeding gums, gingivitis, tooth loss attributed to vitamin C deficiency
Extremity exam	Extremity point to nutritional deficits in particular. vitamin C for Arthralgia and thiamin for Calf pain
Mental status/nervous system exam	Findings on the neurological and mental systems point to nutrient deficits. Thiamin treats ophthalmoplegia and foot drop Thiamin, biotin, and vitamin B12 for paresthesia Depressed posture and vibratory senses due to vitamin B12 deficiency Niacin treats anxiety, depression, and delusions vitamin B12 for memory problems Loss of the lower extremities and hyporeflexia vitamin B12 and thiamin for deep tendon responses With severe thiamin deficiency, Wernicke-Korsakoff syndrome may be seen.
Functional Assessment	Gait, chair stands, stair steps, and balance are among the physical abilities that should be observed and tested. These offer sophisticated assessments of combined neurological health, balance, and strength.

Table 3. Historical data assessment

Parameters	
Body weight	weight loss of 10% of usual body weight last 6 month Wt. loss >5% usual body weight last 3 month Wt. loss >20%. usual body weight t any time
Medical and surgical conditions; chronic disease	Critical condition, serious burns, major abdominal surgery, multi-trauma, closed head injury, adult respiratory distress syndrome, mild to moderate chronic HF, IBD, and cystic fibrosis are some of the medical conditions that can cause death.
signs/symptoms	Tachycardia Fever or hypothermia
Disorder GIT Eating difficulties	diarrhea, constipation Vomiting, nausea
Medication use	Adverse drug effect. Examine probable interactions between drugs and nutrients
Dietary practices	weight reduction, vegetarian
Influences on nutritional	alcohol or substance abuse dependency, caregivers Ask about ADL, IADL,

Clinical Signs

Fever or hypothermia are two examples of clinical markers of inflammation, as well as other generalized symptoms like tachycardia.

Laboratory Tests

Protein biochemical markers traditionally used in nutrition assessment. Albumin, prealbumin, transferrin, and retinol-binding protein are the most common visceral proteins used to assess nutritional status. These proteins are produced by the liver and often reflect hepatic synthetic capability. When hepatic insufficiency develops or when intake of substrates is inadequate for synthesis of proteins, the serum concentration of visceral proteins decreases. Critical judgment should be used when analyzing laboratory indications of inflammatory response and potential protein deficiency (albumin, prealbumin). Other helpful test markers for glucose, WBC count, and CRP. The presence of a systemic inflammatory response may also be supported by a negative nitrogen balance and high REE.

No single test or group of tests can be recommended as a routine or reliable indicator of protein status. It is a combination of measures—biochemical, anthropometric, dietary, and clinical findings—that produce a more complete picture of protein status.

Methods to Determine Energy Expenditure

A foundational goal of nutrition support is to preserve lean body mass and maintain immune function while avoiding complications related to under- or overfeeding. Many predictive equations for estimating expenditure have been described in the literature. The traditional method of assessing energy expenditure is the basal energy expenditure (BEE): the amount of energy (kilocalories) needed to support basic metabolic functions in a state of complete rest, shortly after awakening, and after a 12-hour fast. BEE refers to the metabolic activity necessary to sustain life (i.e., respiration, pulse, body temperature BEE is most commonly calculated using the Harris–Benedict equations.

Basal metabolic rate (BMR) is the energy expended in the postabsorptive state, approximately 2 hours after a meal. BMR is approximately 10% greater than BEE. Calculations of BEE or BMR do not include additional energy required as a result of stress or activity. The Harris–Benedict equations can be modified to include stress and physical activity factors, or these variables are estimated at 20 to 35 kcal/kg/day for moderate-to-severe stress. Only one factor should be used (i.e., do not add multiple factors) Select the factor that corresponds to the patient's dominant situation. (See Table 4 & 5).

Direct Calorimetry

A direct measurement of the amount of heat generated by the body within a structure large enough to permit moderate amounts of activity. These structures are called whole-room calorimeters. Urine is also collected and measured to account for the small amount of chemical energy lost in urea excretion in urine. The technique is not practical in the patient care because the individual must remain alone in the chamber for an extended time without caregivers or medical equipment (both of which produce heat).

Indirect Calorimetry

The most accurate method for determining resting energy expenditure (REE) for hospitalized individuals. *Indirect calorimetry* is a technique that measures inspired and expired gas flows, volumes and concentrations of O2 and CO2 to estimated metabolic rate. The equipment used is also known as a metabolic cart.

Indirect calorimeters have many advantages over direct calorimeters in terms of smaller size, lower cost, easier measurement and maintenance, shorter measurement periods, and minimal interruption of patient care. Subjects do not need to be isolated inside of room-size chambers as long as their respiratory gases can be completely captured for approximately 30 minutes.

Table 4. Estimation of energy expenditure

Basal Energy Expenditure (BEE)	
Harris–Benedict (HB) equations BEE men (kcal/day) = 66.47 + 13.75 Wt. in Kg + 5.0 ht in cm – 6.76 A BEE women (kcal/day) = 655.10 + 9.56 Wt. in Kg + 1.85 ht in cm – 4.68 A	
Or	
Energy Requirements	
Hospitalized patient, mild stress	20–25 kcal/kg/day
Moderate stress, malnourished	25–30 kcal/kg/day
Severe stress, critically ill	30–35 kcal/kg/day

Table 5. HB Equation activity/stress factor according to physical activity and clinical condition

Physical activity	Stress factor	Clinical condition	Stress factor
Strictly bed rested	1.2	Fever	1+0.13/C
Out of bed or/shivering	1.3	Elective surgical procedures	1-1.2
Quadriparesis	0.8	Peritonitis/ or multiple fractures	1.2-1.5
Paralysis	0.9	Head injury	1.5-1.8
Hemiparesis	1.2-1.3	Infection (severe)/sepsis	1.4-2.5
		Cancer	1.1-1.3
		COPD	1.2-1.3
		Burns	1.5-2
		AIDS	1.5-1.8

Estimation of Protein Goal, Fluid and Micronutrients

Protein Needs

Estimation of protein needs is necessary in nutritional assessment. Protein needs are calculated based on body weight, degree of stress, and disease state. The initial estimation is often made with a degree of subjectivity and clinical judgment, with adjustments made based on patient response. The usual recommended daily protein allowances are 0.8 g-1.5 /kg for adults. Well-nourished, hospitalized patients with minimal stress need 1 to 1.2 g of protein/kg/day to maintain lean body mass. The requirement for protein intake may be as high as 2 g/kg/day for a patient in a hypermetabolic, hypercatabolic state secondary to trauma or burns. Daily protein requirements for children and preterm infants 1-3g/kg /day.

Guidelines for Adult and children and preterm infants' protein needs are summarized in Tables 6 and 7.

Table 6. TPN macronutrients and micronutrients

Nutritional components of TPN	
Dextrose	70% (contains 3.4Kcal/g
Fat emulsion	10% or 20% (contains about 10Kcal/g
Amino acids (AAs)	3-20% and provide 4 Kcal/g
Electrolytes	Added to adjust and maintain the normal physiologic serum concentrations
Multivitamins and trace elements	Added according to the daily amount recommendations

Table 7. Protein requirements in different age group

	Protein requirement (g/Kg/day)
Very low birth weight	3-4
Preterm	2.5-3
Infant/neonate	2-2.5
Infant	1.5-2
Preschool/school age	1-1.5
Adolescent	0.8-1.5

Fluids

Various approaches are used to estimate fluid requirements in adults. Formulas used to calculate daily fluid requirements should account for the patient's weight, age, and clinical status. Water is needed to support an individual's LBM, which fluctuates with weight and decreases with age.

Some practitioners have found clinical success by calculating fluid needs (mL/d) with the following 2 formulas and then using the average of the results.

1. Equation (based on body weight and age):
   - 9 Ages 18–55 years: 35 mL × Body Weight (kg)
   - Ages 56–75 years: 30 mL × Body Weight (kg)
   - Ages >75 years: 25 mL × Body Weight (kg)
   - Fluid-restricted adults (eg, those with kidney disease, cardiac disease, or fluid overload states): ≤25 mL × Body Weight (kg)

2. Equation (Holliday-Segar formula adjusted for age):
   - More than 1 month age body wt. 3-10 kg: 100 ml/ Body Weight (kg)
   - Body wt. 10 -20 kg: 1000 ml + 50 ml/ Body Weight (kg) for every kg between 10-20 kg
   - Body wt. more than 20 kg:1500 ml + 20 ml/ Body Weight (kg) for every kg>20 kg
   - 12–14 Ages ≤50 years: 1500 mL for first 20 kg Body Weight + [20 mL × Remaining Body Weight (kg)]
   - Ages >50 years: 1500 mL for first 20 kg Body Weight + [15 mL × Remaining Body Weight (kg)]

3. Equation (based on kcal)
   - 1-1.25 ml per kcal

Additional fluid must be provided for patients such as

1. Severe diarrhea or emesis
2. Large draining wounds
3. Excessive diaphoresis
4. Constant drooling
5. Paracentesis losses
6. Drains
7. High gastric, fistula, and ostomy outputs
8. Persistent fevers (Fluid needs increase by 7% for each °F above normal (13% for each °C above normal)
9. Women who are lactating also have increased fluid requirements

Some fluid losses contain significant amounts of electrolytes, minerals, or proteins that require replacement along with water. Knowledge of the composition of specific body fluids is therefore useful. Table 8 shows the volume of fluid secreted and its electrolyte content throughout the GI tract. Abnormalities in renal excretion and excessive losses from the GI tract (e.g., vomiting, nasogastric suctioning, diarrhea) are often primary contributors to electrolyte imbalances. Identifying the etiology of the electrolyte imbalance is essential to providing safe and effective treatment.

Table 8. GI volume of fluid secreted and its electrolyte content

	Volume	Sodium (Na)	Potassium (K)	Chloride (Cl)	Bicarbonates (HCO3)
Plasma	-	140	5	100	25
Gastric secretions	2500	50	10	80	40
Upper intestinal fluids	3000	140	10	100	25
Bile and pancreatic secretions	1500	140	5	80	60
Mature ileostomy	500	50	5	20	25
Inflammatory diarrhea	-	110	40	100	40
Mixed Gastric aspirate	-	120	10	-	-

Micronutrients

Requirements for micronutrients (i.e., electrolytes, trace elements, and vitamins) vary with age, gender, route of administration, and underlying clinical conditions. A complete assessment will include identification of risks for deficiencies or toxicities with micronutrients based on the patient's specific nutritional status and concurrent disease processes. Symptoms of certain trace elements & Vitamins deficiencies and toxicities are listed Table 9 & 10.

Table 9. Trace element deficiency and toxicity symptoms

Trace Elements	Deficiency	Toxicity
Manganese (Mn)	-Carbohydrate and lipid metabolism impairment -protein synthesis impairment	Extrapyramidal neurological manifestations with signals hyperintensity on magnetic resonance imaging in basal ganglia.
Selenium (Se)	Cardiomyopathy, myalgia, skeletal myopathy and nails discoloration	Alopecia, brittle hair and nails, rashes "garlic" breath like odor and neurological manifestations
Zinc (Zn)	Dermatitis, anorexia, alopecia, impaired immune function and wound healing, glucose intolerance	Anemia, nervous system abnormalities in patients with renal disorders.
Chromium (Cr)	Glucose intolerance, neuropathy encephalopathy and hyperlipidemia	No known toxicities
Copper (Cu)	Anemia (hypochromic microcytic), leukopenia, thrombocytopenia (rare)	Hepatocellular damage since it accumulates in liver
Iron (Fe)	Anemia (hypochromic microcytic),), pallor, tiredness	Accumulate in liver, hemosiderosis, hemochromatosis, can be fatal
Iodine	Hypothyroidism cause weakness, cold intolerance, increased body weight and hair thinning	Thyroiditis, enlarged thyroid gland, hypo/hyperthyroidism, iodermia

Table 10. Lipid-soluble vitamins deficiency and toxicity symptoms

Vitamin (Vit.)	Deficiency	Toxicity
Retinol (Vit. A)	Xerophthalmia stages as follows: night blindness, xerosis of conjunctiva, ulceration, iron deficiency, increased infection severity and risk	Increased intracranial pressure, headache, nausea, dizziness, joint pain
Calciferol (Vit. D)	Osteomalacia an rickets, osteoporosis, hypocalcemia, myalgia nd bone pain, generalized weakness	Hypervitaminosis D, hypercalcemia, with manifestations of nausea, dehydration and constipation, kidney stones may also occur due to hypercalciuria
Tocopherols, tocotrienols (Vit. E)	Rare, may include neuropathy, myalgia, ataxia, hemolytic anemia, and retinopathy	Hemorrhage, coagulopathy, skeletal muscle weakness, diarrhea, nausea and fatigue
Phylloquinones (Vit K1) Menaquinones (Vit. K2)	Bleeding, prolonged prothrombin time, osteoporosis	No toxicities associated with Vit. K supplements or food sources, interferes with anticoagulant oral therapy

Question 1: Which of the following is most suggestive of malnutrition?

a) 10th percentile of triceps skinfold thickness
b) Voluntary body mass index change from 30 to 25 over 6 month
c) Involuntary weight loss of 10% usual body weight over six months
d) Albumin decrease from 4.0 to 3.5

Answer c.

Question 2: A patient with alcoholism is admitted with small bowel obstruction and is started on PN providing 400 grams of dextrose. If, after 3 days, the patient develops mental status changes Wernicke-Korsakoff syndrome it is most likely due deficiency of:

a) pyridoxine
b) thiamin
c) cyanocobalamin.
d) niacin.

Answer c.

Question 3: Which parameter is measured when using IC?

a) Heat loss
b) Catabolic rate
c) Gas exchange
d) Free energy balance

Answer c.

Enteral Nutrition

Enteral nutrition (EN) delivers nutrients by tube or mouth into the GI tract. EN is preferred method for the feeding and advantage over parenteral nutrition if the gut works. It is thought to be more physiological, and more effect by utilizing the normal route of digestion and absorption nutrients, maintain gut structure and function, fewer metabolic, infectious and technical complication; and less costly.

EN is indicated for the patient who cannot or will not eat enough to meet nutritional requirements and who has a functioning GI tract and a method of enteral access. Potential indications include neoplastic disease, organ failure, hypermetabolic states, GI disease, and neurologic impairment.

Contradictions of Enteral Feedings

- Expected resumption of unrestricted oral intake in less 7 days
- Bowel obstruction
- Terminal condition, no aggressive treatment
- Major hemorrhages in upper GI tract
- Hemodynamic instability
- Inability to gain access
- High output fistulas (>500mL/d)
- Significant bowel wall edema

EN should begin as soon as possible ideally within 24 to 48 hours of ICU admission because this approach appears to decrease infectious complications and reduce mortality. Only if the Patients who have a functional GI tract and are hemodynamically stable ought to be fed right away. EN initiation can be delayed until 7 to 14 days in well-nourished none critically ill Patients with insufficient oral intake.

Table 11. Enteral feeding route

	Nasogastric	Nasoenteric	Gastrostomy	jejunostomy
Indication	Inserted when short-term access is indicated.		Long-term access (>4 weeks)	
Site	- Nasogastric: nose into the stomach - Nasoduodenal: nose through the pylorus into the duodenum - Nasojejunal: nose through the pylorus into the jejunum past the ligament of Treitz		Percutaneous endoscopic gastrostomy (PEG)	-Direct percutaneous endoscopic jejunostomy (DPEJ) -Direct percutaneous endoscopic gastrojejunostomy (PEGJ)
Access and confirmation of access	PH step up, capnography, radiography is still the gold standard		Endoscopic, fluoroscopic, or surgical methods	
Contraindication	-Obstructing head, neck, and esophageal pathology or injury preventing safe insertion.		-Obstruction of the GI tract proximal to the stomach and the inability to transilluminate the abdominal wall for identification of a safe abdominal access site	
Advantages	Easy to insert, inexpensive, multiple commercially available tubes and sizes		Long term lower morbidity and cost, large-bore tubes less likely to clog, multiple commercially available tubes and sizes	Potential reduced aspiration risk, multiple commercially available tubes and sizes, low-profile buttons available
	Nasogastric Nasoenteric		Gastrostomy	jejunostomy
Complication	Misplacement to the bronchopulmonary leading to pneumothorax Tube dislodgement, tube malfunction, tube occlusion, tube feeding aspiration, and intestinal ischemia.		Complications can be divided into procedural and post procedural events. Procedure related complications are uncommon such as intraprocedural aspiration, hemorrhage, perforation of the GI lumen, and prolonged ileus. Pneumoperitoneum, as a result of the percutaneous insertion procedure Buried bumper syndrome results from growth of the gastric mucosa over the internal bumper.	

Table 12. Types of Enteral Nutrition administration

Characteristics	Continuous	Cyclic	Intermit	Bolus
	Preferred for initiation	Provides formula at a continuous rate for less than 24 hours daily Used for patients who need supplemental nutrition	Similar to bolus feedings in the amount and frequency of feedings to be administered. Intermittent feedings differ from bolus feedings in that each feeding is administered over a half an hour to an hour period	Large volume feedings that are administered rapidly. Long-term care residents who have a gastrostomy
Rate	20 to 50 mL/hour 1 to 2 mL/kg/hour for children	Over 8 to 12 hours	Volumes can range from 240 to 720 mL (1 to 3 cups) over 30 to 60 minutes from 4 to 6 times per day Using a feeding container or bag, with or without an enteral pump	Started with 100 till 240 mL of formula over a 4- to 10-minute time-frame with infusions 3 to 6 times per day Using gravity administration via a syringe 2 to 4 mL/kg per bolus for children
Advantage	Preferred for initiation Well tolerated Appropriate in certain settings (e.g., ICU) Decreased risks of gastric distension and aspiration Used with any route of feeding, Intragastric, direct into duodenum or jejunum	Allowing breaks from the infusion system Increasing mobility Commonly used for patients who need supplemental nutrition	Improves tolerability Mimics normal eating patterns. Protocols outline	Short administration time (eg, 5–10 min) Minimal equipment (eg, a syringe) Mimics normal eating patterns. Protocols outline
Disadvantage	Cost and inconvenience associated with pump and administration sets			Cramping, nausea, vomiting, aspiration, and diarrhea

Access [2]

EN can be administered through four routes, which have different indications, tube placement options, advantages, and disadvantages. The selection depends on the anticipated duration of use and GI motility (See Table 11) [2].

Administration Method

EN can be administered by continuous, cyclic, bolus, and intermittent methods. The choice depends on the feeding tube location, patient's clinical condition, intestinal function, residence environment, and tolerance to tube feeding (See Table 12).

Protocols outlining initiation and advancement criteria are a useful strategy to optimize achievement of nutrient goals based on GI tolerance. Clinical signs of intolerance include abdominal distention or cramping, high gastric residual volumes, aspiration, and diarrhea [3].

Dosing of Enteral Nutrition

- The A.S.P.E.N. guidelines stated that, in order to derive clinical benefit from EEN, it is preferred to consume between 50% and 65% of target calories during the first week of hospitalization.
- Effective EN delivery as consistent infusion of 90% of a calculated caloric goal.

Timing of Enteral Nutrition

Critically ill: EN should begin as soon as possible ideally within 24 to 48 hours of ICU admission. Patients who have a functional GI tract and are hemodynamically stable ought to be fed right away. Well-nourished none critically ill Patients with insufficient oral intake for 7 to 14 days, patients in whom a 7- to 14-day period of insufficient oral intake is anticipated [4].

Formula

EN formulations were created to provide essential nutrients, including macronutrients (eg, carbohydrates, fats, and proteins) and micronutrients (eg, electrolytes, trace elements, vitamins, and water). Over time, formulations have been enhanced to improve tolerance and meet specific patient needs.

There are also disease-specific formulas. In selecting an appropriate enteral formula, the following items should be considered:

- Functioning capabilities of the GI tract.
- Adequacy of PO intake.
- Estimated calorie and protein needs.
- Fluid status and fluid needs.
- Site of feeding administration.
- Diagnoses and medical status.
- Anticipated length of feeding (short-term vs. long-term).

Categorizing formulas as listed in Table 13 simplifies the formula selection process. Soluble and insoluble fiber has been added to several EN formulations. Potential benefits of soluble fiber include trophic effects on colonic mucosa, promotion of sodium and water absorption, and regulation of bowel function.

Table 13. Types of EN formula [5]

Formula	Indications	Examples
Standard	Well-tolerated feeding, with normal GI function and fluid needs	Osmolite Promote Nutren Replete
Standard with fiber content	Long-term needs for enteral tube feeding and/or constipation	Jevity Promote with fibers Nutren with fibers Replete with fibers
Standard-Nutrient dense (high nitrogen or calorie)	Increased wound healing	Osmolite 1.2, 1.5 Jevity 1.2, 1.5 Isosource 1.5
Fluid restricted	Restricted fluid allowance	Two Cal HN Nutren 2.0
Peptide-based with hydrolyzed (partially) whey proteins	Impaired digestive function	Peptamen Peptamen 1.5w/prebio Vital Vital 1.5
Amino acid based (100% free amino acids)	Impaired digestive function	Vivonex T.E.N
Immune enhanced	Stress or trauma	Impact Oxepa Pivot
Renal	Kidney function disorder, restricted potassium, phosphorus, and fluid	Nepro Suplena novosource renal
Diabetes	Moderate carbohydrate, fiber enhanced	Glytrol Diabetisource
Pulmonary	High fat content, moderate-low carbohydrate	Pulmocare Nutrenpulmonary
Hepatic	-High branched chain amino acids -Low aromatic amino acids	Nutrihep

Enteral Order Sets and Protocols

These order sets can be designed to meet the needs of the institution and can be paper- or computer-based protocols. They should include the four elements of

1. Patient identifier
2. Formula name
3. Enteral access device and site
4. Administration method and rate.

Protocols and order sets should include strategies to reduce the danger of enteral feeding contamination and the risk of regurgitation and aspiration.

- The protocol should be evidence-based and should explicitly state what the nurse should do in various clinical settings in order to optimize effective EN administration and maximize tolerance.
- A crucial part of a nurse-driven procedure would be starting EN and moving on to the target, for instance. A nurse may be given the ability to make changes to better deliver EN if more recent evidence-based suggestions are included. Order sets can help with decision-making by Permitting a more regular gastric residual volume (GRV) of two consecutive checks of 250 mL or one check of more over 500 mL before EN is stopped.
- They could incorporate prokinetics if a patient is experiencing persistently elevated GRV [6].

Transitional Feeding

- Enteral feedings can be transitioned from continuous feedings to bolus or intermittent feedings. This is usually done through a series of steps to evaluate if the patient can tolerate a larger volume given periodically while still providing adequate nutrition with limited continuous feedings
- continuous feedings to cyclic feedings. This may be accomplished by increasing the rate while decreasing the hours of infusion
- transitioning from enteral feeding to an oral diet
- EN may be discontinued if receive 70% goal caloric requirements from oral rout.

Gastric Feeding If normal gastric function is presumed, then gastric feedings are generally used. One advantage of gastric feedings is that they are more physiologic. The stomach acts as a natural reservoir for nutrients, so gastric placement of the feeding tube more closely mimics how the body receives nutrients.12 It also allows for intermittent and bolus feeds, which have both metabolic and lifestyle benefits.

Small-bowel Feeding Duodenal or jejunal feeding may be preferred if a patient has gastroparesis or reflux, or is diagnosed with aspiration risk. It may also accommodate early satiety problems. They decrease the risk of microaspiration, as well as of aspiration pneumonia.

Complications and Monitoring

Appropriate monitoring of patients receiving EN is essential to recognize and prevent complications. Complications can be divided into three groups: mechanical, metabolic, and GI.

Aspiration is a common complication associated with tube feeding. It occurs when a patient inhales a substance, such as water or tube feed, into the airway, which causes dyspnea and coughing. Prolonged aspiration is dangerous because it can lead to pneumonia. Head of bed elevation is the primary measure to prevent aspiration. Monitor gastric residual volume.

Nausea/Vomiting are common complications to enteral feeding and increase the risk of aspiration and pneumonia. There are many possible causes of nausea or vomiting. Both gastric retention and rapid infusion of hyperosmolar formula can cause nausea/vomiting. In these cases, a clinician must reduce the rate of feeding, but if the patient is vomiting, feedings should be held. The fat content of feeds also affects a patient's tolerance, with feedings that are lower in fat being generally better tolerated.

Abdominal Distention is the accumulation of air or liquid in a patient's abdomen and can cause major discomfort to the patient. Abdominal distention can be diagnosed by observing an increase in abdominal girth (about 8-10 cm) and/ or palpating the abdomen patient's report of symptoms such as bloating and cramping can also indicate abdominal distention. Rapid bolus or intermittent feeds of cold formula can cause abdominal distention, continuous feed can treated this.

Constipation - certain medications can cause constipation. It is therefore important to have a proactive bowel regime. Dehydration and lack of fiber are also frequent causes of constipation. Adding additional fluid to the formula in addition to fiber can prevent waste buildup. Fecal impaction or obstruction is a type of stool accumulation that can be diagnosed by a rectal exam. Fecal implantation can be alleviated by rectal exam if it is close to the rectum, but surgical or endoscopic methods may have to be used if the impaction is higher in the colon.

Diarrhea is higher stool frequency, volume, and water content. Most causes of diarrhea are not incidental to tube feeding. Certain medications, especially those containing magnesium, phosphorus, and sorbitol, can be hyperosmolar, causing diarrhea. Diarrhea can also be due to bacterial growth. Prolonged antibiotic use creates an imbalance in gut microflora, resulting in antibiotic associated diarrhea. Despite the fact that Clostridium difficile, a bacteria that causes diarrhea, is only one of the possible causes, a stool culture is often done to confirm antibiotic-induced diarrhea. Use of pre- and probiotics promotes proliferation and can restore the patient's microbiota to resolve diarrhea associated with harmful bacterial overgrowth (6).

Hyperglycemia Monitor serum glucose every 6 hours, correct glucose level before initiation tube feeding, treat underlying disease.

Electrolyte disturbance Monitor closely for hypo or hyper, treat underlying cause.

Fluid imbalance Monitor input and output daily, change in body wt. more than 2 kg reflect ECF volume or diuretic therapy [7].

Drug Nutrients Interaction

- Drugs cannot be crushed not to add Nasogastric feeding Enteric coated Tablets to protect drugs from gastric acid or the stomach from an irritating drug, long-acting products to reduce the number of daily doses. Crushing may cause immediate release of the total drug dose, increasing the risk of toxicity and reducing efficacy. For example, a 200-mg extended-release morphine capsule is designed to gradually release drug over 24 hours. When crushed or dissolved before administration, the full 200-mg dose is immediately released, resulting in increased risk of respiratory depression and potentially respiratory arrest.
- Drugs that contain initials such as CD, CR, ER, LA, SA, SR, TR, XL, and XR following the name generally need to be taken intact and should not be crushed or dissolved for administration.
- Specific drug interaction Phenytoin, Fluoroquinolones,: Holding administration of the EN formulation for at least 1 hour, and possibly 2 hours, before and after phenytoin administration seems to produce the most consistent results Table 14.

Table 14. Medications with special considerations for enteral feeding

Drug	Interactions	Recommendations
Phenytoin	-Decreased bioavailability with tube feeding -Possible binding with protein hydrolysates or with calcium caseinates	Consider holding of tube feeding 1-2 hrs before and after phenytoin. Adjust the rate of tube feeding Monitor clinical response ad phenytoin serum concentration and consider IV phenytoin if serum concentration not achieved.
Fluoroquinolones Tetracyclines	Decreased bioavailability due to the potential of complex formation with divalent and trivalent cations	Consider holding of tube feeding about 1hr before and after drug use. Avoid jejunal ciprofloxacin use and monitor clinical response
Warfarin	Decreased warfarin absorption; it therapeutic efficacy antagonized by vitamin K in enteral feeding formula	Consider tube holding about 1 hr before and after drug use. Adjust dose based on INR. The dose may require to be increased with starting tube feeding and decrease when enteral feeding is stopped.
Omeprazole Lansoprazole	Administration by enteral feeding complicated by acid-labile drugs within delayed release, base-labile granules	Granules may become moistened with water and occlude tubes. A liquid can be prepared extemporaneously for oral use through the feeding tube

Question 1: What is the most important intervention to reduce the risk of pulmonary aspiration during gastric tube feedings?

a) Turn the tube feeding off when repositioning the patient.
b) Hold tube feedings for a gastric residual > 200 mL
c) Elevate the head of bed 30 to 45 degrees.
d) Provide mouth care every 2 to 4 hours.

Answer c.

Question 2: Which of the following medications would be appropriate to crush and deliver via an enteral feeding tube?

a) Nifedipine XL
b) Metoprolol immediate release
c) Enteric coated aspirin
d) Diltiazem CD

Answer b.

Question 3: A 55-year-old critically ill patient has been tolerating a standard 1 cal /mL feeding formula well over the past week. She begins having frequent bouts of loose stools. What should be the clinician's next suggestion?

a) Change to a peptide-based formula
b) Determine the cause of diarrhea

c) Add pre- and probiotics
d) Change to a fiber-supplemented formula

Answer b.

Parenteral Nutrition

Parenteral nutrition is a sort of nutrition support that involves giving nutrients intravenously to people who cannot or won't consume enough food orally or enterally. In order to meet needs, PN can be added to an oral diet or enteral nutrition (EN), used as the only source of nutrition while recovering from a gastrointestinal (GI) tract infection or injury, or as a long-term life-sustaining treatment for patients whose ability to enterally absorb nutrients has been compromised. and multiple trace minerals (zinc, copper, manganese, chromium, selenium). It can also be used as a vehicle to provide certain medications. The principal forms of PN are central and peripheral—which describes the venous route of delivery.

Early versus Late Parenteral Nutrition A.S.P.E.N. currently recommends delaying administration of PN for 7 to 10 days in seriously sever ill adult patients where enteral nutrition is not feasible, unless they are severely malnourished or at high nutritional risk. Similarly, their recommendations state that in both low- and high-risk patients who are unable to meet greater than 60% of their goal by EN, supplemental PN should be delayed 7 to 10 days. These guidelines are based on evidence that despite an increase in energy and protein intake, there is a lack of clinical benefit associated with early parenteral supplementation. Studies such as that by Heyland confirm the risk of PN use by demonstrating increased infection rates and intensive care unit length of stay as well as cost. However, studies have shown that PN can be used safely. In their study, Doig and colleagues demonstrated that PN use can be safe and also less days spent on ventilation, although length of intensive care and hospital stay were not improved. When providing nutrition support therapy, critical review of a patient's nutritional risk and status as well as clinical condition must accompany guidelines for PN use. Central Parenteral nutrition given is delivered through a high flow vein, typically the right atrium's superior vena cava when the Expected duration is more than 10 days or limited peripheral venous access or nutrient needs are large or fluid restriction is required. The high concertation of dextrose (20%-30%) and amino acid (5%-10%) for administration through the central vein. Central venous access devices include Groshong®, Hickman®, Hohn®, multiple lumen catheters, peripherally inserted central catheter (PICC) lines, and implanted intravenous port devices Peripheral: is a form of intravenous feeding that is injected into a vein in a body part other than the heart, called total parenteral nutrition (TPN), Osmolarity <900 mOsm/L, Expected duration <2 weeks.

Indications and Contraindications

When evaluating whether a patient is eligible for PN, consider that PN carries a high risk of serious complications. It is also a costly therapy, due to the expense of vascular access devices, monitoring laboratory values, and treating potential complications. While PN has been shown to improve markers of nutritional status, it does not consistently improve clinical outcomes. PN is only clearly suggested for a specific subset of illness conditions and situations and should not be used as a first treatment option for nutrition support. For these reasons, the expected benefits of PN therapy should outweigh the risks.

Despite the preference for EN from a clinical perspective, there are circumstances in which PN would be indicated, EN has been tried, including with several tube positions, but it hasn't worked. A compromised GI tract makes EN contraindicated. A paralytic ileus, mesenteric ischemia, small-bowel obstruction, a GI fistula distal to the feeding tube tip, and a GI fistula with outputs of more than 500 mL/day are all potential causes of GI tract dysfunction. The patient's preference should always be considered. Some patients who are prescribed EN may refuse to have a tube placed and prefer to be fed via the parenteral route [8].

TPN Components

PN formulations are complex mixtures containing up to 40 different nutrient components, including macronutrients which energy substrates such as carbohydrate (dextrose), protein (amino acids), and fat (lipid or IV fat emulsion), along with micronutrients such water, electrolytes, vitamins, and trace minerals.

Macronutrients

Carbohydrates

Dextrose should make up 40% to 60% of your daily calorie needs as standard formulation.

- GIR (glucose infusion rate) is everything, provides 3.4 kcal/g, in its hydrated form, compared with dietary carbohydrate which provides 4 kcal/g
  - Adult 3-5 mg/kg/min/ Pediatric Initially 4-8 mg/kg/min/ typical max of 11-14 mg/kg/min/ Advance by 1-2 mg/kg/min as glucose tolerates

The recommended dose listed in Table 15. Adult recommendation as follow

- 2-3 g/kg/d (minimum).
- 4-5 g/kg/d (Optimum).
- < 7 g/kg/d (Maximum)

Start max-

- 150 - 200 g/day (general)
- 100 – 150 g/d (diabetic or stress hyperglycemia)
- Increase to goal when blood glucose less than 180 mg/dl (10 mmol/L)

Table 15. Advantages and disadvantages of 2-in-1 and 3-in-1 parenteral nutrition

2-in-1 PN	3-in-1 (TNA)
• Enhanced overall stability. • Better flexibility in concentrating dextrose and amino acids • More flexibility for higher concentrations of electrolytes to be added. • Improved medication compatibility. • Minimized risk of bacterial growth because of acidic pH and high osmolarity. • Better visualization • Allow the use of bacterial retention filter (0.22-micron) • Decreased risk of catheter tubes occlusion if IVFE is not used daily.	• Aseptically compounded by the pharmacy. • Simplified regimen especially for patients at home with less supply and equipment cost. • Less nursing time needed for administration • Reduced risk of contamination • Inhibited bacterial growth versus separate IVFE Minimize infusion-related reactions from IVFE because of slower infusion rate. • Improve lipid clearance because of slower infusion rate Decreased risk of phlebitis with PPN
• Higher administration costs and time when lipids are infused separately Increased risk of touch contamination • Increased phlebitis risk, particularly if PPN is not coinfused with IV lipid emulsion • IVFE given in a piggyback manner is limited to a maximum hang time of 12 hours.	• Impaired visualization of particulate matter or precipitate because of opacity of IVFE admixture • IVFE is less stable—more prone to lipid separation. • Admixture is less stable with concentrated electrolyte additives larger particle size of IVFE admixture. • Must use 1.2-micron. Cannot use 0.22-micron bacterial retention filter. • Limited compatibility with medications. • Containers with diethylhexyl phthalate should be avoided because this toxic material may be extracted by the lipid and may harm patients.

Amino Acids

Nitrogen and energy source for protein synthesis (provides 4 kcal/g).

Premature neonates: 3-4 g/kg/day / Term neonates & infants: 2.5-3 g/kg/day shown in Table 7.

Amino acids are classified into three groups: essential, nonessential, and semi-essential amino acids. Essential amino acids mean that our bodies cannot manufacture them, so they must be obtained exogenously, while nonessential means that our bodies can produce the amino acid from available carbon and nitrogen precursors Figure 1 and Table 16.

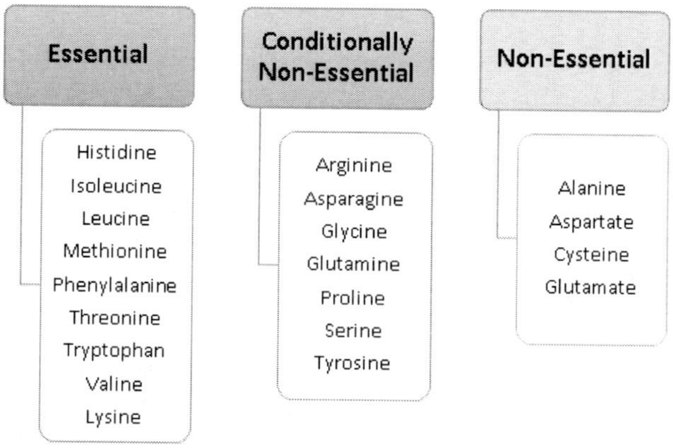

Figure 1. Classifications of amino acids.

Table 16. The approximate protein requirements in different disease group

Patients	Calorie/ Energy requirements	Protein requirements
Healthy, well-nourished, maintenance	20 to 25 kcal/kg/day	0.8-1g/kg/day
Generally under-nourished, critically ill, major surgery, trauma, burns, sepsis, metabolic stress	25 to 30 kcal/kg/day and up to 35 kcal/kg/day in specific situations	1.2-2 g/kg/day, and up to 2.5 g/kg/day in specific situations
Acute kidney injury, chronic kidney disease	25 to 30 kcal/kg/day, and up to 35 kcal/kg/day in specific situations	IHD: 1.2-1.5 g/kg/day CRRT: 1.5-2.5 g/kg/day PD: 1.2 -1.3 g/kg/day
Obese patients with critical illness (BMI >30kg/m2) (Hypocaloric feeding)	11 to 14 kcal/kg/day ABW Or 22-25kcal/kg/day IBW	BMI 30-40kg/m2: more than 1.5-2 g/kg/day IBW BMI >40kg/m2: more than 2-2.5g/kg/day

Lipids

Composition Abbreviation	Intralipid 20% SO	Lipofundin 20% MCT/LCT	ClinOleic 20% OO/SO	SMOFlipid 20% SMOF	Omegaven 10% FO Not available in SA	Lipoplus 20% MCT/LCT/FO Not available in SA
Oil source %						
Soy bean	100	50	20	30	0	40
MCT	0	50	0	30	0	50
Olive	0	0	80	25	0	0
Fish	0	0	0	15	100	10
% Fatty acids						
Linoleic	53	50	18.7	21.4	4.4	25.7
Arachidonic	0.1	0.2	0.5	1.0	2.1	NA
α-Linolenic	8	7	2.3	2.5	1.8	3.4
EPA	0	0	0	4.7	19.2	3.7
DHA	0	0	0	4.4	12.1	2.5
ω6 – ω3 ratio	7:1	7:1	9:1	2.5:1	1:8	2.7:1
Phytosterols (mg/l)	348 ± 33	NA	327 ± 8	47.6	0	NA
Phytosterols (mg/l) (44)	439 ± 5.7	278 ± 5.09	274 ± 2.6	207	NA	NA
α-tocopherol (mg/l)	38	85 ± 20	32 or 180	200	150-296	190 ± 30
Osmolarity (mOsm/L)	260	380	270	380	308-376	NA

Abbreviations: SO: Soybean oil; MCT: Medium Chain Triglycerides; OO: Olive Oil; FO: Fish oil; EPA: Eicosapentaenoic Acid; DHA: Docosahexaenoic acid

Patients in intensive care units frequently have energy deficiency, which is a major issue that is linked to higher rates of complications, hospital stays, and mortality. The infusion of lipid injectable emulsions (ILEs) provides a high energy supply, contributes to the prevention of high glucose infusion rates, and is indispensable for supplying the body with essential fatty acids (EFAs). In the United States, ILE components include an oil source, egg yolk phospholipid as an emulsifier, Glycerin makes the formulation isotonic, while sodium hydroxide raises the pH to a range of 6 to 9 in the final product. Historically, the most common oil sources used in ILEs have been soybean oil and safflower oil, which contain long chain triglycerides (LCTs). These oils were used because they are relatively inexpensive, abundant on the market, and effectively deliver non glucose energy to the body. A disadvantage of soybean and safflower oils is their high levels of omega-6 fatty acid and low levels of omega-3 fatty acid, a ratio that is known to promote systemic inflammation. In an effort to alleviate concerns about lipid emulsions made from soybean oil, alternative sources of fatty acids were and continue to be investigated.20 In 2016, the Food and Drug Administration approved SMOFlipid, which is comprised of four different oils: 30% soybean, 30% medium-chain triglycerides derived from coconut oil, 25% olive oil, and 15% fish oil. SMOFlipid, and others like it, have an improved omega-3:omega-6 ratio that may reduce the risk of harmful changes to the liver, such as parenteral nutrition associated liver disease (PNALD) and hepatic steatosis, and may preserve antioxidant capacity in severely ill patients. Ideally, this can contribute to better health outcomes such as shorter ICU stays.

Essential Fatty Acid Deficiency

Essential fatty acids (EFA) are linoleic and linolenic acids, cannot be synthesized by the body. The most notable clinical change are dry flaky skin and desquamation, poor wound healing, sparse hair growth, Eczematoid dermatosis of the face and neck, and anemia, thrombocytopenia, and enlarged fatty liver.

Micronutrients

Electrolytes Parenteral solutions represent a significant portion, if not all, of total daily fluid and electrolyte intake. Depending on the patient's specific needs, different electrolytes are added in maintenance or therapeutic doses to PN formulations. Acetate and chloride do not have specific ranges for intake; rather, they are adjusted as needed to maintain acid– base balance.

For administration in PN, calcium gluconate and magnesium sulfate are the preferred forms of these electrolytes compared to calcium chloride and magnesium chloride because they are less likely to produce physicochemical incompatibilities, which are physical or chemical changes that can occur in PN leading to precipitation, color changes, or chemical degradation that can compromise the solution as shown in Table 17.

Trace Elements, the need for trace elements in long-term parenteral nutrition was realized when patients began to develop deficiency symptoms that were alleviated through trace element supplementation. Some of the deficiencies that developed were copper, zinc, manganese, selenium, chromium, and molybdenum. Of these, copper, zinc, manganese, selenium, and chromium are the most commonly supplemented trace elements in PN formulations. These trace minerals are available in both individual form and various trace element combinations at concentrations safe for use in neonates, pediatrics, and adults.14 The American Medical Association and A.S.P.E.N. have published recommendations for daily parenteral dose of selenium, zinc, copper, manganese, and chromium, as seen Table 18.

Table 17. ASPEN recommendation electrolytes requirements in parenteral nutrition in different age groups [9]

Micronutrient	Standard daily requirements			
	Preterm neonates	Infants/Children	Adolescent and children >50kg	Adults
*Sodium	2-5/kg	2-5/kg	1-2/kg	1-2/kg
*Potassium	2-4/kg	2-4/kg	1-2/kg	1-2/kg
Chloride and acetate	As needed according to acid-base balance			
*Calcium	2-4/kg	0.5-4/kg	10-20/kg	10-15/kg
#Phosphorus mmol	1-2/kg	0.5-2/kg	10-40/kg	20-40/kg
*Magnesium	0.3-0.5/kg	0.3-0.5/kg	10-30/kg	8-20/kg

*: amount in mEq, #: amount in mmol.

Table 18. Trace elements dose for pediatrics and neonate in parenteral nutrition [10]

Trace elements	Standard daily requirements				
	Preterm neonates	Term neonates (3-10kg)	Children (10-40kg)	Adolescents >40kg	Adults
Zinc	400 mcg/kg	250 mcg/kg	50 mcg/kg (max 5000mcg/day)	2-5mg	3-5 mg
Copper	20 mcg/kg	20mcg/kg	20 mcg/kg (max 500mcg/day)	200-500mcg	0.3-0.5 mg
Manganese	1 mcg/kg	1 mcg/kg	1 mcg/kg (max 55 mcg/day)	40-100 mcg	55 mcg
Chromium	0.05-0.3 mcg/kg	0.2 mcg/kg	0.2 mcg/kg (max 5 mcg/day)	5-15 mcg	<1 mg
Selenium	2 mcg/kg	2 mcg/kg	2 mcg/kg (max 100 mcg/day)	40-60 mcg	60-100 mcg

N.B.: Full daily dose is recommended unless the patient is able to ingest or absorb enterally/ orally.

Table 19. Vitamins requirements in parenteral nutrition for adults

Vitamin	Standard requirements	Vitamin	Standard requirements
Ascorbic acid	200 mg	Niacinamide	40 mg
Vitamin A	3300 IU	Pantothenate	15 mg
Vitamin D	200 IU	Biotin	60 mcg
Vitamin E	10 IU	Folic acid	600 mcg
Thiamine/ pyridoxine	6 mg	Vitamin B12	5 mcg
Riboflavin	3.6 mg		

Table 20. Multivitamin dose for neonates and children in parenteral nutrition

*Manufacturers recommendations		#NAG-AMA recommendations	
Body weight (Kg)	Dose (ml)	Body weight (Kg)	Dose (ml)
Less than 1	1.5	Less than 2.5	2 ml/kg
1 to less than 3	3.25	≥ 2.5	5 ml
> 3	5		

*Infuvite Pediatric (Baxter) and M.V.I. Pediatric (Hospira).
Nutrition Advisory Group-American Medical Association.

Multivitamins In addition to macronutrients and electrolytes, patients receiving PN require vitamins to prevent deficiency and promote optimal health. Clinical practice guidelines include the justification, dosage, and the route of delivery for inclusion of vitamins in patients receiving PN. Guideline adherence ensures optimum nutrition care and improves patient outcomes. Commercially available vitamin products for parenteral nutrition supplementation include both single and multivitamin infusion products. In 2000, the Food and Drug Administration issued parenteral multivitamin dosing requirements. In accordance with these requirements, parenteral multivitamins include vitamin A, vitamin D, vitamin E, vitamin K, vitamin B1, vitamin B2, vitamin B6, vitamin B12, niacin, folic acid, pantothenic acid, biotin, and vitamin C. One parenteral multivitamin product is available without vitamin K for patients on warfarin anticoagulant therapy. The standard requirements of vitamins for adults and neonates are summarized in Tables 19 and 20. Single vitamins are used when a patient requires more of a vitamin than a parenteral multivitamin provides. Currently, there are no single vitamin products available for biotin, pantothenic acid, riboflavin, vitamin A, vitamin D or vitamin E as shown in Table 20.

PN Formulation Type

PN formulations may be prepared in one of two ways:

- A dextrose–amino acid (2- in-1) mixture in which IV fat emulsion (IVFE) is administered separately as a piggybacked infusion.
- A total nutrient admixture (TNA or 3-in-1) in which the dextrose, amino acids, and IVFE are combined in solution in the same bag.

Premixed PN solutions are also available commercially in different percentages of dextrose and amino acid preparations. Premixed PN solutions are sterile products that have a longer shelf life; however, these formulations limit the ability to customize the final product to meet individual patient needs.

Both systems are available to the practicing clinician, and each has advantages as well as disadvantages. These are reviewed in Table 15.

Order of Mixing for 3 in 1 TNA

1. First Add dextrose then amino acids AAs mix well then add sterile water.
2. Start with phosphate electrolyte which is first to be added, mix well.
3. Add other electrolytes (except Ca) and trace minerals.
4. Mix thoroughly to spread the phosphate evenly and avoid precipitate with the calcium.
5. Add Calcium
6. Keep a close eye for precipitates or contaminants.
7. Add lipid if 3-in-1 formulation. ((Note: Avoid mixing dextrose and lipids together directly as the low pH of dextrose may cause the lipid emulsion to become unstable).
8. Add vitamins last, as close to the time of PN administration as possible in acute care settings, or just before infusion in patients receiving home PN. see Table 21.

Table 21. ASPEN guidelines recommendation in TPN [11]

	Initiation		Advance by		Goals	
Infants (<1y)	Preterm	Term	Preterm	Term	Preterm	Term
Protein g/kg/day*	3-4	2.5-3	-	-	3-4	2.5-3
Dextrose mg/kg/min	6-8	6-8	1.4-1.7	3.5	10-14 (max 14-18)	10-14 (max up to 18)
Fat g/kg/day	0.5-1	0.5-1	0.5-1	0.5-1	3 (max 0.15 g/kg/h)	2.5-3 (0.15 g/kg/h)
Children (1-10y)						
Protein g/kg/day	1.5-2.5		-		1.5-2.5	
Dextrose mg/kg/min	3-6		2-3		8-10	
Fat g/kg/day	1-2		0.5-1		2-2.5	
Adolescents						
Protein g/kg/day	0.8-2		-		0.8-2	
Dextrose mg/kg/min	2.5-3		1.2		5-6	
Fat g/kg/day	1		1		1-2	

* The dose of protein doesn't need titration; protein requirements will be increased with critical illness

N.B. Glucose infusion rate (mg/kg/min) = [dextrose (g/d)x1000]/[24(h/d)x body weight (kg)].

Initiation of PN

PN generally should begin with dextrose, AA and lipid at goal unless the patient is at high risk of refeeding syndrome or suboptimal tolerance is anticipated (e.g., brittle diabetic). If intolerance is expected, initiate PN on the first day with fewer calories from dextrose and total calories should be limited to 50 – 75% of estimated calorie requirements [12].

Monitoring

Routine monitoring and evaluation of nutritional status and the metabolic effects of therapy are required for patients receiving PN therapy. Nutritional goals established in the patient care plan are estimates of a patient's nutritional requirements and must be evaluated regularly to assess adequacy of therapy. Daily monitoring parameters include vital signs, body weight, temperature, serum chemistries, hematologic indices, nutrition intake, and fluid intake and output (see Table 22) [10].

Table 22. Routine monitoring parameters for parenteral nutrition

Parameter	Baseline	Initiation	Critical illness	Stable inpatient	Stable at Home
CBC	√		Weekly	Weekly	as electrolytes schedule
BUN, creatinine, Electrolytes (Na, K, Cl, Co2) & Glucose (BG)	√	Daily x 7 days	Daily	1-3/week	Every other week for 1-3 months then every month and as needed
Mg, Po4, ICa	√	Daily x 3 days	Daily	1-2/week	as electrolytes schedule
Finger-stick BG		Every 6 hrs	Every 6 hrs	Every 6 hrs	If getting ill or at risk of glucose intolerance
Triglycerides	√		Weekly	Weekly	as electrolytes schedule, then every 6-12 months
Liver function tests	√		Weekly	Weekly	as electrolytes schedule

Discontinuation of PN

Rebound hypoglycemia upon discontinuation of PN is rare. Patients requiring large doses of insulin have a greater propensity for rebound hypoglycemia, but predicting which patients will experience rebound hypoglycemia is difficult. To reduce the risk of rebound hypoglycemia in high-risk patients, a 1-to-2-hour taper down of the infusion may be necessary. If a PN solution must be discontinued suddenly or unexpectedly in patients sensitive to abrupt discontinuation, 5-10% dextrose-containing IV fluid should be infused for 1 or 2 hours to avoid a possible rebound hypoglycemia [13].

Complications

Micronutrient-Related Complications Adult Patients Receiving PN

Should receive a standard daily dose of parenteral multivitamins. Excessive intake of lipid-soluble vitamins A, D, E, and K has the potential for accumulation therefore, the potential for toxicity. Vitamin A toxicity in patients with chronic renal failure receiving PN. Reducing the frequency of fat-soluble vitamin administration to twice per week in renal failure patients. Other PN related complications shown in Table 23.

Table 23. PN related complications

Problem	Possible Causes	Prevention or Therapy
Metabolic complication		
Hyperglycemia	• Stress-associated Hyperglycemia in acutely ill and septic patients • Excess carbohydrate administration • Chromium deficiency	• Maintained blood glucose between 150 to 180 mg/dl • Initiated at half of the estimated energy needs, or approximately 150 to 200 g dextrose, for the first 24 hours. Carbohydrate administration should not exceed a rate of 4 to 5 mg/kg/min • Monitor response via serum and capillary glucose levels every 6 to 8 hours • Initial insulin therapy • add 0.05 to 0.1 units per gram of dextrose in the PN solution, or 0.15 to 0.2 units per gram of dextrose may be used in patients who are already hyperglycemic. • Supplemental short-acting or rapid-acting insulin may be administered (using a sliding scale) • Increasing the chromium dose in the PN formulation beyond the standard amount commercially prepared multiple trace in element injections may be necessary subcutaneously if needed
Hypoglycemia	• Excessive or erroneous administration of insulin • Abrupt discontinuation of PN solutions	• Initiation of a 10% dextrose infusion, administration of an ampule of 50% dextrose, and/or stopping any source of insulin administration. • A 1- to 2-hour taper down of the infusion, or half the infusion rate
	•	• Blood glucose concentration 30 minutes to 1 hour after the PN solution is discontinued
Refeeding syndrome	• Aggressive nutrition support Nutrition repletion of a malnourished patient;	• Energy and fluid should be initiated and advanced slowly • Replace electrolyte abnormalities
Hypertriglyceridemia	• rapid administration rates of IVFE more than (0.11 g/kg/hr).	• ILE intake should be not exceeded than 30% of total energy, or 1 g/kg/d • Infused over infused at least 8 to 10 hours (if ILE is administered separately) • avoided ILE infusing if TG serum triglyceride concentrations >400 mg/Dl
Azotemia	• Prerenal azotemia (Excessive protein, inadequate nonprotein calories, dehydration, hepatic encephalopathy, or hyperammonemia)	• Decreased amino acids provided • (use of high branched-chain, or low aromatic amino acid formulations) in hepatic failure and hepatic encephalopathy patient • When calculating lipid requirements, account for any drugs mixed in a lipid emulsion (e.g., propofol, clevidipine)
Metabolic Bone Disease (Osteoporosis and osteomalacia)	• long-term PN use • Inadequate Ca and P intake	• PN formulation should be designed to: • Minimize hypercalciuria, • Provide adequate vitamin K, Mg, Ca, and P, • Avoid metabolic acidosis,

Table 23. (Continued)

Problem	Possible Causes	Prevention or Therapy
Metabolic complication		
	• Higher AA doses (2 g/kg/d as compared to 1 g/kg/d) in PN formulations • Chronic metabolic acidosis • Cyclic PN • Vitamin d deficiency • Vitamin d toxicity • Aluminum toxicity • Mg deficiency • Copper deficiency • Vitamin K deficiency	• Provide appropriate amino acid dose, vitamins and trace elements, • Minimize aluminum contamination
Hepatobiliary disorders (Steatosis, cholestasis, and gallbladder sludge/stones)	• Overfeeding • Long-term PN • Lack of enteral stimulation • Choline or carnitine deficiency • Aluminum toxicity	• Rule out non-PN etiologies. • Decreasing dextrose, Decreasing ILE • Cyclic PN infusion • Encourage oral diet • Prevent/treat bacterial overgrowth by using antibiotic • Treat pruritus with cholestyramine, rifampin, or phenobarbital
occlusion, thrombosis, and breakage	• Thrombotic Occlusion The risk of venous thrombosis is greater if patients have had prolonged bed rest, have venous stasis, have sepsis, or have hypercoagulation, or morbid obesity, smoking, or ongoing estrogen therapy, certain malignancies. • Non thrombotic Occlusion Drug-heparin interactions, PN formulations with inappropriate calcium-to-phosphate ratios, and lipid residue, Lipid occlusions may slowly accumulate	• Use thrombolytics • Low-dose anticoagulation therapy might have a prophylactic benefit in patients at risk for catheter-related thrombosis • Use of a 0.9% normal saline flush between all IV medications, infusions, and heparin is the key to prevention
Pneumothorax Vascular injury with hemothorax Brachial plexus injury Cardiac arrhythmia	• Improper placement	• Catheter position established with a chest x-ray prior to initiating therapy. • TPN line should not be used for other purposes such as measuring central venous pressure, administering blood products, or the infusion of other medications
Infectious complications		
Sepsis, line infections	• Infection rates associated with PN were clearly much higher during the days of overfeeding (historically referred to as hyperalimentation) • Poor glucose control • Poor hygiene • Contaminations	• Used Skin antiseptic agent is 0.5% chlorhexidine in alcohol solution, or alternative antisepsis solutions include iodine, iodophor (povidone-iodine), and 70% alcohol in case contraindication for chlorhexidine • Changing the dressing routinely (every 48-72 hours) • Changing the TPN intravenous tubing every 48 hours. A 0.22- in-line filter should be used whenever fat is not being infused and 1.2 with lipid infused • Inspecting the site for tenderness, erythema, edema, loose sutures, or drainage • Glycemic control between 140 and 180 mg/dl

Central Parenteral Nutrition Calculations

1. Determine caloric requirements:
    - BMI <30 kg/m2, administer 25-35kcal/kg/day based on body weight (BW)

Example: if patient BW is 70 kg: 30kcal x 70 = 2100kcal needed

- Underfeeding involves that the patient administer about 80% of caloric needs.

2. Determine fluid requirements:
    - Administer 1500ml plus 20ml/kg for kilograms over 20kg

Example: if patient BW is 70 kg: 1500+ (20x50) = 2500 ml/day

3. Determine protein (AAs) requirements:
    - Maintenance 0.8-1g/kg/day
    - Moderate stress 1.3-1.5 g/kg/day
    - Severe stress 1.5-2 g/kg/day

Example: if patient BW is 70 kg: 1.5g x 70=105g x 4 kcal=420 kcal from protein

4. Administer about 20% to 30% of total calories as lipids
    - Administer 25% as lipid. Example: 2100 x 25%= 500kcal
    - 1g lipid contain 10 kcal; so to get 500kcal need 50 grams

5. Determine remaining calories and administer as dextrose

Example: 2100- (420 + 500) = 1180 kcal

- 1gram dextrose contain 3.4 kcal; 1180/3.4=350 gram dextrose
- Dextrose maximal rate is 4-6mh/kg/minute

6. Estimate the daily maintenance amounts of electrolytes, vitamins and trace elements.

Stability and Compatibility of PN

The deterioration of nutritional components that modifies their original properties is referred to as the stability of PN formulations. The ability of PN additives, such as pharmaceuticals, to preserve their chemical integrity and pharmacological function is another definition of stability. Some vitamins, such as cyanocobalamin, folic acid, phytonadione, pyridoxine, riboflavin, thiamin, and retinol, are lost due to photodegradation caused by exposure to light, especially fluorescent light. On the other hand, problems with PN formulation compatibility typically include the production of precipitates. These precipitates could be liquid or solid, such crystalline materials or the phase separation of water and oil in a TNA. In contrast, compatibility relates to problems with PN formulations that typically include the production of precipitates. The following are the main issues with stability and compatibility:

- The stability of the lipid emulsion, of 3-in-1 PN solutions
- The potential for Ca P precipitation,
- The stability of vitamins and trace elements
- Another important factor is pH; Ca P solubility increases as pH decreases.

For maximal stability, TNA should maintain final concentrations of amino acid ≥4%, dextrose, ≥10%, and ILE ≥2% to more likely remain stable for up to 30 hours at room temperature (25°C) or for 9 days refrigerated (5°C) followed by 24 hours at room temperature Medications [14].

Calcium and Phosphate

When Ca and P salts are used in PN formulations in excess, crystalline precipitates, pulmonary emboli, and catheter blockage are all possible consequences. The major compatibility issue with PN formulations and variables is Ca and P solubility. Table 24 lists those influences [15].

Table 24. Factors that influence calcium and phosphorus compatibility

Increased risk of calcium phosphate precipitation: • Increased calcium concentration • Increased phosphate concentration (including amino acids with phosphorus content) • Calcium chloride salt use (vs calcium gluconate) • Increased temperature of PN admixture
Increased calcium phosphate solubility: • Increased amino acid concentration • Increased dextrose concentration • Lower pH of the PN admixture

Drugs and PN

Medications should not be added to PN formulations unless there is clear evidence from the literature or standard references to support stability, compatibility, and maintenance of pharmacological and therapeutic efficacy that is specific to the nutrient composition in the PN to be dispensed. Formulations that appear stable when refrigerated could form precipitates at room temperature. Certain drugs that are compatible with the PN can be given via Y-site administration (piggyback drug delivery system). A review is available elsewhere [16].

Insulin

Hyperglycemia is the most common complication of PN. Regular human insulin is only added to PN to aid in blood glucose control [17].

H2-Antagonists

H2 antagonists are often added to the PN admixture in patients requiring gastrointestinal stress ulcer prophylaxis. Famotidine is a common additive and has been shown to be stable in 3-in-1 admixtures of various compositions for at least 72 hours.

Heparin

Adding heparin offers the following advantages: Reduces fibrin sheath formation around the catheter, prevents catheter occlusion, reduces phlebitis in patients receiving TPN via a peripheral vein, and Enhances lipid emulsion clearance by enhancing lipoprotein lipase stimulation (LPL) activity.

Zinc

Zinc (Zn) is involved in numerous aspects of cellular metabolism. A reduced gastric acidity can decrease zinc availability for absorption. More than 95% of the body's zinc content is intracellular. Extra amount is needed for patients with severe stress, diarrhea, ileostomy output.

Iron

Iron dextran has been used in 2-in-1 PN formulations. However, the addition of iron to 3-in-1 PN admixtures has not been well studied and reports of incompatibilities exist.

Question 1: A pregnant patient is admitted with hyperemesis gravidarium (HG). Which of the following is a clinical indication for PN use?

a) Vomiting NOT controlled with supportive care within 48 hours
b) Intolerance to EN trial and supportive care measures
c) Patient refusal of EN tube placement
d) Fluid and electrolyte imbalances

Answer b.

Question 2: What is the most common complication associated with PN administration?

a) Hypophosphatemia
b) Hyperkalemia
c) Hyponatremia
d) Hyperglycemia

Answer d.

Question 3: What is the smallest pore size filter that is recommended for TNA?

a) 0.22 μm
b) 0.5 μm
c) 1.2 μm
d) 5 μm

Answer c.

References

[1] Mueller, C., C. Compher, D. M. Ellen, A. S. f. Parenteral, E. N. B. o. D. J. J. o. Parenteral, and E. Nutrition, *ASPEN clinical guidelines: nutrition screening, assessment, and intervention in adults.* 2011. 35(1): p. 16-24.

[2] Gopalan, S., S. J. C. O. i. C. N. Khanna, and M. Care, *Enteral nutrition delivery technique.* 2003. 6(3): p. 313-317.

[3] Gorman, R., J. J. C. N. E. Morris, and P. Tube Feeding. 3ª Ed. Saunders, *Minimally invasive access to the gastrointestinal tract.* 1997: p. 174-192.

[4] Li, J. Y., T. Yu, G. C. Chen, Y. H. Yuan, W. Zhong, L. N. Zhao, and Q. K. J. P. o. Chen, *Enteral nutrition within 48 hours of admission improves clinical outcomes of acute pancreatitis by reducing complications: a meta-analysis.* 2013. 8(6): p. e64926.

[5] Kane, K. and K. Prelack, *Advanced Medical Nutrition Therapy.* 2018: Jones & Bartlett Learning.

[6] Martindale, R. G., M. J. C. O. i. C. N. Warren, and M. Care, *Should enteral nutrition be started in the first week of critical illness?* 2015. 18(2): p. 202-206.

[7] Pancorbo-Hidalgo, P. L., F. P. García-Fernandez, and C. J. J. o. c. n. Ramírez-Pérez, *Complications associated with enteral nutrition by nasogastric tube in an internal medicine unit.* 2001. 10(4): p. 482-490.

[8] Worthington, P., J. Balint, M. Bechtold, A. Bingham, L. N. Chan, S. Durfee, A. K. Jevenn, A. Malone, M. Mascarenhas, D. T. J. J. o. P. Robinson, and E. Nutrition, *When is parenteral nutrition appropriate?* 2017. 41(3): p. 324-377.

[9] McClave, S., R. Martindale, V. Vanek, M. McCarthy, P. Roberts, B. Taylor, J. Ochoa, L. Napolitano, and G. J. A. C. o. C. C. M. Cresci, *ASPEN Board of Directors.* 2016: p. 277-316.

[10] Nakasaki, H., T. Katayama, S. Yokoyama, T. Tajima, T. Mitomi, M. Tsuda, T. Suga, K. J. J. o. P. Fuj, and E. Nutrition, *Complication of parenteral nutrition composed of essential amino acids and histidine in adults with renal failure.* 1993. 17(1): p. 86-90.

[11] Corkins, M. R., *The ASPEN pediatric nutrition support core curriculum.* 2015: American Society for Parenteral and Enteral Nutrition.

[12] Kraft, M. D., I. F. Btaiche, and G. S. J. N. i. c. p. Sacks, *Review of the refeeding syndrome.* 2005. 20(6): p. 625-633.

[13] Mundi, M. S., E. M. Nystrom, D. L. Hurley, M. M. J. J. o. P. McMahon, and E. Nutrition, *Management of parenteral nutrition in hospitalized adult patients.* 2017. 41(4): p. 535-549.

[14] Robinson, C. A., J. E. J. T. J. o. P. P. Sawyer, and Therapeutics, *Y-site compatibility of medications with parenteral nutrition.* 2009. 14(1): p. 48-56.

[15] Maswoswe, J., A. Okpara, and M. J. H. P. Hilliard, *An old nemesis: calcium and phosphate interaction in TPN admixtures.* 1995. 30: p. 579-579.

[16] Sacks, G. S. J. P. G., *Drug-nutrient considerations in patients receiving parenteral and enteral nutrition.* 2004. 28(7): p. 39-49.

[17] Marcuard, S. P., B. Dunham, A. Hobbs, J. F. J. J. o. P. Caro, and E. Nutrition, *Availability of insulin from total parenteral nutrition solutions.* 1990. 14(3): p. 262-264.

Chapter 5

The Hospital Pharmacy

Mohammed Almeziny[1,*]
Yasmin M. Madney[2]
Mohammed Saad Althanyan[3]
Ahmed Abdulrahman A. Alotaibi[4]
Raghad Ali Alkhodair[5]
Abeer Alibrahim[5]
Ahad Abed M. Almutairi[5]
Mohammed Hamdan Alharbi[5]
Salah M. Seif[2]
Basma M. E. Mohamed[2]
and Mohamed Emam Abdelmobdy Abdelrahim[2]
[1]Prince Sultan Military Medical City (PSMMC),
Riyadh, Saudi Arabia
[2]Clinical Pharmacy Department, Faculty of Pharmacy, Beni-Suef University,
Beni Suef, Egypt
[3]Medical Services for Ministry of Interior, Riyadh, Saudi Arabia
[4]King Faisal Specialist Hospital and Research Center, Riyadh, Saudi Arabia
[5]Prince Sultan Military Medical City, Riyadh, Saudi Arabia

Learning Objectives

After completing this chapter, the reader would be able to:

- Understand the role of a pharmacist within a healthcare setting and distinguish inpatient and ambulatory services provided by the pharmacist
- Distinguish different types of pharmaceutical compounding preparations and understand precautions that should be followed during their preparation.

---

* Corresponding Author's Email: meziny@hotmail.com.

In: Clinical Pharmacist Tools to Deliver Rational Medication Use
Editor: Mohamed Emam Abdelmobdy Abdelrahim
ISBN: 979-8-88697-857-5

- Summarize the requirements according to USP chapters for sterile compounding and non-sterile preparations.
- Be familiar with safe handling of hazardous drugs.
- Understand the role of the pharmacist in operating room.
- Distinguish different types of drug distribution systems.
- Be familiar with continuous quality improvement activities and the role of Key Performance Indicators (KPI) to enhance patient care and increase pharmaceutical services efficiency.
- Be familiar with role of pharmacy automation to enhance patient care, medication safety and increase pharmaceutical services efficiency.
- Be familiar with ambulatory, clinical pharmacy services and drug information center.
- Be familiar with services which are provided by the pharmacist such therapeutic drug monitoring (TDM), antimicrobial stewardship, medication reconciliation, medication use evaluation, investigational drug (ID) and patient counseling.
- Understand the role of the medication safety officer to ensure patient safety.
- Understand the role of the pharmacist within hospital committees.
- Being familiar with commune terminology used in pharmacy practice such as biosimilar, counterfeit medication as well as counterfeit medication.

Introduction

As society's healthcare needs have changed and expanded, there has been an increased emphasis on the provision of care through organized healthcare settings. As a result, an increased number of pharmacists now practice in hospitals. As members of the healthcare team composed of physicians and nurses, among others, institutional pharmacists have an opportunity for direct involvement with patient care. The knowledge and clinical skills that the pharmacist possesses make this individual an authoritative source of drug information for all healthcare professionals, and patients. In addition to direct patient care involvement, pharmacists in hospitals are responsible for systems, which control drug distribution and are designed to assure that each patient receives the appropriate medication, in the correct form and dosage and at the correct time. Hospital pharmacists maintain records on each patient, using them not only to fill medication orders but also to screen for drug allergies and adverse drug effects. Also, pharmacists provide clinical services, included but not limited to adult medicine, pediatrics, oncology, ambulatory care, and psychiatry. The nature and size of the hospital help to determine the extent to which these specific services are needed. Because of the diversity of activities involved in pharmacy departments, there is also demand for management expertise, including finance and budgeting, personnel administration, systems development, and planning.

The Role of Pharmacist

The practice of pharmacy has undergone dramatic changes in recent years as it has evolved from an apothecary focusing on drug products to a healthcare provider focusing on patients [1].

This new vision for professional practice in the pharmacy known as pharmaceutical care following the publication of Hepler and Strand (1990) [2]. As a result of this practice model, pharmacists were promoted as key members of the healthcare team, who were responsible for the therapeutic outcomes of medications [3]. The purpose of pharmaceutical care is to provide patients with direct, responsible medication-related care that improves their health and quality of life [4]. Consequently, the pharmacist must be able to perform a wide variety of activities in order to fulfill this obligation [5]. Pharmacy practice can be classified into three primary areas: community, clinical, and hospital pharmacy [6]. In hospitals, pharmacists have a variety of clinical and non-clinical responsibilities depending on the organization and the clinical needs. Among their responsibilities is ensuring the effective and safe use of medicines through: (review and interpret physician orders in order to prepare medications, assisting other health professionals, such as physicians and nurses with medicines-related issues, preparation, packaging, and labeling of pharmaceutical products for the purpose of the dispensing of medications, preparation of medicines when there is not a ready-made preparation available, assessment of medication records, monitoring of therapeutic drugs, and the management of adverse drug reactions in order to ensure that medicines are working effectively, carrying out medication reconciliation on admissions and during changes in the level of care, as this can help reduce medication errors and hospital readmissions, thus improving patient satisfaction, coordinate comprehensive counseling for patients after they are discharged from hospital, and participating in hospital-wide governance activities related to medication safety and quality such as Drug Use Evaluation (DUE) and developing stewardship programs for high-risk medicines. However, number of activities are carried out beyond clinical patient care, including: providing education and training to healthcare providers at all levels and to patients regarding medicine management, common drug interactions, and appropriate use of medicines, coordinates the activities of pharmacy technicians, ensuring their workflow, ensuring that pharmaceuticals items are prepared and labeled appropriately, provision of services in drug information, supply, and quality control, and engaging in clinical trials to examine new medicines and bring them to market [7]. The pharmacist also performs a leadership role in healthcare system by making decisions, communicating, and managing effectively [4].

Hospital Pharmacy Services

In-Patient Pharmacy Services

Providing inpatient services is one of the hospital pharmacist's key responsibilities. These services include therapeutic drug monitoring, total parental nutrition (TPN), and sterile preparations. Pharmaceutical compounding preparation is one of the most important roles of the inpatient hospital pharmacy. Compounding provides medication for patients who may not be able to use commercially available formulations due to dosage requirements, allergies, or rare diseases. Medications that must be sterile include those administered by injection, intravenous infusions (IV), intraocular injections, intrathecal injections or ophthalmic preparations. Understanding the risks associated with sterile compounding and incorporating established standards is critical to patient safety. Without the direction of standards, compounded pharmaceuticals could be sub-potent, over-potent, or contaminated, exposing patients to serious risks of side effects or even death.

United States Pharmacopeia (USP) creates guidelines for compounding drugs in order to protect patients and lower risks like contamination, infection, and improper dosing. The USP compounding chapters include USP 797 (Sterile Compounding), USP 795 (Non-Sterile Compounding), USP 800 (Handling Hazardous Drugs) and USP 825 (Radiopharmaceuticals) [8]. USP standards apply to all who engage in compounding (pharmacy staff, nurses, and physicians) and all practice settings (hospitals, other healthcare institutions, clinics, and pharmacies) [9]. USP published revisions to chapters 795 and 797 in June 2019 [10]. They are currently being appealed and are not yet finalized. USP 795 (2014) and USP 797 (2008) will remain in use until further notice from USP [10].

The compounding staff is responsible for ensuring that compounded sterile preparations (CSPs) are accurately identified, measured, diluted, and mixed as well as correctly purified, sterilized, packaged, sealed, labeled, stored, dispensed, and distributed. These requirements include sustaining proper standards of cleanliness and providing labeling and further advice for the proper clinical administration of CSPs. When supervising the compounding and dispensing of CSPs, qualified certified healthcare practitioners must ensure the following objectives are met:

- Compounding staff members are appropriately qualified, educated, instructed, and competent to carry out and document the work associated with their sterile compounding responsibilities [9].
- Opened or partially used packages of ingredients for subsequent use in CSPs are adequately stored in the compounding facility under restricted access settings [9].
- Sterilization procedures ensure CSPs sterility while preserving the labeled strength of active ingredients and the physical integrity of the packaging [9].
- Ingredients are accurate in their identity, quality, and purity [9].
- Measuring, mixing, diluting, purifying, sterilizing, packaging, and labeling procedures follow the correct sequence and quality standards established for the specified CSP [9].
- Compounding, packaging, labeling, quality testing, and inspection deficiencies should be quickly detected and corrected [9].

Sterile Compounding

Sterile compounding must be performed according to strict procedures to keep products free from contamination. Drugs injected into the blood or administered into specific other body sites must be free of microorganisms (e.g., viruses, bacteria, fungi) and contaminants (e.g., precipitates, glass shards, particles).

Sterile compounding is used to prepare: Intravenous (IV) drugs (e.g., 1 gram of Ceftriaxone taken from a vial and injected into a 50 mL D5W IV bag), Intramuscular (IM) and subcutaneous (SQ) drugs. Eye drops (e.g., Vancomycin and Cyclosporine eye drops), irrigations, radiopharmaceuticals, pulmonary inhalations (excluding nasal inhalations). It is important for healthcare professional to understand the terminology used by USP as mentioned below as shown in Figure 1.

Definitions

Ante-Area — An International Standards Organization (ISO) Class 8 (see Table 1) or better area where personnel hand hygiene and garbing procedures, staging of components, order entry, CSP labeling, and other high-particulate- generating activities are performed [9].

Buffer Area — An area where the primary engineering control (PEC) is physically located. Activities that occur in this area include the preparation and staging of components and supplies used when compounding CSPs [9].

Primary Engineering Control (PEC) — A device or room that provides an ISO Class 5 (see Table 1) environment for the exposure of critical sites when compounding CSPs. Such devices include, but may not be limited to, laminar airflow work benches (LAFWs), biological safety cabinets (BSCs), compounding aseptic isolators (CAIs), and compounding aseptic containment isolators (CACIs) [9].

Aseptic Processing — A mode of processing pharmaceutical and medical products that involves the separate sterilization of the product and of the package (containers–closures or packaging material for medical devices) and the transfer of the product into the container and its closure under at least ISO Class 5 (see Table 1) conditions [9].

Table 1. ISO classification of particulate matter in room air

Compounding Area	ISO Rating	Particles/m3
Primary engineering control (PEC, called the sterile hood, or isolator, if using a glove box).	5	3,520
Secondary engineering control (SEC, called the buffer room or buffer area). Anteroom, if it opens into a negative pressure SEC (same ISO# as the SEC).	7	352,000
Anteroom, if it opens into a positive pressure SEC.	8	3,520,000

(Limits are in particles of 0.5 µm and larger per cubic meter [current ISO] and cubic feet [former Federal Standard No. 209E, FS 209E])

Beyond-Use Date (BUD) — For the purpose of this chapter, the date or time after which a CSP shall not be stored or transported. The date is determined from the date or time the preparation is compounded [9].

Preparation — A preparation, or a CSP, that is a sterile drug or nutrient compounded in a licensed pharmacy or other healthcare-related facility pursuant to the order of a licensed prescriber; the article may or may not contain sterile products [9].

Sterile — Completely clean and free from pyrogens and contaminations [9].

Stability — the extent to which a drug substance or product retains, within specified limits and throughout its period of storage and use, the same properties and characteristics that it possessed at the time of stability testing [11].

Pyrogen — A substance (infectious organisms or their product toxins or cytokines) that provokes fever [12].

Product — A commercially manufactured sterile drug or nutrient that has been evaluated for safety and efficacy by the FDA [9].

Positive Pressure Room — A room that is at a higher pressure than the adjacent spaces and, therefore, the net airflow is out of the room [9].

Negative Pressure Room — A room that is at a lower pressure than the adjacent spaces and, there- fore, the net flow of air is into the room [9].

Single-Dose Container — A single-dose container is a single-unit container for articles (see General Notices and Requirements) or preparations intended for parenteral administration only [9].

Multiple-Dose Container — A multiple-unit container for articles or preparations intended for parenteral administration only and usually containing antimicrobial preservatives. The beyond-use date (BUD) for an opened or entered (e.g., needle-punctured) multiple-dose container with antimicrobial preservatives is 28 days, unless otherwise specified by the manufacturer [9].

USP 797 Space Requirements for Sterile Compounding

The risk of contamination is decreased by clean air in the compounding area. The ISO establishes standards for air quality based on the quantity and size of airborne particles [13]. The air quality increases with decreasing particle counts. The air quality must be at least ISO 5 in crucial regions closest to exposed sterile medications and containers, such as within the sterile hood PEC [9]. If a particle is 0.5 microns (micrometers) or bigger, it is counted in this measurement. Also, the maximum number of particles per cubic meter should be less than 3,520 particles [9, 13].

The air becomes dirtier the further you are from the PEC. The buffer area or SEC which contains PECs needs to be at least ISO 7. The anteroom, which is the space next to the SEC where hand washing and garbing take place, has to be at least ISO 8 if it opens into a positive-pressure buffer area (non-hazardous drug sterile compounding), or at least ISO 7 if it opens into a negative-pressure buffer area (hazardous drug sterile compounding) [9].

The PEC includes a high-efficiency particulate air (HEPA) filter, which filters particles as the air passes through it. With a 99.97% efficiency, HEPA filters remove particles as small as 0.3 microns in diameter or bigger, including bacteria, viruses, fungi, and dust [9]. The HEPA filter is at the top of the sterile hood of a vertical airflow biological safety cabinet (BSC) or C-PEC. The HEPA filter in a laminar airflow workbench (LAFW) or PEC is located at the back of the sterile hood (horizontal airflow) [9].

The filter eliminates contaminants before the air reaches the PEC. Compounding must be performed in the cleanest air possible, which is the air directly from the HEPA filter. The HEPA filter must be recertified by an expert every six months or if a PEC is relocated. In addition to the ISO air quality in a space, the air pressure in the area relative to the adjacent area is essential [9].

Because air is not harmful when it enters the surrounding area, the air pressure inside the PEC and SEC is positive during non-hazardous compounding [9]. The compounded sterile preparation (CSP) is protected against contamination by positive pressure. With hazardous compounding, negative pressure is required in the containment PEC (C-PEC) and the containment SEC (C-SEC) to isolate and exhaust the space's hazardous air [9, 14]. The compounding staff is protected by negative air pressure [9, 14].

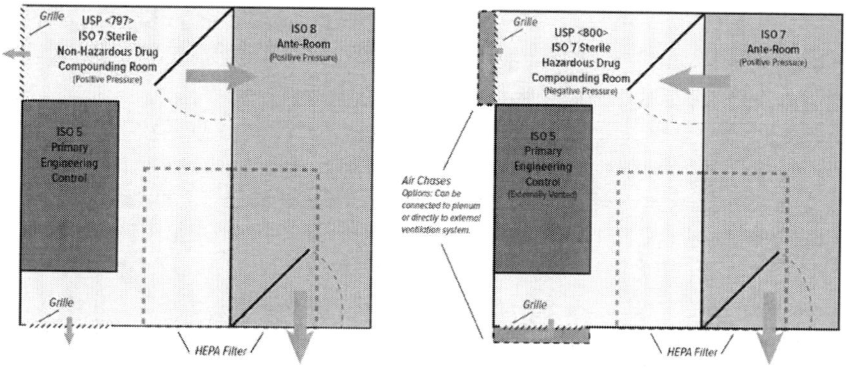

Figure 1. Infrastructure design facilities of USP 797 & 800 rooms [15].

Environmental Quality and Control

Environmental conditions are essential as the quality status of the components, process used, and personnel performance to achieve and maintain sterility and freedom from contamination.

Temperature, air and surface sampling, humidity, and air pressure all through the facility are the environmental elements that must be monitored during the procedure [9].

Temperatures must be maintained within the proper range and recorded on the temperature log sheet. The SEC (buffer room) should be examined once per day and kept at 20°C or below. Unless they contain vaccines, which require twice-day monitoring, the refrigerator and freezer should be inspected daily. The refrigerator temperature should be between 2 and 8 degrees Celsius. According to USP797, if a freezer only contains CSPs (no vaccines), the freezer temperature should be between -25 and -10°C. If the freezer also contains vaccines, the CDC recommends a freezer temperature of -50 to -15°C [16]. Action must be taken and documented if the temperature is out of range [9].

Air sampling is used to identify contaminants in the air. A certified air sampling technician or a trained compounding staff member should conduct it at least once every six months. Additionally, surfaces must be checked on a regular basis, according to USP. The testing should occur at the end of the day when the surfaces are at their dirtiest. All surfaces that are regularly in contact with employees such as inside PECs and other work surfaces, door handles, and equipment should be inspected [9].

Air pressure testing ensures the proper difference between two areas and guarantees that the airflow is unidirectional. Pressure measuring instruments are placed in the cleanroom area and are monitored at least once daily or every work shift [9].

Excess moisture in the sterile compounding area can contribute to bacterial growth; thus, humidity must be carefully monitored. The humidity should be kept below 60% and inspected at least once daily [9].

CSPs Microbial Contamination Risk Levels

The more complex preparation the greatest chance to get contaminated. The contamination risk levels assigned according to the probability of CSPs to get contaminated. There are three contamination levels during compounding, which are low, medium, and high risk to cause would subject patients to the risk of harm, including death [9].

Low-risk level CSPs are preparations manipulated within ISO Class 5 using sterile nonhazardous ingredients, not more than three sterile products, and not more than two entries into one package (ex., bag or vial), and only simple manipulations like transfer, measuring, and mixing. Reconstitution and transfer of Ceftriaxone into one sterile diluent IV bag is an example of a low-risk level of CSPs [9].

Medium-risk level CSPs are preparations manipulated within ISO Class 5 using sterile nonhazardous ingredients; multiple individual sterile products that are combined or pooled to prepare CSPs for multiple patients, like doing stocks of sterile preparations to use them in other sterile preparations; and complex manipulation for more than three sterile products and more than two entries into one package, like total parenteral nutrition (TPN) preparations [9].

High-risk level CSPs are preparations if manipulated in air worse than ISO Class 5 for more than one hour, if using nonsterile ingredients or devices, and if improperly grabbed and gloved as an emergency requiring urgent IV preparations to save the patient's life [9].

In addition, there are two categories. The first one is a Low-Risk Level with 12 hr or less BUD and Immediate Use. Low-risk Level with a BUD of 12 hours or less CSPs are intended to accommodate satellite pharmacies compounding only low-risk level CSPs [9]. Compounding of hazardous drugs is not permitted. These low-risk CSPs do not require an ISO Class 7 clean room or buffer area, instead requiring only an ISO Class 5 hood [9]. Furthermore, these low-risk level compounding areas need to be segregated from other parts of the pharmacy and designated for use as a compounding area. Personnel shall follow cleaning and garbing requirements. Sinks shall not be placed adjacent to the ISO Class 5 hood.

Immediate Use CSPs are exempt from ALL requirements in USP 797 and are intended for situations where there is a need for emergency or direct patient administration such as cardiopulmonary resuscitation, emergency room treatment, and preparation of diagnostic agents [9].

Table 2. Compounding sterile preparations beyond use date based on their microbial contamination risk level

Risk Category	Room Temp (20-30°C)	Refrigerated (2-8°C)	Frozen (< -20°C)
Immediate-Use	1 hour	1 hour	N/A
Low-Risk	48 hours	14 days	45 days
Low-Risk with 12-hour BUD	12 hours	12 hours	N/A
Medium-Risk	30 hours	9 days	45 days
High Risk	24 hours	72 hours	45 days

Low-risk CSPs may qualify for immediate use when only simple aseptic measuring and transfer are needed, only non-hazardous products or diagnostic radiopharmaceutical products are used, not more than two entries into any one container or package are prepared, the aseptic technique is followed during preparation, and administration begins within 1 hour of the start of preparation [9]. In addition, the immediate use provisions mean that once the compounding begins, there are no delays or interruptions in the process of administration to the patient.

Other conditions of the immediate use category are that the dose must be discarded if the administration has not begun within 1 hour, and the dose must be labeled if not administered by the preparer. All CSPs must be prepared in an ISO class 5 environment except for the immediate use category. Table 2 summarizes all CSPs BUD according to their microbial contamination risk levels [9].

Garbing for Sterile Compounding

The fundamental first step in minimizing microbiological contamination in CSPs is the careful hand- and arm-washing of compounding staff members and the appropriate wearing of personal protective equipment (PPE) [9]. The human body usually sheds squamous cells at a rate of 106 or more each hour, and those skin particles are contaminated with microorganisms that may contaminate the sterile products [17, 18].

The following steps will describe how to get ready to start to prepare a sterile product in the compounding area inside the IV room:

- The compounder should don garb in the ante area. The order in which the compounder should don the garb is from dirtiest to cleanest.
- Remove coats, rings, watches, bracelets, and cosmetics before entering the ante-area. Artificial or long nails are not allowed.
- Don head and facial hair covers and face masks, then shoe covers while stepping over the borderline of dividing and separating the dirty side of the anteroom from the clean side. The second pair of shoe covers are required for compounding hazardous drugs (HD).
- The ante area should have a mirror that is used to check that the hair is completely covered. Except when preparing an HDs, using an eye shield is optional.
- Wash your hands with soap and warm water. The hands are the primary source of CSPs contamination.
- Clean under fingernails with warm water to eliminate debris.
- For 30 seconds, wash vigorously in circular motions from the fingertips to the elbows.
- Use paper towels that are lint-free to dry your hands and forearms.
- Don a non-shedding gown that fits snugly around the wrists and has an enclosure at the neck. Disposable gowns are required for HD compounding and preferred for non-HD compounding. If gowns are reusable, they must be laundered before being reused.
- Enter the buffer area.
- Use an alcohol-based surgical hand scrub with antimicrobial activity for the required time per manufacturer and allow it to dry.
- Pick appropriate-sized sterile gloves, ensuring that there is a tight fit with no excess glove material at the fingertips.
- Put on sterile, powder-free gloves. For chemotherapy compounding, two pairs of ASTM D6978 (chemotherapy)-rated gloves are required for compounding HDs. Tuck one pair under the cuffs of the gown and the second pair goes over the cuffs.

- Whenever gloves come into contact with non-sterile surfaces during compounding, sanitize them with 70% isopropyl alcohol (IPA). Do not resume compounding until the alcohol has dried. Continually inspect gloves for tears.
- When the compounding is completed and the compounding personnel leaves the compounding area, all garb except the gown goes into the disposal container. If the gown is not visibly dirty, it can be taken off and kept on the clean side of the anteroom to be re-worn for the current work shift.
- The gown cannot leave the ante area if it is going to be re-worn.
- Removes shoe covers one at a time, ensuring that the uncovered foot is placed on the dirty side of the line of demarcation.
- Hand hygiene is repeated, and all other garb is replaced when re-entering the compounding area.

Handling Hazardous Drugs in Healthcare Settings

Handling hazardous drugs (HDs) by healthcare professionals can result in toxicity. This includes unloading the medications at the receiving dock, stocking the shelves, preparing the drugs in the pharmacy, administering the medications to the patients, and obtaining and cleaning up body fluids with hazardous drug residues. HDs require workspaces, equipment, and devices that have been developed to reduce exposure of the drug to the staff. The United State Pharmacopeia 800 chapter establishes the guidelines for managing HDs and the National Institute for Occupational Safety and Health (NIOSH) specifies which drugs are hazardous. NIOSH keeps a list of all HDs called the NIOSH List of Antineoplastic and Other Hazardous Drugs in Healthcare Settings [9, 19]. Drugs are considered dangerous by NIOSH if they are teratogenic, genotoxic, carcinogenic, toxic to organs at low doses, or labeled by the manufacturer with specific handling [19].

The risk term is defined differently in USP 797 and 800. The risk in USP 797 is based on the risk of the sterile product getting contaminated, while USP 800 the term indicates the probability of harming the personnel who are exposed to the drug. Sterile and non-sterile hazardous compounds must be prepared in a containment-primary engineering control C-PEC located in a Containment-secondary engineering control (C-SEC) or containment-segregated compounding area (C-SCA). Negative air pressure is required for C-PECs, C-SECs, and C-SCAs. Because of the negative air pressure in the C-PEC, air flows into the C-PEC away from the person standing in front of the hood. The biological safety cabinet is an example of C-PEC. It has vertical laminar airflow from the HEPA filter at the top of the hood and negative air pressure, which prevents workers from being exposed to the HDs they are working with [14].

The air in spaces used for HDs compounding can get contaminated and needs to be regularly refreshed. The air changes per hour (ACPH) is the number of times each hour the air in the room is changed. The air in a sterile C-SEC must be replaced at least 30 times each hour. A C-SCA must have at least 12 ACPH. There must be at least 12 ACPH in a place where non-sterile HDs are compounded. These HDs must be kept in a negative-pressure, externally ventilated room with at least 12 air changes per hour.

All places and equipment used to handle HDs must be sterilized at least once daily, which includes deactivating, decontaminating, and cleaning. Two percent (2%) bleach (sodium hypochlorite) or peroxide can be utilized to reduce HD toxicity and remove HD residues for deactivation and decontamination. For cleaning, germicidal detergents such as ammonium, and phenolics can be utilized to remove dirt and microbiological contamination. Sterile 70% isopropyl alcohol (IPA) is used in sterile compounding to inhibit or eradicate microorganisms for disinfection.

Spill kits must be kept in places where HDs are prepared, stored, and administered. Spill kits must be easily obtainable wherever HDs travel, as this is where they can spill. In addition, only staff who are trained in spill management and the use of PPE and NIOSH-certified respirators should be handling the spill incident. If a spill happens, limit the access to the area as soon as possible, and place warning signs around the spill's borders. Several notifications may be required if more than one entry enters the room with the spill. Pregnant women should not participate in cleaning procedures and leave the area immediately. Specific protocols should be kept in the pharmacy, and the staff involved in cleaning should consult the safety data sheet (SDS) for guidance on spill clean-up procedures. For more details, USP 800 chapter provides guidelines on handling HD and how to manage spill incidents safely.

Non-Sterile Preparations

Non-sterile compounding is most commonly used to prepare a dose or formulation that is not commercially available, such as converting a solid tablet to a liquid for a patient who cannot swallow the tablet, avoiding an excipient, creating a 12.5% ointment with only 10% and 20% available and adding a flavor to the medication to make it more palatable. Non-sterile preparations are those that are given by mouth, through a tube, vaginally, rectally, topically, nasally, or in the ear [20].

According to complexity, USP 795 classifies non-sterile compounding into three groups: Simple: requires the healthcare professionals only to follow the instructions in a USP monograph, a compounding kit, or a product preparation manual [20]. Moderate: requires advanced calculations or techniques or the formulation with no documented stability data, like mixing two or more produced cream products when the preparation's stability is unknown [20]. Complex: Making a preparation that needs specialized training, a unique setting, instruments, and protocols to achieve the intended therapeutic effects. Transdermal dose forms, modified-release medications, and suppositories with systemic effects are examples of possible complex preparation types [20].

Non-sterile compounding can be performed in room air, but it must be kept separate from the pharmacy's dispensing area [20]. Appropriate space is needed to prevent the mixing up of substances, containers, and other components. Shelving and storage should be provided in this space. All equipment and containers should be kept off the floor. The area should be clean and well-lighted. To prevent drug deterioration, heating, ventilation, and air conditioning systems must be controlled [20].

Operating Room Satellite Pharmacy

Previously, pharmacy participation in perioperative settings mainly consisted of supplying medication stock for operating room (OR) staff access, ensuring adequate storage conditions, checking expiry dates, and maintaining controlled substance accountability. In the early 1980s, pharmacists realized the importance of increasing engagement, and OR satellite pharmacies began to appear primarily in academic associations [21]. Since then, the presence of the pharmacist has had a crucial and unique function in the operating room satellite pharmacy, covering the demands of patients, nurses, and physicians.

The OR is a complicated, dynamic, time-sensitive, and sometimes disorganized environment. For example, the following are the most common types of anesthetic drug errors: wrong dosage due to a dose, concentration, or infusion rate error [22, 23, 24]. Using the incorrect syringe or vial during medication preparation results in administering the wrong drug [22, 24]. Extra dose [22]. Omission of a dose/failure to act [22, 23]. Many of these medication errors might be avoided by utilizing satellite pharmacy services and implementing strategies to reduce and eliminate errors. Satellite pharmacy services include assign a pharmacist to assist the OR or perioperative team, make sure that a pharmacist is reachable for inquiries around-the-clock, participates in continuing education, and the OR pharmacist receives specific training on basic OR principles [22]. Moreover, stock and maintain medication trays for anesthesia and other medications, and notify staff, particularly anesthesia care providers, of any changes to how drugs are provided, such as new labels or concentrations [22].

Drug Distribution Systems

The majority of patients in hospitals require medicine as part of their treatment. Prescription, preparation, dispensing, administration and monitoring of medication of the patient are all parts of the medication-use process [25]. these processes are all error-prone. Several technology-based solutions, such as patient Bar Coding (BC) systems and Computerized Provider Order Entry (CPOE), have been implemented in hospitals to optimize pharmaceutical administration and medication delivery [25–27]. Drug distribution systems play an essential role in the medication delivery process, which is classified as centralized, decentralized, and Hybrid distribution systems.

In decentralized systems, automated dispensing cabinets (ADCs), such as Pyxis® MedStation® one type of automated drug dispensing system (ADDS) that is used to assist nurses in dispensing medications in an inpatient facility [28]. These systems primarily involve computer-controlled medication dispensing, tracking, and storage [29]. Carousel dispensing technology (CDT) such as Swisslog Pillpick® system and robotic medication picking systems are used in centralized drug dispensing systems, which are hospital pharmacy-based to dispense medications for inpatients [30]. Additionally, there are hospitals where a hybrid approach combining centralization and decentralization is used [31].

The floor system is successfully operated in some hospitals as a decentralized pharmacy under the direct supervision of a pharmacist. This system offers some advantages, such as the availability of medications needed on the floor, eliminating any drug returns, and decreasing the need for drug order transcriptions for the pharmacy. Unfortunately, this system has many disadvantages as increasing the incidence of medication errors and unnoticed drug deterioration, expanding drug inventory on the pavilions, and lack of storage facilities in nursing units.

In individual prescription orders, all medications are dispensed by the pharmacist after the separate prescription order is sent to the pharmacy. This system is usually applicable in small hospitals. It offers the advantages of reviewing all prescriptions by the pharmacist, lowering the incidence of dispensing medication errors, improving communication between pharmacists, nurses, and physicians, and limiting the drug supply to ensure that the treatment will not be continued without review. The main disadvantages associated with this system are increasing the incidence of administration errors, increased potential for drug loss due to waste and deterioration, and the increased need for excessive nursing human resources.

The unit dose system is an approach for distributing and managing medications in managed healthcare environments that are coordinated between pharmacies and medical wards. With the help of this system, medical professionals can ensure that patients get the appropriate dosage of medicine for their conditions. The medications in this system are prepackaged in single individual doses and are in the most suitable form for administration. At any given time, the patient care area never has more than a 24-hour supply of doses on hand [32]. The unit dose system reduces medication errors, medication costs, drug control, drug use monitoring, patient-care drug inventories, and adaptability to computerized and automated systems [32].

Best pharmaceutical practices require all prescriptions to be reviewed for appropriateness by a pharmacist unless there is an urgent situation when the resulting delay would harm the patient. A medication ward stock and override list was created to give a licensed practitioner the privilege to dispense and administer medication to the patient in an emergency. Usually, each hospital has a committee for ward stock and overrides medications. This committee is responsible for specifying the ward stock. Finally, the utilization of professional resources and pharmacy and nursing personnel decreases the incidence of medication errors, improves drug control and monitoring by the pharmacist, and reduces drug inventories in wards.

Ambulatory Services

Provision of healthcare services to patients who are not confined to beds is known as ambulatory care which can be classified into primary, secondary, or even tertiary care. The location of the outpatient pharmacy should be present nearby the normal patient traffic flow. In all cases, a waiting area should be available. A pharmacist should be the director of the outpatient pharmacy and other pharmacists have the responsibilities of ensuring the correct choice of drugs, doses, and routes of administration. Correct and complete labeling and packaging according to standards of pharmacy practice should be offered to all medications dispensed to patients. All drugs in the outpatient area should be properly controlled. The dispensing pattern carried within this unit is identical to that carried on by community pharmacies. The directions and other information are placed on the label, ancillary labels are affixed, the proper medications are then placed in the container, a check for accuracy is conducted, and finally, the prepared prescription is wrapped and dispensed. The outpatient prescription label should bear minimum information as patient's full name, prescription identification number, specific directions for use, date of issue, name or initials of dispenser, name of prescribing physician, strength of preparation, dispensing time, source and batch identifying a number and name, address, and telephone number of hospital.

Clinical Pharmacy Services

The clinical pharmacy is a healthcare specialty which describes the activities and services that made by clinical pharmacists to improve the rational and proper use of medications. Applying specific pharmacology, pharmacokinetics, pharmaceutics, and therapeutics knowledge to patient care is part of the clinical pharmacy process [33].

The education requirements for clinical pharmacist are a Master of Clinical Pharmacy or postgraduate pharmacy practice residency training programs [33].

Standards of Practice for Clinical Pharmacists

- *Qualifications:* licensed pharmacists with specialized advanced education and training [34].
- *Process of Care:* consists first of the assessment of the patient by (reviewing the medical record, meeting with the patient and/or caregivers to gather and record all the patient's current medications (including dosages and administration routes), adherence, allergies, attitudes toward, and experiences with, drug therapy. Also obtaining, compiling, and analyzing patient data and prioritizing patient problems and needs connected to medication.) then evaluation of medication therapy, Development and implementation of a plan of care, and follow-up and monitoring of the medication [34].
- *Documentation:* the essential components to include in the document-tation are:
  - Medication history.
  - Active problem list with assessment of each problem.
  - Plan of care to enhance medication regimen and improve patient outcomes [34].
- Collaborative, Team-Based Practice and Privileging.

  Clinical pharmacists collaborate with other healthcare professional as part of the healthcare team to deliver high-quality, coordinated treatment that is centered on the needs of the patient. Clinical pharmacists collaborate with other healthcare specialists as part of the healthcare team to deliver high-quality, coordinated treatment that is centered on the needs of the patient [34].
- Professional Development and Maintenance of Competence: Clinical pharmacists continue their proficiency by:
  A. Certification in the proper specialization that is important to their profession, and maintenance of certification, covering the specialties acknowledged by the Board of Pharmacy Specialties (BPS).
  B. Regular participation in Continuing Professional Development (CPD) activities to improve practice skills for providing direct patient care
  C. Maintaining an active license through the relevant state board(s) of pharmacy, including participating in the mandatory Continuing Pharmacy Education (CPE) requirements [34].
- *Professionalism and Ethics:* Clinical pharmacists demonstrate professionalism by being accountable, dedicated to excellence, respectful of others, honest, caring and compassionate [34].

- *Other responsibility:* may also serve as educators, researchers, clinical preceptors/ mentors, administrators, managers, policy developers, and consultants [34].

Drug Information Centers

Drug information (DI) is defined as "The provision of unbiased, well-referenced, and critically evaluated information on any aspect of pharmacy practice" [1].

The first Drug information center (DIC) was established in 1962 in the United States. Its main objective was to provide DI services and educational purposes. Furthermore, it was concerned with medication use evaluations (MUEs), Adverse drug reactions (ADRs), and formulary management.

Many DICs developed since then, gaining attention to training pharmacy students regarding the necessary DI skills. Moreover, there was corresponding increased accessibility to medical and pharmaceutical databases. (This section will be discussed in detail in separate chapter).

Therapeutic Drug Monitoring

In the early 1970s a number published articles emphasis on individualizing of therapy by the monitoring of medication concentration and appropriate adjustment of dose led to improve of patient outcomes [35].

Therapeutic Drug Monitoring (TDM) aims to individualise medication therapy and to prevent both subtherapeutic and toxic medication concentrations. TDM uses medication concentration in body fluids to adjust the dosage of medications according to the characteristics of the patient being treated and the response obtained. TDM is recognised in improving of therapy outcomes with these agents [35].

A number of factors effect drug concentration and a single sample will only represent the concentration at the sampling time. When a new drug is started, 'steady state' generally will not be reached after four elimination half-lives. Sampling prior to steady state may not be accurate therefore, it not be done unless a problem is anticipated (e.g., non-compliance or toxicity). Results must be interpreted accordance with clinical observations and other relevant information. Usually, the TDM services are provided incorporation between the pharmacy and the laboratory departments. The roles of pharmacy are interpretation of measured plasma drug concentrations and provide the assistance for drug dose selection, while, the role of clinical laboratory is analysing the body fluid sample for medications levels [36].

Due to its expenses and time consuming, TDM is not performed for medications with pharmacological response that can be easily established by clinical means (e.g., majority of antibiotic, analgesics etc.) or by laboratory values (e.g., anticoagulants, antidiabetic agents, statins drugs, thyroid abnormalities medications) or for medications with wide therapeutic window (e.g., penicillins). On the other hand, it is wised to perform TDM for medications with narrow therapeutic window and the drug's action cannot readily be assessed clinically (e.g., antiepileptic immune suppression) [36]. (This section will be discussed in detail in separate chapter).

Continuous Quality Improvement

Continuous quality improvement (CQI) is defined as "a culture of sustained improvement targeting the elimination of waste in all systems and processes of an organization [37]. CQI has started in automobiles manufacturing: by Ford and enhanced upon by Japan's Toyota, or Lean manufacturing, in the 1930s. There are many CQI methodologies, such as Total Quality Management (TQM), the Model for Improvement (MFI), and Six Sigma [37]. The of Many sophisticated methodologies has been development, which resulted in a additional comprehensive CQI toolbox that has been used across a variety of systems beyond manufacturing [37].

In the public health context, quality improvement (QI) is defined as "the use of a deliberate and defined improvement process... which is focused on activities that are responsive to community needs and improving population health" [37]. Quality has been defined in the context of three domains: safety, effectiveness and patient experience [38].

Adoption of CQI in healthcare sectors has significantly increased. CQI continues to be a beneficial tool for bridging research evidence with direct service as result, patients' health outcomes are improved [37].

Commitment to CQI's potential for enhancing both clinical and population outcomes has led to the institutionalization of QI in healthcare education. Currently, in many healthcare disciplines, CQI is as a required rotation during residency [37].

In pharmacy practices, CQI aims to enhanced patient safety through a reduction in medication errors, quality-related events (QREs) and improve patient outcomes [39].

As result for CQI important, ISMP Canada recommended that each pharmacy manager shall designate a licensed pharmacist or pharmacy technician at that pharmacy as the Quality Improvement Coordinator (QIC) [40].

The tasks of QIC included but not limited to initiating and monitoring of a Continuous Quality Improvement plan.

Coordinate with pharmacy staff and hospital CQI department about Quality Related Events.

Key Performance Indicators (KPI)

Key performance indicators (KPIs) are measurable tools used by an organization to evaluate the progress of a specific task. KPIs by themselves do not inform the reason(s) of changes in performance or measure the quality, instead they act as alarms to warn of opportunities for improvement in the process and patient outcome [41].

KPIs play a role in improving practice. They allow practician to track their performance over period of time. The metrics provide bench marks for continuous quality improvement initiatives [38].

These metrics presented for example the percentage of reconciled medicines within 24 hours of admission. This would reflect the added value of pharmacy services. KPIs should be evidence-based ,reflect continuous improving in practice, clear and easy to measure. In addition, the impact of the KPIs on patient outcomes should be easily understandable to patients and clinicians. In pharmacy there are two types of KPIs [41]. These KPIs reflect the clinical and process of services. For example, an KPI might be the average time taken to dispense medicines, while the clinical KPI should reflect professional activates such as number of medication errors and adverse drug reactions (ADR) etc. Examples of clinical KIPs admission drug histories, participation in medical round, ADR management number of drug protocol initiated with corporation with clinical pharmacist, number drug information inquires, in-service education for other healthcare professionals CPR participation [38].

Medication Safety

Enhancing a patient's quality of life while reducing medication risk is the major objective of medication therapy. However, the common risks of medication use in humans include medication error and Adverse drug reaction (ADR) [42]. According to National Coordinating Council for Medication Error Reporting and Prevention (NCC MERP) medication error "is any preventable event that may cause or lead to inappropriate medication use or patient harm while the medication is in the control of the healthcare professional, patient, or consumer" [43]. Medication error has a great impact on the healthcare system. Therefore, it can cause harm to patient health including hospitalization, increased length of stay, disability, and mortality. Moreover, medication error leads to compromised patient confidence in the healthcare system and increases healthcare costs. Medication error can occur at any stage of the medication use process (MUP) [42]. There are many ways to classify medication errors the most famous method is MUP. The MUP includes the following: prescribing, transcribing, Dispensing, administering, and Monitoring [44]. Additionally, many factors can contribute to medication errors including incomplete patient information, polypharmacy, inexperienced or untrained staff, shortage of staff or workload, environmental factors (poor lighting, noise), poor communication between healthcare providers, confusing drug packaging (look-alike), poor handwriting or use inappropriate abbreviations, verbal orders, and lack of effective policies and procedures [42].

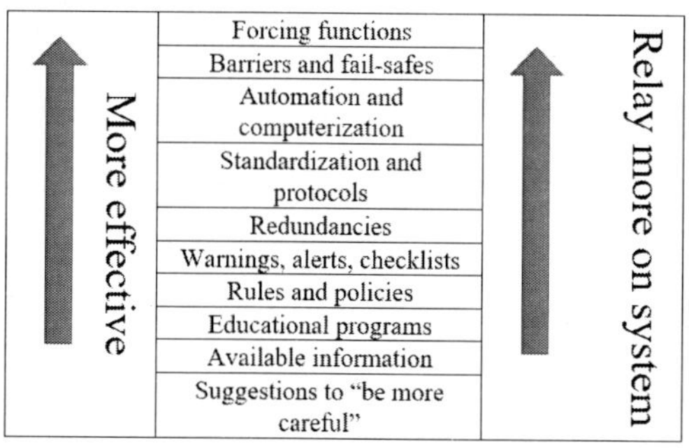

Figure 2. ISMP hierarchy of risk-reduction strategies [46].

Medical errors can be classified into two major types, errors of omission and errors of the commission. To further explain, errors of omission can occur as a result of actions not taken e.g., if a patient does not receive treatment due to an unjustified reason. While errors of the commission can occur as a result of the wrong action taken e.g., wrong dose, wrong patient, etc. [45]. The Institute for Safe Medication Practices (ISMP) suggested a rank order of error reduction strategies as follow from most effective to the lowest as showed in Figure 2 [42].

Starting with forcing functions and constraints, automation and computerization, simplifying and standardizing, reminders, checklists and double-checking systems, rules and policies, education, and lastly, information.

Pharmacists play a pivotal role in the medication safety field such as making efforts to prevent, detect, and resolve any medication-related problems. In addition, collaborate with other healthcare professionals to ensure the best use of medication [42]. The NCC MERP classified medication errors according to the severity of the outcome from (A to I). Firstly, category A defined as the situation or event that can cause an error. However, the error occurred in category B but did not reach the patient. While the error in category C occurred without causing any harm, the error in category D required monitoring. Despite those uncounted errors in categories E, F, G, and H resulted in temporary harm and required intervention, required hospitalization, permanent patient harm, and required intervention to sustain life respectively. Finally, in Category I the error led to patient death [47]. Aside from medication error, the World Health Organization (WHO) described ADR as "A response to a drug which is noxious and unintended, and which occurs at doses normally used in man for prophylaxis, diagnosis, or therapy of disease or modification of physiological function" [48]. The pharmacovigilance department in drug regulatory authority agencies is responsible for receiving all ADR. The Pharmacovigilance term is defined by European Medicines Agency (EMA) as "the science and activities relating to the detection, assessment, understanding, and prevention of ADR or any other medicine-related problem" [49].

Antimicrobial Stewardship

For decades microbes, specifically bacteria, have become increasingly resistant to various antimicrobials. The World Health Assembly's endorsement of the Global Action Plan on Antimicrobial Resistance (AMR). in May 2015, the Political Declaration of the High-Level Meeting of the General Assembly on AMR. In September 2017, both recognize AMR as a global threat to public health. These policy initiatives admit overuse and misuse of antimicrobials as a main reason for development of resistance, as well as a need to improve the use of antimicrobials.

Antimicrobial stewardship (ASP) optimizes the use of antimicrobials, optimize patient outcomes, decrease AMR and health-care-associated infections, and save healthcare expenses amongst others. Stewardship is defined as "the careful and responsible management of something entrusted to one's care". It was originally applied in the healthcare setting as a tool for enhancing antimicrobial use, termed ASP [50].

Today, ASP is one of three "pillars" of an integrated approach to healthcare systems augmentation. The other two are infection prevention and control (IPC) and medication and patient safety [50].

ASP principles also apply to the use of antimicrobials in the veterinary and agriculture sectors, typically with an stress on the responsible and prudent use of these medications. Although the growing levels of viral, fungal and parasite resistance to antimicrobials are of concern [50].

ASPs become very commune in health systems, due in large part to both the current Joint Commission standards (JCI) requiring ASPs in healthcare setting, as well as the Infectious

Diseases Society of America (IDSA) guidelines on implementing ASPs. ASPs often differ in structure and scop depending on the nature and size of the healthcare setting, local antimicrobial issues identified, and the depth and extent of resources available to support the program. Irrespective of the approach selected, every ASP should collect data to evaluate the program's impact through process and outcome measures. Regardless accreditation requirements and national guidelines supporting ASPs.

Goals of an ASP

Standardized validated key performance indicators (KPIs) for ASP does not currently exist; however, programs should use an approach that meet several goals:

- Track and review antimicrobial utilizations.
- Benchmark data.
- Recognize trends.
- Disseminate results to targeted population in order to generate feedback and optimize ASP results.

To meet these goals, collaboration between the ASP team and IC team may be beneficial, as the focuses of these groups overlap; taking a collaborative method can help both entities in accomplishing their goals. Furthermore, working with information technology (IT) is crucial for every ASP to specify how to best utilize information and the electronic health record (EHR) to run reports and track KPIs. KPIs should be selected based on available ASP resources and the reporting abilities of the health informatic system. Developing a positive work averment with the laboratory will enhance ASP outcomes. Finally, in order for the ASP to success and develop, open communication and administrative supports are essential [51].

Intravenous to Oral Conversion

Most patients who initially need IV therapy for a serious infection can switch to oral medication after 24 to 48 hours if their clinical condition is improving and they can tolerate an oral formulation [52].

Advantages of oral over IV rout:

- Reduction in the incidence of infected IV lines acquired in health facilities.
- Potential reduction in the risk of side effects; parenteral drug preparation errors are much more common than with oral formulations.
- Improve mobility for patients, minimizes their discomfort, and may even lead to an earlier hospital discharge.
- Saves time for both nurses and doctors.
- Possible decrease in treatment expenses, allowing funds to be used more wisely elsewhere [53].

Note: In critically ill patients who need IV antimicrobials or in individuals who are unable to absorb medications after oral administration, IV to oral switch therapy is NOT recommended [52].

Types of IV to oral switch:

- *Sequential therapy:* Conversion from IV administration to oral medication using exactly the same compound and dosage.
- *Switch therapy:* Switching IV medication with oral equivalent using a different compound in the same class of drugs and potency.
- *Step down therapy:* Replacement of IV medication with an oral one which may be a different drug class, or within the same class but with a different dosage and frequency [53].

Medication Reconciliation

Medication Reconciliation is the process of providing the most complete list of all medications a patient is taking together with drug name, dosage, frequency, and route and linking that list towards the doctor's admission, transfer, and/or discharge orders, with the aim of giving the patient the appropriate drugs at all hospital transitional points [54]. The main objective is to prevent medication errors and drug interactions. The pharmacist plays key roles in medication reconciliation. Through establishing and monitoring medication reconciliation procedures that are oriented on the patient and educating patients and their healthcare professionals about the advantages and limitations of drug reconciliation approaches. For the creation of information systems, continuing competency assurance, training, therapeutic expertise, and ongoing quality improvement are all essential [55].

Procedure:

1. Develop a list of current medications.
2. Develop a list of medications to be prescribed.
3. Compare the medications on the two lists.
4. Make clinical decisions based on the comparison.
5. Communicate the new list to appropriate caregivers and to the patient [56].

Hospital Committee

Pharmacy and Therapeutic Committee

The Pharmacy and Therapeutics (P&T) committee is an advisory group of the medical staff and serves as the organizational line of communication between the medical staff and the pharmacy department. This committee is composed of physicians, pharmacists, and other healthcare professionals selected with the guidance of the medical staff. This committee should be composed of at least 3 physicians, pharmacists, and a representative of the nursing staff. The committee should meet regularly, at least 6 times per year, and when necessary. It can invite to its meetings persons within or outside the hospital who can contribute specialized or unique knowledge, skills, and judgments [57].

Generally, this committee has the responsibility for the development and surveillance of all drug utilization policies and practices within the hospital to assure optimum clinical results and minimum potential for hazard. The Committee shall assist in the formulation of broad professional policies regarding the evaluation, appraisal, selection, procurement, storage, distribution, use, safety procedures, and all other matters relating to drugs in the hospital [57].

A formulary is a list of drugs and related information that is updated regularly and represents the clinical judgement of pharmacists, physicians, and other specialists. Among other things, a formulary includes a list of drugs and items or equipment connected to medications, and drug usage policies, vital pharmacological auxiliary information, decision-support resources, and implementation guidelines [57].

Infection Control Committee

A multidisciplinary committee is responsible for infection control programs. The committee aims to Improving patient outcomes in the different practice settings of health systems requires identifying and lowering the risks of acquiring and transmitting infections among patients, healthcare professionals, and others [58].

The infection control committee typically creates organizational guidelines and practices addressing:

1. The administration and delivery of healthcare services for patients and workers.
2. Infection prevention and control education for employees, patients, families, and other caregivers.
3. Monitoring tools to track the development and spread of diseases.
4. Monitoring tools to monitor the application of antibiotics and the emergence of resistance [58].

Pharmacist Role in Infection Control Committee:

1. Minimizing the spread of infections: by developing pharmacy infection control policy.
2. Promoting the Optimal Use of Antimicrobials [58].

Institutional Review Board (IRB)

The Institutional Review Board (IRB) is a panel that has been explicitly assigned the task of reviewing and regulating human subject's medical research.

The goal of IRB review is to ensure that sufficient measures are taken to protect the rights and welfare of those who are participating as research subjects, both in advance and through periodic evaluation [59].

Medication Use Evaluation

Medication use evaluation (MUE) is defended as "an ongoing, systematic, and interdisciplinary performance improvement method that has an overarching goal of optimizing patient outcomes through evaluation and improvement of medication-use processes" [60]. MUE can be viewed as a part of a performance improvement program. Among the primary goals of MUE are to improve patient outcomes and quality of life via a multidisciplinary strategy that assesses clinical outcomes, as well as focusing on the factors of optimal medication usage and process aspects (e.g., prescribing, dispensing) [61]. It can refer to a drug or therapeutic class, a health condition, or a medication-use process (Prescribing, transcription, preparing, dispensing, administration, and monitoring). The five objectives of the MUE program are: optimizing medication therapy, enhancing patient safety, standardizing processes so that unnecessary variation will be reduced, determining the value of innovative practices, complying with regulatory or quality requirements, and reducing costs [62]. There are a variety of roles that pharmacists and other healthcare professionals may play in MUE, depending on the practice setting, organizational goals, and resources available. The organizational body (e.g., quality management or quality improvement (QI) committee, pharmacy and therapeutics committee) overseeing the MUE process generally consists of at a minimum a prescriber, pharmacist, nurse, and an administrator or health system representative. Additionally, pharmacy technicians, pharmacy students, and pharmacy residents, can be involved in conducting MUEs in healthcare facilities and healthcare systems, if possible. Furthermore, there is a need for additional healthcare professionals to contribute their perspectives when the evaluation and improvement processes address their areas of specialty and accountability. However, the pharmacists are the primary healthcare professionals responsible for the development and coordination of MUEs because they are considered to be the most qualified and experienced healthcare professionals in this regard due to their expertise and mission to ensure appropriate medication use. There are several steps involved in the MUE process which follow the Find Organize Clarify Understand Select Plan Do Check Act (FOCUS-PDCA) model, including:(*F*ind a process that needs to be improved, *O*rganize the team that is familiar with the process, *C*larify existing knowledge about the process., *U*nderstand what causes variation in processes, *S*elect process improvement, *P*lan: Establish a solution, *D*o: Implement improvements, *C*heck: Assess the outcome, *A*ct: Determine what changes are necessary and implement them. In order to determine if an MUE process is successful, it should be evaluated in terms of improved patient outcomes and decrease in expenditures [60].

Investigational Drug (ID)

Investigational Drug (ID) defined as a pharmaceutical form of an active medication or placebo being examined or used as a reference in a clinical trial, including products already with a marketing authorization but used or assembled (formulated or packaged) in a way different from the authorized form, or when used for an unauthorized indication, or when used to gain further information about the authorized form. The terms "investigational drug", "investigational new drug" and "investigational medicinal product" are considered to be synonymous [63].

Each institute that uses ID MUST establish guidelines to comply with governmental regulations for ID. The aim of these guidelines is to confirm that the clinical trials which are conducted in human population are designed and performed at the highest scientific and ethical standards. Compliance with these guidelines provides public assurance that the rights, safety and well-being of the trial human subject are secured, comply with the principles stated in the Declaration of Helsinki, and that the clinical trial data are credible [63].

Counterfeit Medication

The WHO defined this type of medication as "one which is deliberately and fraudulently mislabeled concerning the identity and/or source"64. Counterfeiting can apply to both branded and generic products and may contain correct or wrong ingredients, without active ingredients, insufficient active ingredients, or with fake packaging. In some countries, the occurrence of counterfeiting relates to expensive hormones, steroids, and anticancer medicines, but in others, it may relate to inexpensive generic medicines. The counterfeit medication causes serious harm to human health. That leads to a loss of public confidence in the healthcare system. And effect on the reputation and financial standing of the original manufacturer. Various factors can facilitate the production and distribution of counterfeit medication including weak or absent national drug regulatory authority, lack or inadequate enforcement of legislation and weak penal sanctions, shortage or high price of the original drug, lack of control for exporting drugs, and increase international trade in pharmaceuticals through the Internet [64].

Pharmacists play a crucial part in preventing counterfeit medications by reporting suspected counterfeit medications, implementing international recommendations to ensure the integrity of the supply chain, purchasing medications from reliable sources, educating patients about the dangers of purchasing medications through the Internet, and monitor for counterfeit product alerts [65].

Brand and Generic Medications

FDA defined brand name product as" the original/innovator product that has passed rigorous tests and evaluations". while generic name product defined "as drug that has the same active ingredient, dosage, safety, effectiveness, strength, stability, and quality as their brand-name drug". innovator company has sole right to manufacture and distribution for a period of time. The common reasons for increasing the availability of generic drugs are to make treatment more affordable and increase access to healthcare all over the world. FDA approved generic product that pass a rigorous scientific review process that ensures provides the same clinical benefit and risk as the brand name drug. however, Generic drugs can look different in color, shape, and size and may contain different inactive ingredients. Generic drugs are cheaper than their brand-name drugs because they do not have to repeat studies that are required for brand-name drugs to demonstrate safety and effectiveness [66].

Biosimilar

The FDA defined biosimilar as "a biological product that is highly similar to the reference product and has no clinically meaningful differences in term of safety, purity, and potency". Biological products are large and complex molecules produced in living sources such as bacteria, yeast, and animal, used to diagnose, prevent, treat several diseases. There are several types of biological products approved to use all over the world include protein, vaccine, blood components, allergenic products and monoclonal antibodies. Biosimilar drug approved by FDA after rigorous evaluation to assure safety, efficacy and quality. Therefore, the manufacturer should provide Analytical and comparative clinical studies, toxicity and immunogenicity evaluation to demonstrate drug's potency, purity, and safety. Furthermore, additional data on the impact of switching between the biosimilar and the reference product are required. A biosimilar is considered an interchangeable product when it meets the requirements and can be used in place of the reference product without the prescriber's intervention [67].

Pharmacy Automation

Healthcare organizations can benefit from automated systems by reducing the occurrence of errors, increasing efficiency, reducing the time required for validating medications, and facilitating the accessibility of medicines in healthcare units [68]. In pharmacy practice, automation offers great promise. Pharmacy practice seeks to provide pharmaceutical care, and by using reengineering techniques and automating the pharmacy process, this goal can be achieved [69]. In 1999, The Institute of Medicine (IOM) published the landmark report "To Err is Human: Building a Safer Health System" which raised awareness about medication errors in particular. Medication errors (MEs) are a subset of medication errors that can be defined as "any preventable event occurring in the medication-use process" [70]. Medications travel from the pharmacy to the patient through a medication use process (MUP), which includes (1) prescribing, (2) transcribing and documenting, (3) dispensing, (4) administering, and (5) monitoring [71]. Many health systems currently employ a variety of automations across all phases of the medication use process in an effort to improve safety and effectiveness. In the MUP, technologies such as clinical decision support software (CDS) and computerized provider order entry (CPOE) are utilized [72]. Generally, CDS is a type of application that analyzes data in order to assist healthcare providers in making clinical decisions. This is meant to help increase the quality of care among geographically separated members of the same health care team, reducing medical errors, increasing efficiency, ensuring proper drug compliance, and ensuring proper prevention [73]. CPOE is a software application for entering electronic medication orders, lab tests, admissions, radiology requests, referrals, and procedure orders within inpatient and outpatient settings. In addition, this component provides real-time information on diagnostics and treatments and tools that aim to enhance patient care and reduce medical errors and costs [74]. The dispensing process involves the use of automated pharmacy carousel systems, central robotic dispensing technology, centralized narcotic dispensing and inventory tracking devices, decentralized automated dispensing devices, Intravenous and total parental nutrition compounding devices, pneumatic tube delivery systems and unit dose medication repacking systems [72]. An automated pharmacy carousel systems allow safe and compact storage of medications within pharmacies (carousels) or automated dispensing cabinet (ADC) [70]. Further, drug distribution system automates the storage, dispensing, return, restocking, and crediting of unit-dose, bar-coded inpatient medications [75]. Additionally, development of intravenous compounding robotic systems has been made to improve both the safety of patients and pharmacy staff when compounding high-risk IV medications. Moreover, it is intended that these systems will improve the compounding accuracy when compare robotic systems over manual preparations as well as reduce the risk of pharmacy staff exposure to hazardous medication [70]. Further, pneumatic tube systems in the pharmacy provide safe, rapid, and efficient delivery of specific medications [76]. Unit dose medication repacking systems is the practice of transferring a finished drug product from the original container in which it was distributed to another container without further manipulation of the drug [77]. As part of the administration process, barcode medication administration technology (BCMA) and CDS support based infusion pumps (smart pump) have been developed [72]. It is important to note that BCMA systems are able to successfully reduce medication errors by electronically ensuring the '3 rights' of medication administration right patient, right drug, and right time, at the patient's bed side. Thereafter, the system automatically enters the information about the administration of the medication into an electronic medication administration record (eMAR) [78]. A significant improvement in medication safety has been achieved with smart pump devices. Smart pumps are infusion systems that perform a test of reasonableness, as they are referred to by the Institute for Safe Medication Practices (ISMP). Infusion rates and dosage concentrations are monitored using these devices to ensure that the pump programming is within pre-defined, institutionally defined upper and lower limits. On the other hand, there is a potential medication error, such as under or over-delivery of a medication dose, a risky order, or an incorrectly calculated infusion rate [79]. Aside from that, the use of electronic clinical documentation systems as well as the use of web-based tracking programs for compliance and disease management are being used as part of the monitoring process [72].

Patient Counseling

Patient counseling refers to the provision of medication information to patients or their representatives, in either an oral or written form, or to the provision of instructions for use, advice on side effects, storage, diet, and lifestyle modifications. During this process, a pharmacist and patient or caregiver interact one-on-one [80]. The basis of successful therapeutic outcomes depends on the interaction between the patient and the healthcare provider. Pharmacists who engage in an interactive approach to communication are capable of finding meaning, responding reflectively, and assessing understanding [81]. There are a number of federal regulations that provide pharmacies with guidance on how to handle pharmaceuticals, however, the Omnibus Budget Reconciliation Act of 1990 (OBRA-90), which was implemented in 1993, imposes expectations on pharmacists in relation to interactions with their patients [3, 4]. The primary purpose of OBRA-90 was saving federal government money by enhancing therapeutic outcomes [82]. In order to achieve this, the pharmacist must perform the following three duties when dispensing a prescription under OBRA-90. First is to obtain and maintain a patient medication record (PMR) for each patient. After the patient's PMR has been reviewed, conduct a prospective drug use review (ProDUR) when filling or refilling a prescription. Finally, counsel the patient or the patient's representative on the drug being prescribed [83]. It is important that a patient's PMR contains all the required information about the patient including: (full name, address, and phone number, date of birth, age, gender, drug profile, pharmacist comments, chronic conditions, allergies, and adverse drug reactions) [83]. However, ProDUR should include the following reviews:(Overuse/underuse, Therapeutic duplication, drug-disease interactions, drug-drug interactions, drug-pregnancy interactions, incorrect dose or duration of treatment, drug-allergy interactions, misuse/abuse of medications, conditions for early refills, ingredient duplication, and contraindications to drugs based on the patient's age [83]. Moreover, an examination of the PMR by the pharmacist is necessary to determine whether any of these potential conflicts are present. When conflicts rise, pharmacists must use clinical judgment to decide whether to dispense a prescription, consulting with the physician if needed or talking to the patient [83]. As part of the counseling process, pharmacists should keep in mind a several of points, including: (medication's name, dosage form, dose, route of administration, duration of treatment, special directions and precautions for (preparation, administration, and use by the patient), the most common severe side effects and adverse effects or interactions that may occur, as well as therapeutic contraindications that may be faced, self-monitoring techniques, storage instructions, information for refilling, and steps to be taken in case of missed doses [83]. Last but not least, in order to ensure patients' knowledge and understanding of how to use their medications, ask them to describe or demonstrate how they will use their medications and identify their effects [84].

References

[1] Khan, N., McGarry, K., Naqvi, A. A., Iqbal, M. S., & Haider, Z. (2020). Pharmacists' viewpoint towards their professional role in healthcare system: a survey of hospital settings of Pakistan. *BMC Health Services Research,* 20(1), 610. https://doi.org/10.1186/s12913-020-05459-0

[2] Mohiuddin, AK. (2020). The excellence of pharmacy practice. *Innovations in Pharmacy*, 11(1), 3. https://doi.org/10.24926/iip.v11i1.1662

[3] Thamby, S. A., & Subramani, P. (2014). Seven-star pharmacist concept by World Health Organization. *Journal of Young Pharmacists: JYP,* 6(2), 1–3. https://doi.org/10.5530/jyp.2014.2.1

[4] ASHP statement on pharmaceutical care. (1993). *American Journal of Health-System Pharmacy: AJHP: Official Journal of the American Society of Health-System Pharmacists,* 50(8), 1720–1723. https://doi.org/10.1093/ajhp/50.8.1720

[5] Wiedenmayer, K., Summers, R. S., Mackie, C. A., Gous, A. G. S., Everard, M., & Tromp, D. (n.d.). *Developing pharmacy practice A focus on patient care* Handbook -2006 Edition. Who.int. Retrieved October 16, 2022, from http://apps.who.int/iris/bitstream/handle/10665/69399/?sequence=1

[6] Mohiuddin, AK. (2020). The excellence of pharmacy practice. *Innovations in Pharmacy,* 11(1), 3. https://doi.org/10.24926/iip.v11i1.1662

[7] Bond Software. (n.d.). *About hospital pharmacy.* Org.au. Retrieved October 16, 2022, from https://shpa.org.au/about-shpa/about-hospital-pharmacy

[8] *USP Compounding Compendium.;* 2022. Accessed September 21, 2022. https://www.usp.org/sites/default/files/usp/document/products-services/products/usp-compounding-compendium-june-2022-toc.pdf

[9] *The United States Pharmacopeial Convention.* General Chapter <797> Pharmaceutical compounding–sterile preparations.

[10] *USP Compounding Standards and Beyond-Use Dates (BUDs).*; 2019. Accessed September 21, 2022. https://www.usp.org/sites/default/files/usp/document/our-work/compounding/usp-bud-factsheet.pdf

[11] Wong AW, Datla A. Assay and Stability Testing. *Sep Sci Technol.* 2005; 6(C):335-358. doi:10.1016/S0149-6395(05)80057-1

[12] Wood WB, Kaiser HK. Pathogenesis of fever. *Medizinische Klinik (1947).* 1962;57:873-874. doi:10.1007/978-3-319-92336-9_3

[13] *Cleanrooms and Associated Controlled Environments-Part 1: Classification of Air Cleanliness by Particle Concentration.*; 2015. www.iso.org

[14] *The United States Pharmacopeial Convention. Briefing: <800> Hazardous Drugs–Handling in Healthcare Settings.*; 2014.

[15] Production Automation Corporation. Differences Between USP 795, 797, and 800 Cleanrooms. Accessed September 24, 2022. https://www.cleanroomproducts.com/art-cr-usp-795-797-800-differences

[16] CDC, Ncird. *Temperature Monitoring Best Practices for Frozen Vaccines-Celsius (C) Frozen Vaccines 3 Take Action If out of Range!*; 2018. www.cdc.gov/vaccines/SandH

[17] Eaton, T. Microbial Risk Assessment for Aseptically Prepared Products. Am Pharm Rev. 2005; 8 (5, Sep/Oct): 46–51..

[18] Agalloco, J, Akers JE. *Aseptic Processing: A Vision of the Future.*; 2005.

[19] *Occupational Exposure to Antineoplastic Agents. Centers for Disease Control and Prevention Web.*; 2004. www.cdc.gov/niosh

[20] The United States Pharmacopeial Convention. General Chapter <795> Pharmaceutical compounding non-sterile preparations.

[21] Keicher, PA, McAllister, JC. Comprehensive pharmaceutical services in the surgical suite and recovery room. *American Journal of Health-System Pharmacy.* 1985;42(11):2454-2462. doi:10.1093/ajhp/42.11.2454

[22] Wahr, JA, Abernathy, JH, Lazarra, EH. Medication safety in the operating room: Literature and expert-based recommendations. *Br J Anaesth.* 2017;118(1):32-43. doi:10.1093/BJA/AEW379

[23] Nanji KC, Patel A, Shaikh S, Seger DL, Bates DW. Evaluation of Perioperative Medication Errors and Adverse Drug Events. *Anesthesiology.* 2016;124(1):25-34. doi:10.1097/ALN.0000000000000904

[24] Lobaugh LMY, Martin LD, Schleelein LE, Tyler DC, Litman RS. Medication Errors in Pediatric Anesthesia. *Anesth Analg.* 2017;125(3):936-942. doi:10.1213/ANE.0000000000002279

[25] Belén Jiménez Muñoz, A, Muiño Miguez, A, Paz Rodriguez Pérez, M, Esther Durán Garcia, M, Sanjurjo Saez, M. Comparison of medication error rates and clinical effects in three medication prescription-dispensation systems. *Int J Health Care Qual Assur.* 2011;24(3):238-248. doi:10.1108/09526861111116679

[26] Poon, EG, Keohane, CA, Yoon, CS. Effect of Bar-Code Technology on the Safety of Medication Administration. *New England Journal of Medicine.* 2010; 362(18): 1698-1707. doi:10.1056/NEJMsa0907115

[27] Paoletti, RD, Suess, TM, Lesko, MG. Using bar-code technology and medication observation methodology for safer medication administration. *American Journal of Health-System Pharmacy.* 2007;64(5):536-543. doi:10.2146/ajhp060140

[28] ASHP Guidelines on the Safe Use of Automated Dispensing Devices. *American Journal of Health-System Pharmacy.* 2010;67(6):483-490. doi:10.2146/sp100004

[29] Zaidan, M, Rustom, F, Kassem, N, al Yafei, S, Peters, L, Ibrahim MIM. Nurses' perceptions of and satisfaction with the use of automated dispensing cabinets at the Heart and Cancer Centers in Qatar: a cross-sectional study. *BMC Nurs.* 2016;15(1):4. doi:10.1186/s12912-015-0121-7

[30] Acheampong, F, Anto, BP, Koffuor, GA. Medication safety strategies in hospitals – A systematic review. *International Journal of Risk & Safety in Medicine.* 2014;26(3):117-131. doi:10.3233/JRS-140623

[31] Gray, JP, Ludwig, B, Temple, J, Melby, M, Rough, S. Comparison of a hybrid medication distribution system to simulated decentralized distribution models. *American Journal of Health-System Pharmacy.* 2013;70(15):1322-1335. doi:10.2146/ajhp120512

[32] American Society of Hospital Pharmacists. ASHP technical assistance bulletin on hospital drug distribution and control. *Am J Hosp Pharm.* 1980; 37:1097– 1103.

[33] Korayem, GB, Badreldin, HA, Eljaaly, K, Aldemerdash, A, Al-Suhaibani, LK, Joharji, H, Aljuhani, O, Al-Omari, BA, Almudaiheem, HY, Alhifany, AA, Alawagi, M, Al-Mowaina, SM, Al-Jazairi, AS, Albekairy, AM, Al-Jedai A. Clinical pharmacy definition, required education, training and practice in Saudi Arabia: A position statement by the Saudi society of clinical pharmacy. *Saudi Pharm J.* 2021 Nov;29(11):1343-1347. doi: 10.1016/j.jsps.2021.09.008. Epub 2021 Sep 21. PMID: 34819795; PMCID: PMC8596147.

[34] American College of Clinical Pharmacy. Standards of Practice for Clinical Pharmacists. *Pharmacotherapy* 2014;34(8):794–797. Available from http://www.accp.com/docs/positions/guidelines/StndrsPracClinPharm_Pharmaco8-14.pdf.

[35] Marks, V. A historical introduction. In: Widdop B, ed. *Ther Drug Monit.* Edinburgh: Churchill Livingstone; 1985:3-15.

[36] Hallworth, Mike. *Therapeutic drug monitoring Clinical Guide fourth edition abbott.*

[37] Loper, AC, Jensen, TM, Farley, AB, Morgan, JD, Metz, AJ. A Systematic Review of Approaches for Continuous Quality Improvement Capacity-Building. *Journal of Public Health Management and Practice*. 2022 Mar;28(2):E354.

[38] Ibrahim, N. How to Improve Clinical Pharmacy Practice Using Key Performance Indicators. *Glob J Med Therap.* 2020;2(1):10-4.

[39] Hincapie, AL. Continuous quality improvement regulations for community pharmacy practice in the United States. *J Am Pharm Assoc* (2003). 2021 Jul-Aug;61(4):470-475.e2. doi: 10.1016/j.japh.2021.02.008. Epub 2021 Feb 19. Erratum in: *J Am Pharm Assoc* (2003). 2022 Jan-Feb;62(1):285. PMID: 33722542.

[40] *Saskatchewan college of pharmacy professionals. Quality Improvement, Coordinator Manual: A Guide to Continuous Quality Improvement.* Canada, ISMP. Available https://saskpharm.ca/document/3910/COMPASS_QI_Coordinator_Manual.pdf

[41] Slavik, Richard S. *Making Progress: National Clinical Pharmacy Key Performance Indicators (cp KPI).* Canadian Society of Hospital Pharmacists 2015.

[42] Billstein-Leber, Molly, COL Jorge D. Carrillo, Angela T. Cassano, & Jennifer J. Robertson, "ASHP Guidelines on Preventing Medication Errors in Hospitals." *American Journal of Health-System Pharmacy* 75 (2018): 1493–1517.

[43] About medication errors. *NCC MERP.* https://www.nccmerp.org/about-medication-errors. Published January 30, 2015. Accessed October 6, 2022 .

[44] Leape, LL, Bates, DW, Cullen, DJ, Cooper, J, Demonaco, HJ, Gallivan, T, & Edmondson, A. (1995). Systems analysis of adverse drug events. *JAMA,* 274(1), 35-43.

[45] Rodziewicz, Thomas L, Houseman, Benjamin and Hipskind, John E. "Medical error reduction and prevention." *StatPearls* [Internet].(2022)

[46] Canda, ISMP. *Rank Order of Error Reduction Strategies.* https://www.ismp canada.org/Jul17C-Sylvia/tsld014.htm. Published July 2017. Accessed October 23,2022.

[47] *Taxonomy of medication errors.* NCC MERP.https://www.nccmerp.org/taxonomy-medication-errors. Published July 18, 2014. Accessed October 7, 2022 .

[48] *Safety of Medicines* - World Health Organization. https://apps.who.int/iris/bitstream/handle/10665/67378/WHO_EDM_QSM_2002.2.pdf Published February 2002. Accessed October 4, 2022 .

[49] *Pharmacovigilance: Overview.* European Medicines Agency.https://www.ema.europa.eu/en/human-regulatory/overview/pharmacovigilance-overview. Published October 27, 2022. Accessed October 5, 2022.

[50] World Health Organization. (2019). *Antimicrobial stewardship programmes in health-care facilities in low- and middle-income countries: a WHO practical toolkit.* World Health Organization. https://apps.who.int/iris/handle/10665/329404. License: CC BY-NC-SA 3.0 IGO

[51] *Zeitler, Kristen. Measure the Performance of Antimicrobial Stewardship Programs Pharmacy Purchasing & Products.* November 2018 - Vol.15 No. 11 - Page #64

[52] Cyriac, JM, James, E. Switch over from intravenous to oral therapy: A concise overview. *J Pharmacol Pharmacother.* 2014 Apr;5(2):83-7. doi: 10.4103/0976-500X.130042. PMID: 24799810; PMCID: PMC4008927.

[53] https://www.nhsgrampian.org/service-hub/medicines-management/antimicrobial/hospital--acute-care/iv-to-oral-switch/
[54] Lester, PE, Sahansra, S, Shen, M, Becker, M, Islam, S. *Medication Reconcili-ation: An Educational Module. MedEdPORTAL.* 2019 Nov 1;15:10852. doi: 10.15766/mep_2374-8265.10852. PMID: 31934615; PMCID: PMC6952281.
[55] Patel, E, Pevnick, JM, Kennelty, KA. *Pharmacists and medication reconciliation: a review of recent literature. Integr Pharm Res Pract.* 2019 Apr 30;8:39-45. doi: 10.2147/IPRP.S169727. PMID: 31119096; PMCID: PMC6500442.
[56] Barnsteiner, JH. Medication Reconciliation. In: Hughes RG, editor. *Patient Safety and Quality: An Evidence-Based Handbook for Nurses.* Rockville (MD): Agency for Healthcare Research and Quality (US); 2008 Apr. Chapter 38. Available from: https://www.ncbi.nlm.nih.gov/books/NBK2648/
[57] American Society of Health-System Pharmacists. ASHP statement on the pharmacy and therapeutics committee and the formulary system. *Am J Health-Syst Pharm.* 2008; 65:2384–6.
[58] American Society of Health-System Pharmacists. ASHP statement on the pharmacist's role in infection control. *Am J Health-Syst Pharm.* 1998; 55:1724–6.
[59] *IRB-FAQs. Institutional Review Boards Frequently Asked Questions* | FDA (2019), (available at https://www.fda.gov/regulatory-information/search-fda-guidance-documents/institutional-review-boards-frequently-asked-questions).
[60] Afanasjeva, J, Burk, M., Cunningham, FF, Fanikos, J, Gabay, M, Hayes, GJ, Masters, PL, Rodriguez, R, & Sinnett, MJ. (2021). *ASHP guidelines on medication-use evaluation.*
[61] *American Journal of Health-System Pharmacy: AJHP: Official Journal of the American Society of Health-System Pharmacists*, 78(2), 168–175. https://doi.org/10.1093/ajhp/zxaa393
[62] *VA Pharmacy Benefits Management Services [PBM] & Center for Medication Safety* [VA MedSAFE]. (2012). VA Medication Use Evaluation (MUE) Toolkit. https://www.pbm.va.gov/PBM/vacenterfor medicationsafety/tools/MUEToolkit.pdf
[63] *Saudi Food & Drug Authority Guidelines for Investigational New Drugs (IND)* Requirements Riyadh Saudi Arabia SFDA 01/09/2010 https://www.sfda.gov.sa/sites/default/files/2021-03/Guidelinesfor InvestigationalNewDrug_IND__v11-EN.pdf
[64] *Guidelines for the development of measure combat counterfeit drugs.* world health organization. https://apps.who.int/iris/bitstream/handle/10665/65892/WHO_EDM_QSM_99.1.pdf. Published January 1999. Accessed October 1, 2022.
[65] Chambliss WG, Carroll WA, Kennedy D. *Role of the pharmacist in preventing distribution of counterfeit medications. J Am Pharm Assoc (2003).* 2012;52(2):195-199. doi:10.1331/JAPhA.2012.11085
[66] *Overview & Basics.* U.S. Food and Drug Administration. https://www.fda.gov/drugs/generic-drugs/overview-basics. Published September 2017. Accessed October 4, 2022.
[67] *About biosimilars and interchangeable products.* U.S. Food and Drug Administration. https://www.fda.gov/drugs/biosimilars/biosimilar-and-interchangeable-products. Published October 2017. Accessed October 6, 2022.
[68] Bagattini, ÂM, Borges, JLA, Riera, R, & de Carvalho, DCMF. (2022). Automation of a tertiary hospital pharmacy drug dispensing system in a lower-middle-income country: A case study and preliminary results. *Exploratory Research in Clinical and Social Pharmacy,* 6(100151), 100151. https://doi.org/10.1016/j.rcsop.2022.100151.
[69] Lee, MP. (1995). Automation and the future practice of pharmacy--changing the focus of pharmacy. *Pharmacy Practice Management Quarterly,* 15(3), 23–35.
[70] Boyd, MA., & W Chaffee, B. (2019). *Critical evaluation of pharmacy automation and robotic systems: A call to action. Hospital Pharmacy,* 54(1), 4–11. https://doi.org/10.1177/0018578718786942.
[71] Vogenberg, FR, & Benjamin, D. (2011). The medication-use process and the importance of mastering fundamentals. *P & T: A Peer-Reviewed Journal for Formulary Management,* 36(10), 651–652.
[72] Barker, KN. (2005). *Handbook of institutional pharmacy practice* (T. R. Brown, Ed.; 4th ed.). American Society of Health-System Pharmacists.
[73] Karnik, K. (2014). FDA regulation of clinical decision support software. *Journal of Law and the Biosciences,* 1(2), 202–208. https://doi.org/10.1093/jlb/lsu004.

[74] Qian, S. (2021). Computerized Provider Order Entry. In *Encyclopedia of Gerontology and Population Aging* (pp. 1126–1131). Springer International Publishing.

[75] *Faculty By Department, & Find a Physician.* (n.d.). Robotics. Rochester.edu. Retrieved October 16, 2022, from https://www.urmc.rochester.edu/pharmacy/about/safety/robotics.aspx

[76] *Delivery of pharmaceutical products via the pneumatic tube system procedure.* (2020). Gov.au. https://www.wacountry.health.wa.gov.au/~/media/WACHS/Documents/About-us/Policies/Delivery-of-Pharmaceutical-Products-via-the-Pneumatic-Tube-System-Procedure.PDF?thn=0.

[77] *Pharmacy services policy C-020 repackaging medications.* (2020). https://health.uconn.edu/policies/wp-content/uploads/sites/28/2021/02/C020-Repackaging_Medications.pdf.

[78] Shah, K, Lo, C, Babich, M, Tsao, NW, & Bansback, NJ. (2016). Bar code medication administration technology: A systematic review of impact on patient safety when used with computerized prescriber order entry and automated dispensing devices. *The Canadian Journal of Hospital Pharmacy,* 69(5), 394–402. https://doi.org/10.4212/cjhp.v69i5.1594.

[79] Nessim, D. (n.d.). *Decision Support Infusion Devices: Technology with intelligence :* December 2004 - pharmacy purchasing & products Magazine. Pppmag.com. Retrieved October 16, 2022, from https://www.pppmag.com/article/163.

[80] ASHP guidelines on pharmacist-conducted patient education and counseling. (1997). *American Journal of Health-System Pharmacy: AJHP: Official Journal of the American Society of Health-System Pharmacists,* 54(4), 431–434. https://doi.org/10.1093/ajhp/54.4.431.

[81] *Communication Skills*: Dr. Hisham S. abou-Auda. (n.d.). Scribd. Retrieved October 16, 2022, from https://www.scribd.com/document/50813889/Communication-Skills-Hisham

[82] Omnibus budget reconciliation act of 1990 - Rx-wiki. (n.d.). Rx-wiki.org. Retrieved October 31, 2022, from http://rx-wiki.org/index.php?title=Omnibus_Budget_Reconciliation_Act_of_1990

[83] OBRA 1990. (n.d.). Hawaii.gov. Retrieved October 31, 2022, from https://medquest.hawaii.gov/en/plans-providers/pharmacy/produr/obra-1990.html

[84] Palaian, S, Prabhu, M, & Shankar, PR. (2006). Patient counseling by pharmacist - a focus on chronic illness. *Pakistan Journal of Pharmaceutical Sciences,* 19(1), 65–72.

Chapter 6

Drug Information

Amira B. Kassem[1]
Haitham Saeed[2]
Mashal Maslah Aljead[3]
Gehad Hassoub[1]
Asmaa A. Elsayed[5]
Mohamed Emam Abdelmobdy Abdelrahim[2]
and Hoda Rabea[2,*]

[1]Clinical Pharmacy and Pharmacy Practice Department, Faculty of Pharmacy, Damanhour University, Egypt
[2]Clinical Pharmacy Department, Faculty of Pharmacy, Beni-Suef University, Beni Suef, Egypt
[3]Toxicology Management Specialist, Drug and Poison Information Center, Prince Sultan Militarily Medical City (PSMMC), Riyadh, Saudi Arabia
[4]Pharmaceutical Services Department Research Coordinator, King Hamad University Hospital, Bahrain
[5]Clinical Pharmacy Department, Faculty of Pharmacy, Sohag University, Sohag, Egypt

Learning Objectives

After completing this chapter, the reader would be able to:

- Identify and apply the concept and principles of evidence-based medicine (EBM).
- Describe the advantages and difficulties of EBM and its role in improving decision-making.
- Identify searching strategies to obtain more precise search results and choose the best resources for a specific information inquiry.
- Review and evaluate Primary, secondary, and tertiary information resources and Explore online evidence-based medicine resources.

---

* Corresponding Author's Email: Hoda.ahmed@pharm.bsu.edu.eg.

In: Clinical Pharmacist Tools to Deliver Rational Medication Use
Editor: Mohamed Emam Abdelmobdy Abdelrahim
ISBN: 979-8-88697-857-5

- Understand the role of the pharmacist in drug information centers.
- Learn how to assess literature and clinical guidelines and how to apply a systematic approach to answer drug-related questions.

Drug Information Centers

Drug information (DI) is defined as "The provision of unbiased, well-referenced, and critically evaluated information on any aspect of pharmacy practice [1]."

The first Drug information center (DIC) was established in 1962 in the United States. Its main objective was to provide DI services and educational purposes. Furthermore, it was concerned with medication use evaluations (MUEs), Adverse drug reactions (ADRs), and formulary management.

Many DICs developed since then, gaining attention to training pharmacy students regarding the necessary DI skills. Moreover, there was corresponding increased accessibility to medical and pharmaceutical databases.

Pharmacist's Role in DIC

The main goal of reviewing evidence-based guidelines is to enhance medication use, improve patient care and clinical outcomes, and manage resources.

According to the clinical setting and demands, pharmacists can provide a wide range of DI services. A DI provider should have good communication skills, both orally and written, to anticipate the DI needs of patients or other health care practitioners (HCP), search, retrieve, and evaluate the literature, and finally discuss and document essential knowledge to patient care.

Drug Information Activities

DI specialists can gather, assess, and communicate information more effectively to produce evidence-based recommendations and improve patient care. Also, DI specialists can participate in many drug safety activities and collaborate with bioinformatics experts. Usually, most DI inquiries would be categorized into one of the following:

1. Proper use of drugs
2. Efficacy for a specified disease state
3. Dosing schedules/regimens
4. Drug compatibilities or interactions
5. Use in pregnancy or lactation or special populations
6. Therapeutic drug monitoring (TDM)
7. Pharmacokinetics/Pharmacodynamics
8. Storage conditions/ drug stability
9. Medication availability
10. Adverse drug event
11. Drug product identification

The activities of the DI specialist can be summarized as follows [2]:

1. An expert can contribute DI to patients and HCPs when there is a knowledge gap.
2. Developing and managing a drug formulary based on scientific evidence regarding efficacy and safety, Pharmacoeconomics, and institution-specific considerations.
3. Evaluating the clinical importance of drug safety alerts issued by the FDA or other resources.
4. Integrating Programs to analyze health outcomes and develop clinical decision-making tools. (e.g., pharmacotherapeutic guidelines, medication-use evaluation criteria, and therapeutic interchange protocols).
5. Developing printed and online educational materials for patients and healthcare providers on subjects such as appropriate medication use.
6. Collaborating in quality improvement research projects and drug cost analyses.
7. Participating in institutional review boards (IRBs) and protocol appraisal.
8. Implementing measures to avoid medication errors and ADRs, assuring institutional adherence with Risk Evaluation and Mitigation Strategies (REMS), and directing reporting and analysis systems (e.g., MedWatch).
9. Participating as a peer reviewer and contributing to scientific literature.
10. Participation in Continuing Professional Development (CPD) for HCPs.
11. Developing clinical guidelines such as prescription privileges and alternative treatment.

A DI specialist should follow a systematic approach to properly respond to a DI request. The first systematic approach was proposed by Watanabe, et al. in 1975. Many modifications have been made to ensure that all pertinent information is evaluated before drafting an answer.

The outlines of a 9-step systematic approach can be summarized as follows:

1. *Identify the Inquirer* - Consider the requestor's access to health information and level of expertise to develop a response with an acceptable viewpoint.
2. *Gather Detailed Background Information* - Gather detailed background information, including assessing the patient's medical record, if appropriate, to optimize the reply. This may include; name, age, weight, gender, medical history (including allergies), major organ dysfunction (cardiac, liver, kidney), drug history (dose, regimen, and indication).
3. *Specify the Real Inquiry and the Required Information* - Requestors of information are typically vague in verbalizing their inquiry and provide more specified data only when asked. Ask exploratory questions to reveal the real question and improve the search strategy. For example, "Why is the inquiry being questioned?" and "Does the query relate to a particular patient?" may clarify important details of the true question.
4. *Classify/Categorize Requests* - Categorizing questions would help in the search strategy and evaluate resources (e.g., medications availability, ADRs/contraindications, drug compatibilities, compounding/ formulation, drug interactions, dosage/ administration, pharmacokinetics, pharmacodynamics/ efficacy, safety in pregnancy/lactation, and toxicity/poisoning).
5. *Search Strategy* - The PICOS approach helps to generate searchable terms to help in searching secondary resources such as Pubmed. PICO stands for: Patient/Population,

intervention/Exposure, Comparator/control, Outcomes. Each DICs should develop and maintain a list of search strategies reflecting the nature of their inquiries and the res the resources available

6. *Analysis and Synthesis* - It is the most critical step in formulating responses and recommendations. Evaluate and search tertiary, secondary, and primary resources, including electronic databases. The critical assessment, review, and evaluation of available evidence is known as analysis. Synthesis, on the other hand, is the systematic integration of gathered data to generate a conclusion.
7. *Communicate the Information* - As needed, provide an oral or written answer, or both. Supporting documentation (e.g., primary literature) could be provided when possible. Verbal responses are most suited to conveying a response to a simple uncomplicated query. Assess whether a written response is required following the verbal reply. While written responses may be more appropriate for a more complex inquiry. The systematic written format can be presented as follows;
    a. Request and background information.
    b. Response:
    c. In some cases, a brief introductory paragraph is necessary for clarification of the terminology and issues at hand. Summarize what the literature says about the issue, pointing out any inadequacies or deficiencies in the literature. Be concise and unbiased.
    d. Conclusion.
    e. Summarize the information gathered with the appropriate conclusion.
    f. References
    The response should be appropriately referenced.
8. *Document* - Document all information related to the request for further inquiries. For example, information resources, time spent on the request, and the response.
9. *Follow-Up Assessment* - Assess the quality and appropriateness of the information communicated and if it is reflected in changes in medication use or clinical outcomes. Follow-up can be done by phone, in person, or by mail.

Formulary Management

A formulary is an updated list of drugs and medical devices approved for use in a particular healthcare setting/country. It aims to ensure rational drug use in terms of safety, efficacy, and cost.

The DI pharmacist's role includes:

1. Analyze and evaluate Clinical literature regarding its relevance to the hospital's patient population
2. Conduct unbiased, detailed analyses of drugs that might be included in the formulary to ensure safe, effective, and economical drug use
3. Evaluate DI provided either written or verbally by medical representatives
4. Maintain an up-to-date formulary system of approved drugs and/or drug-use guidelines

5. Examine and update drug libraries, drug policies, and alert systems utilized in technological resources (computerized prescriptions/order entry systems, bar-coding systems, and smart infusion pumps)
6. Collaborate with practitioners who have clinical competence in areas of patient care relevant to the DI being provided.

Educational Support Services

Many DIC pharmacists participate in writing, reviewing, and editing newsletters to educate healthcare practitioners about guidelines, policy and formulary updates, and medication safety issues. DIC pharmacists would provide evidence-based data on drug-related issues by participating in seminars, case studies, or workshops. They provide either In-services for the staff or precepting students/residents on rotation.

Information Documentation and Management

All DI documentation compiled in response to DI requests should be maintained in a safe location that allows periodic retrieval by authorized personnel. Documentation is a critical step that highlights the significance of DICs services and serves as a basis for quality evaluations, performance improvements, and details a systematic approach in case of medico-legal conflicts. As a result, academic or population-based DI activities should be accurately reported.

DICs are expanding their adoption of electronic documentation systems, which have boosted the amount of documentation with increased efficiency and cost savings. Furthermore, an electronic system can support a regulated and systematic method while providing a conveniently retrievable archive that can be used to easily locate previously answered questions.

Documentation of DI services should include components identified through the systematic method. The ASHP Guidelines state that "the professional actions of pharmacists that are intended to ensure safe and effective medication use and that may impact patient outcomes should be documented in the patient medical record [3]." If the DI request is patient-specific, you may document the request and the related response in the patient's medical record.

Filing of Requests and Completed Responses

Requests and completed responses would be filed systematically for potential future use. Before being reused, the filed response must be evaluated and updated, if needed.

Filing System

The DI filing system should be systematic, comprehensive, and up-to-date to allow easy retrieval of individual DI inquiries. The indexing process of the included information in DI files must follow a structured procedure specified in departmental regulations.

For paper and electronic drug files indexing, the American Hospital Formulary System, the therapeutic classification system for numbering drugs, the International Classification of Diseases for classifying diseases, and miscellaneous systems for clinical files may be used. The inclusion and exclusion criteria for filing information will be determined by the scope of services provided and the type of storage system employed. Duplicated information should be avoided.

Records Retention

DI records and responses shall be kept for a minimum of seven years for legislative requirements and retained according to the specific organization's policy.

Culling of Records

The contents of the filing system should be reviewed periodically to exclude outdated records.

Quality Assessment

The quality of the DI service should be continuously evaluated to find whether the information provided was useful and assisted the requester to optimize clinical outcomes.

Currently, there is no standardized method described in the literature to evaluate DIC services despite their importance. For quality evaluation, several DICs have reported using double-check procedures before issuing a response, random retrospective audits by a DI expert, receiving feedback from the requestor, and completing an internal review by a committee.

Evaluating the Structure for Providing DI Services

The structure of the DI services should be assessed as follows:

1. Adequacy of Personnel and suitability of premises and equipment
2. Effectiveness of organizational structure
3. Suitability of services hours
4. Availability of DI resources
5. Development and use of policies and procedures.

Assessment of the Process of Providing DI Services

Evaluating the process for answering DI questions through randomly selecting and auditing the requests, documentation, references used, and the responses provided. This evaluation process would help to improve the quality of DI services provided and consists of the following:

(a) Periodical internal peer reviews
(b) Regular audits
(c) Surveys for requesters to assess their compliance with the service.

Follow-up

If the audit reveals additional information that is relevant to the original DI request, the DI expert should communicate that information to the requestor within a reasonable time frame.

Assessment of the DI Services Outcomes

The outcome of DI provision must be assessed by conducting a survey (in writing or by telephone) designed to determine the following:

1. Requester satisfaction with answer speed and perceived quality
2. The response outcome (for example, order change or dosage adjustment)
3. The influence of the response on patient outcome (such as cure of disease or improvement, resolution, or prevention of symptoms).

Reporting Performance

A performance report should be written and presented to pharmacy management at least twice yearly. This report would aid in documenting, reviewing, and monitoring the DI services' performance. It should contain project priorities, a summary of requester evaluations, and accomplishments (a summary of requests received, response reports, and additional responsibilities). It could also include reports comparing performance to the previous reporting period and unaddressed challenges that may impact the DI service's performance.

Follow-up Action Plan

Pharmacy management and the DI service should formulate a strategy to constantly enhance the DI services as structure, procedure, and outcomes. This strategy should be implemented and modified as needed to ensure that the service fulfills the DI requirements of the requesters.

DI Resources

The quantity of medical literature is growing exponentially. DI resources describe types of literature utilized in the development and provision of DI services. Purchasing DI resources, including electronic subscriptions, should consider the following:

1. Resource features including updates frequency, year of publication, type of information, organization of material, method of delivery, and cost.
2. Practice setting (e.g., needs of HCPs within that institution, and institutional-specific regulatory requirements).
3. Accessibility of the resource (e.g., easily locating print resources, number of users allowed by subscription).

Primary Resources

Primary resources are simply defined as the most up-to-date evidence available in biomedical journals i.e.; original research. Original research includes case reports, case series, clinical trials, letters to the editor, and conference abstracts. All articles are peer-reviewed (single or double-blind) before publication.

Note that review articles are considered as tertiary resources because they are narrative in nature and not provide new information However, systematic reviews and meta-analyses that summarize primary literature and establish new analyses for the data are considered primary resources. The primary literature is growing at an exponential rate. More than 20,000 biomedical journals are published annually, and most of them publish a combination of primary research studies and secondary review articles.

The basic structure of a research article consists of:

I. Title

It should reflect the research question yet be concise and unbiased.

II. Abstract/Summary

Summarize the main points in the study and be consistent with the manuscript. Highlighting study results and the significance of the work consists of the following sections: background, the aim of the study, methods, results, and a conclusion. Keywords are added to help retrieve the article.

III. Introduction

Including background information and history, a review of the previous literature, and a rationale of the present study

IV. Aim of the Work

V. Methods/Patients and Materials

It includes study design, setting, subject selection and recruitment, inclusion and exclusion criteria, primary and secondary outcome measures, follow-up measures, description of analytical techniques, type and time of data collection, and statistical analysis of the data.

VI. Results

This part summarizes findings in tables, charts, and figures. The focus on reviewing results should be on the significance of the outcomes.

VII. Discussion/Conclusion

The authors provide an unbiased interpretation and assessment of the results, not only citing studies with similar results. It consists of comparisons with earlier research findings to appropriately explain the study's relevance. There is also a review of the study's limitations as well as strengths for additional investigation.

VIII. References/Bibliography

Authors should document references cited in the manuscript. It is a great tool to verify the accuracy of the information mentioned in the article.

The main drawback of primary resources is limiting the information to one or two trials and excluding the background and general information found in the tertiary literature.

Some of the most reputable peer-reviewed journals are listed below.

1. New England Journal of Medicine (NEJM)
2. The Lancet
3. Nature
4. Pharmacotherapy: The Journal of Human Pharmacology and Drug Therapy
5. The Journal of American Medical Association (JAMA)

Secondary Resources

The majority of secondary DI resources are electronic indexing and abstracting systems that give a convenient way to search and organize primary literature (Table 1). Because not all secondary resources have the same selection of articles, detailed research requires exploring many databases.

Indexing systems refer to data including bibliographic citations, without access to the abstract. *Abstracting systems* provide not only the citation but also the abstract and a link to the full-text article. A clinical judgment should never be based only on reviewing the abstract.

Common types of Abstracts are; Telegraphic (only string words), Indicative (Structured sentences), and Informative.

Relevant articles should be assessed and reviewed during the clinical decision-making process. One limitation of secondary databases is that there is a time lag between publication and indexing an article into a secondary resource. Also, most secondary resources utilize an advanced search engine, which necessitates the adoption of new terminology and terms. So, analyzing secondary resources requires practicing the structure and terms related to each database.

For example, PubMed searches and retrieves primary literature using Medical Subject Headings (MeSH) keywords. Most secondary resources adopt Boolean operators ("AND"; "OR"; and "NOT") to provide more or fewer articles. "AND" can narrow a search, while "OR" can provide a broader search. Finally, the majority of secondary resources use limits such as language, clinical trial design, publication date, and so on.

Table 1. Common secondary sources (adopted from *Clinical Pharmacy Education, Practice and Research textbook*) [4]

Source	Search Language	Comments
MEDLINE	MeSH	Available through a variety of services: National Library of Medicine (NLM) through PubMed (www.ncbi.nlm.nih.gov/PubMed) (free) Ovid (www.ovid.com) (commercial); allows the search of more than one database at a time; offers other databases, such as those for dentistry and alternative health EBSCO (www.ebscohost.com); allows the search of more than one database at a time; offers other databases, such as those for dentistry and alternative health (commercial)
Excerpta Medica's Embase	Emtree: Contains 58,000 preferred terms (of which more than 28,000 are drugs and chemicals) and more than 240,000 synonyms (with over 150,000 drugs and chemicals) All MeSH terms are included Generic names as referenced by the FDA and European Medicines Agency (EMEA)	Contains more than 7500 titles from mostly peer-reviewed journals, including 2000 not in MEDLINE Includes 800 conference and 260,000 conference abstracts For more information, go to www.embase.com
IDIS (aka IOWA)	Uses the United States Adopted Name (USAN) and the International Classification of Diseases (ICD) coding system Descriptors may differ from MeSH terms	Contains more than 200 peer-reviewed English-language medical and pharmaceutical journals Includes data back to 1966 Full-text articles available electronically from 1988 to the present (articles from 1966 to 1988 on microfiche) For more information, go to www.uiowa.edu/~idis/ idistday.htm
IPA	Descriptors may differ from MeSH terms	Contains information from more than 800 pharmacy and health-related journals published worldwide since 1970 Available through Ovid and EBSCO Concentrates on all aspects of drug development, pharmacy professional meetings, and state pharmacy journals including meeting abstracts For more information, go to http://science.thomsonreuters.com

DI = drug information; FDA = U.S. Food and Drug Administration; IDIS = Iowa Drug Information Service; IPA = International Pharmaceutical Abstracts; MeSH = Medical Subject Heading.

Secondary resources include MEDLINE (through PubMed, EBSCO, Ovid), Academic Search Premier, Cochrane Database of Systematic Reviews, Iowa DI Service (IDIS), International Pharmaceutical Abstracts (IPA), Embase/Excerpta Medica, Biosis Previews/Biological Abstracts, CancerLit, SedBase, Reactions, Clin-Alert, Current Contents, and Toxline.

Tertiary Resources

Tertiary databases simplify and summarize data from the primary literature but do not include original data (Tables 2 and 3). Several tertiary resources synthesize data in tables and figures that are simple to access, utilize, and arrange. Users frequently favor one resource over another depending on the information provided, such as tables, appendices, or special sections.

Table 2. List of tertiary resources by category (adopted from ACCP 2018) [5]

Type of request	Books/Printed resources	Online Resources
ADRs	Meyler's Side Effects of Drugs AHFS Drug Information, ASHP Drug information handbook Drug Facts and Comparisons	Lexicomp Micromedex Clin Alert Online FDA Adverse Event Reporting system Facts and comparisons eAnswers
Biostatistics	Basic and clinical biostatistics Drug Information: A Guide for Pharmacists	Basic and clinical biostatistics (AccessMedicine) Drug Information: A Guide for Pharmacists (AcessPharmacy)
Chemical structure Information	Goodman's and Gilman's: the pharmacological basis of therapeutics Remington: the science and practice of pharmacy Merk Index	Goodman's and Gilman's: the pharmacological basis of therapeutics (AccessMedicine) PubChem USP-NF online
Compounding	Extemporaneous Formulations for Pediatric, Geriatric, and special need patients Trissel's Stability of Compounded Formulations Allen's Compounded Formulations Pediatric Dosage Handbook	www.compoundingtoday.com (international journal of pharmacy compounding)
Comprehensive Medical information	Treatment Guidelines Prescriber's Letters Pharmacist Letters	eMedicine (http://emedicine.medscape.com/) UpToDate (http://www.uptodate.com/) Dynamed (http://www.dynamed.com/) Cleveland Clinic: Disease management project
Drug identification	The Pill book	Facts and comparisons eAnswers Lexi-Drug ID RxList Medscape
Drug Interaction	Drug Interaction Facts Drug Interaction Analysis And Management (Hansten and Horn's)	Facts and comparisons eAnswers Lexicomp Online Micromedex Medscape

These include textbooks, compendia, online databases (e.g., Micromedex, Lexicomp, and Up To Date), and review articles. Tertiary databases are simple to use, whereas online databases can be readily updated with new information. It is regarded as first-line resources when dealing with a DI question, but readers should clinically evaluate and judge the quality of information. If the tertiary resource is not updated or comprehensive, a secondary resource should be reviewed to locate the primary literature. Examining a textbook should consider the date of publication, Author's name, Publisher, presence of references, and alternative resources available.

Major drawbacks of tertiary resources are possible errors in transcription, human bias, missing data, misinterpretation of information, and lack of expertise by authors. Another limitation is the lag time for publication.

Table 3. List of tertiary resources by category

Type of request	Books/Printed resources	Online Resources
Drug Safety		Facts and comparisons eAnswers Lexicomp Online BlackBoxRx
Evidence-based medicine	User's Guide to the Medical Literature: Essentials of Evidence-based clinical Practice (JAMA Evidence)	National Institute for Health and Care Excellence (NICE guidelines)
General Pharmacy Practices	AHFS Drug Information (ASHP) Drug information handbook (Lexicomp) Drug Facts and Comparisons	Lexicomp Micromedex Facts and comparisons eAnswers Medscape
Investigational drug information		FDA website MedlinePlus Manufacturer websites
Pharmacogenomics	Concepts in Pharmacogenomics (ASHP)	The Pharmacogenomics Knowledgebase (https://www.PharmGKB.org/)
Pharmacokinetics	Basic Clinical Pharmacokinetics Applied Biopharmaceutics and Pharmacokinetics	Applied Biopharmaceutics and Pharmacokinetics (AccessPharmacy)
Therapeutics	Goodman's and Gilman's: the pharmacological basis of therapeutics Applied Therapeutics: The Clinical Use of Drugs (Koda-Kimble's) Pharmacotherapy: A Pathophysiologic Approach (Dipiro's)	Pharmacotherapy: A Pathophysiologic Approach (Dipiro's) (AccessPharmacy) UpToDate eMedicine Merk Manual (http://merck.com/mmpe/index.html)
Pediatric dosage recommendations	The Harriet Lane Handbook Pediatric Dosage Handbook Pediatric Pharmacotherapy (ACCP)	Current Diagnosis and Treatment: Pediatrics (AccessMedicine)
International Drug References	Martindale: The Complete Drug Reference Index Nominum International Drug Directory	Lexi-Drug International Martindale: The Complete Drug Reference

When the search for a specific DI question, it is useful to categorize it into specific subject areas (ADRs, drug interactions, and so on).

Internet Resources of DI

Online resources provide a wealth of information that is unfiltered and of varying quality, making it subject to user interpretation. Internet resources are easy to access, and patients use the Internet to search for DI when they do not have access to a qualified healthcare practitioner. [6] Evaluating information presented online should focus on the author's specialization, accuracy and references available, information quality (suitable for the audience, concise, updated, reviewed, and unbiased), and the cost of utilizing this resource. Compared to a DI specialist, patients lack the skills to evaluate the validity of the DI presented on the Internet. The National Library of Medicine (NLM) made a 16-minute video to help patients and healthcare practitioners to identify the suitable internet DI resource available at: (www.nih.gov/MEDLINEplus/webevalu.html).

Common Secondary Online DI Websites

Cochrane Library (www.cochranelibrary.com)

The library contains six databases for systematic reviews and clinical guidelines/protocols. This database is known for systematic reviews and meta-analyses which analyze and summarize multiple RCTs to make a recommendation about a particular DI.

EMBASE (www.embase.com)

It allows access to all DI resources available in MEDLINE and international journals that are not found in other secondary resources.

Google Scholar (www.googlescholar.com)

It is a free online secondary resource that uses keywords (not MESH terms) for articles searches.

International Pharmaceutical Abstracts (IPA)

It is an international resource oriented to pharmacy and pharmacy practice available via EBSCO health (https://health.ebsco.com/products/international-pharmaceuticalabstracts).

It Provides access to both journal articles and meeting abstracts. IPA is very helpful to search for drug compounding, IV drugs, and stability studies.

PubMed

It is the most commonly used free-access secondary resource. It contains over 26 million articles from MEDLINE about biomedicines, life sciences, bioengineering, and more. It is available via the national center for biotechnology information as a part of the U.S. NLM (https://www.ncbi.nlm.nih.gov/pubmed).

Searching PubMed

PubMed is an essential secondary DI resource for pharmacists, including a wide range of scientific journals. MEDLINE (one of the key secondary DI resources) is the main component of PubMed, but it also searches other secondary DI resources and offers links to PubMed Central. PubMed Central offers full-text access to open-access articles as well as a wide range of scientific book chapters and other DI resources.

Searching PubMed Using MeSH Terms

Articles are indexed in MEDLINE using MeSH terms. Using MeSH terms provide more specific and fewer results (more focused results on the topic of interest). Also, it will increase search sensitivity and provide more relevant articles because these terms links with other synonyms. So, searching for the MeSH term "heart failure" will directly relate to a variety of current and past expressions of this term as "congestive heart failure", "myocardial infarction", and "heart decompensation".

Searching MeSH Terms

From the homepage, select "MeSH Database" below the "Explore" menu in the middle, right-hand side of the screen. Terms are individually searched through the MeSH search bar. If an exact MeSH term is searched, the entry will be displayed. However, if it was not an exact match, the MeSH database will provide a list of potential terms. MeSH terms and sub-terms are organized in a hierarchy way to provide extra relevance to the article topics. Sub-term checkboxes can help to customize/specify the search.

Boolean Operators

If more than one term is added to the search, the appropriate Boolean operator should be selected to provide a more effective search.

Using the operator "NOT" can unnecessarily exclude articles relevant to the search. After adding the suitable terms and operators, click "Search PubMed" to provide the search results. Sometimes, wrong terms can omit key articles related to the search topic.

PubMed New Interface

The new interface provides automatic term mapping. Using simple terms, PubMed automatically maps them to MeSH terms and searches in all fields.

(a) This interface combines the benefits of MeSH terms sensitivity (i.e., linking synonyms) with the broadened scope of the "all-fields" search. The operator "AND" is always assumed unless other operators are used. This method saves time and helps retrieve more potentially related articles. However, searching "all fields," may produce fewer specific results.
(b) This method ensures that recently published articles would appear in the search (because MeSH indexing takes 3–6 months), as well as find articles that, for whatever reason, were not indexed to the expected terms. Using the date filters would provide an easy way to retrieve recently published articles. The advanced search tool would help to find articles that were not indexed to the expected terms. This tool combines the simple search with the MeSH search using NOT to prioritize the results from the simple search.

PubMed Filters

PubMed defaults to using a "best match" scheme. PubMed provides several filters for your search to improve the quality and ease of retrieval of relevant literature. These include full-text availability, article types (e.g., clinical studies, clinical guidelines, meta-analyses), language, patient age, and species. Additional filters can be accessed using a button below the filter list. Sometimes, subheadings (e.g., dosing and administration) and MeSH major terms are used together to focus on results.

Advanced Search

PubMed always keeps track of searches so that users can retrieve and reference recent searches by selecting "Advanced" below the search bar. Past searches listed under "History and Search Details" can be included in the query. Also, they can be combined using the Boolean operators.

Common Online Tertiary DI Resources

Clinical Pharmacology

This online resource offers a comparison tool that can retrieve a list of products for a selected allergy or dietary restriction criteria (e.g., sugar-free, alcohol-free, gluten-free, sodium free, dye-free). Most information is referenced with a link to PubMed citations, although other information (e.g., adverse event reporting) is not referenced. It also provides information on product dosage forms, clinical effects, and ADRs.

Facts and Comparisons eAnswers

Facts and Comparisons eAnswers is the online version of the Facts & Comparisons textbook. Abbreviated DI is referenced, but not extensively. This resource offers great features e.g., comparison charts and a daily news update including FDA recalls. Moreover, information on look-alike drugs, sound-alike drugs, and a manufacturer index is available.

Lexicomp (Lexicomp online and the Drug Information Handbook)

Lexicomp is a point-of-service DI resource providing a comprehensive DI. Lexicomp presents a useful DI resource to use when quick retrieval of easy-to-understand data is preferable.

It is acquired by Wolters Kluwer, to add Lexicomp to their other holdings, including UpToDate.

It includes current drug shortages, FDA recalls of dangerous drug abbreviations, therapeutically equivalent generic drugs (Available at www.accessdata.fda.gov/scripts/cder/ob/default.cfm), and extemporaneous drug preparations (Pediatric Dosage Handbook).

Moreover, it focuses on providing information concerning special patient populations, toxicology, allergic reactions, pharmacogenomics, product identification, IV compatibility, and different drug interaction tools. Also, it provides useful information about which guidelines address the appropriate drug issue (available also through UpToDate). References are not always mentioned, and some references are not easily retrievable.

Micromedex

Micromedex is designed to provide information to HCPs in hospitals and academic settings about different clinical information. Micromedex offers comprehensive, easy-to-access, and referenced information about different topics (e.g., poison information, acute care medicine, and patient education). Therapeutic indications are graded and given a rating with usage recommendations.

Micromedex now offers a drug interaction application through iTunes that allows one to search for interactions of 50 medications together. Micromedex provides information about off-label drug uses, pharmacokinetics, pharmacodynamics; drug interaction (especially drug-drug, drug-food, drug-tobacco, and drug-alcohol), IV compatibility, dose adjustments, and toxicology.

This application is divided into two main sections: DRUGDEX and DrugPoints. DRUGDEX provides evidence-based detailed DI that is gathered from the primary literature and summarized by editorial specialists. DrugPoint Summary (formerly known as USP-DI volume I) provides summary information on dosing, drug interactions, ADRs, pregnancy warnings, indications, cautions, therapeutic classes, and brand information.

MD Consult/First Consult

MD Consult is a large resource providing comprehensive clinical information. MD Consult includes weekly summaries of journal articles, full-text reference books, practice guidelines, DI (through Gold Standard), information on what patients are reading in general literature, drug updates, daily medical news, customizable patient handouts, medical images, and continuing education. First Consult, a part of MD Consult, provides information on over 700 medical topics as well as differential diagnoses and procedures. First Consult also offers an iPhone application that provides clinical information available for smartphones and personal digital assistants (PDAs).

UpToDate

UpToDate is an evidence-based, peer-reviewed reference that is available through the Web or by PDA. Content is generated by medical experts in their field and covers more than 16 different medical disciplines and 8300 topics. This database is geared toward prescribers, and all information includes summary documents of evidence-based medicine. UpToDate uses Lexicomp information as the source of point-of-service DI.

Electronic Textbook Databases

There are numerous eTextbook collections available for purchase. These databases contain online textbooks in an electronic format. Large publishers such as McGraw-Hill and Wiley InterScience offer collections of their books in electronic format. These collections are often geared toward a specific subject area (e.g., pharmacy, medicine, nursing). Purchasing collections can be more cost-effective than buying individual titles. An advantage of electronic texts is the availability of content to be updated in a timely fashion. A major disadvantage of these resources is their cost. The contents of two commonly used electronic textbook databases are:

Access Pharmacy

This multimedia database has 25 online textbooks. Case studies, laboratory tests, calculators, videos, and effectiveness statements are also available. Titles include Pharmacotherapy: A Pathophysiologic Approach, Goodman & Gilman's: The Pharmacological Basis of Therapeutics, Harrison's Principles of Internal Medicine, Drug Information: A Guide for Pharmacists, and Goldfrank's Toxicologic Emergencies. AccessPharmacy offers a review for the NAPLEX, Multistate Pharmacy Jurisprudence Examination (MPJE), and Top 200 drugs as well as patient cases. Searching may be done by keyword, curricular topic, or organ system.

STAT!Ref

STAT!Ref contains full-text versions of medical and pharmacy texts including American Hospital Formulary Service (AHFS), Mosby's Drug Consult, Rudolph's Pediatric, Basic and Clinical Pharmacology, and Stedman's Medical Dictionary. Subscription rates are à la carte or by Core Collections. Core Collections are available for dentistry, mental health, nutrition and dietetics, pharmacology, and public health. Searching across all texts is available. In addition to popular texts, STAT!Ref offers a medical newsfeed as well as evidence alert feeds.

Self-Assessment Questions

1. Which of the following activities do DICs at hospitals usually NOT directly participate?
   a. Tracking and reporting of ADRs and medication errors
   b. Training healthcare staff on the safe and effective use of drugs
   c. Formulary management
   d. Quality control of manufactured drugs

2. A physician within a health network sends a message to a clinical pharmacist asking to review a patient's medications for drug-drug interactions with the addition of a new HIV medication. The patient's next visit is in 2 weeks. Which would be the most appropriate form of communication for the pharmacist to use to respond to the physician?
   a. Standard message within the electronic health record.
   b. Urgent message within the electronic health record.
   c. Direct page to the physician with results.
   d. Telephone call to the physician's nurse.

3. Which of the following would be the best resource to find information regarding medication errors and medication safety?
   a. Nature
   b. EMBASE
   c. OSHA
   d. ISMP

4. Pharmacist performs a PubMed search to determine whether any articles describe a true increased risk of major bleeding from interactions involving direct oral anticoagulants (DOACs) and cyclosporine, a CYP3A4 and P-glycoprotein inhibitor in human clinical studies. The pharmacist combines the Medical Subject Headings (MeSH) terms for individual DOACs (combined with OR) with the MeSH terms for drug interactions and cyclosporine. The search results in about 50 articles. Which is the best step the pharmacist could take to narrow the search results?
   a. Activate the clinical studies filter.
   b. Add drug class MeSH terms to the list of DOACs combined with OR.
   c. Add the MeSH term for major bleeding.
   d. Change to a non-MeSH term search approach.

Evidence-Based Medicine

What is Evidence-Based Medicine?

Decision-making based on unreliable evidence, personal opinions, basic theoretical science, and observational studies can't provide optimum therapeutic benefits to the patient. So, an important paradigm of clinical practice emerged 'EBM" evidence-based medicine to provide the best clinical decisions. [7]

Evidence-based medicine is a systematic approach to clinical problem-solving that allows the best available research evidence to be combined with clinical expertise and patient values. This concept is shown in Figure 1.

The EBM movement began in 1981, when a group of clinical epidemiologists at McMaster University, Canada led by David Sackett, published the first of a collection of articles in the Canadian Medical Association Journal advising physicians how to appraise the medical literature. In 1991 the term "evidence-based medicine " Was coined by one of Sackett's mentees: Gordon Guyatt, the Program Director of Internal Medicine at McMaster University.

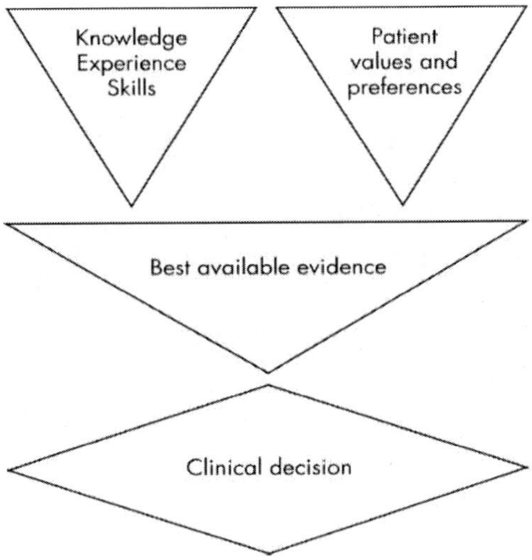

Figure 1. Flow chart of evidence-based medicine.

Evidence-based medicine is the conscientious, explicit, judicious, and reasonable use of the most current best evidence to enhance people's health by making decisions that improve their health-related quality of life and life span. There are three components of EBM: Best available evidence, Expertise with knowledge and experience skills, and patient values and preference as shown in Figure 1.

Principles of EBM

There are two fundamental principles include: [8]

1. Hierarchy of evidence: It states that evidence available in any clinical decision-making can be arranged in descending order of strength based on the likelihood of freedom from error as shown in Figure2.
2. The second key principle of EBM is that evidence alone is never sufficient for decision-making. It must be combined with clinical expertise as well as the expectations and values of patients

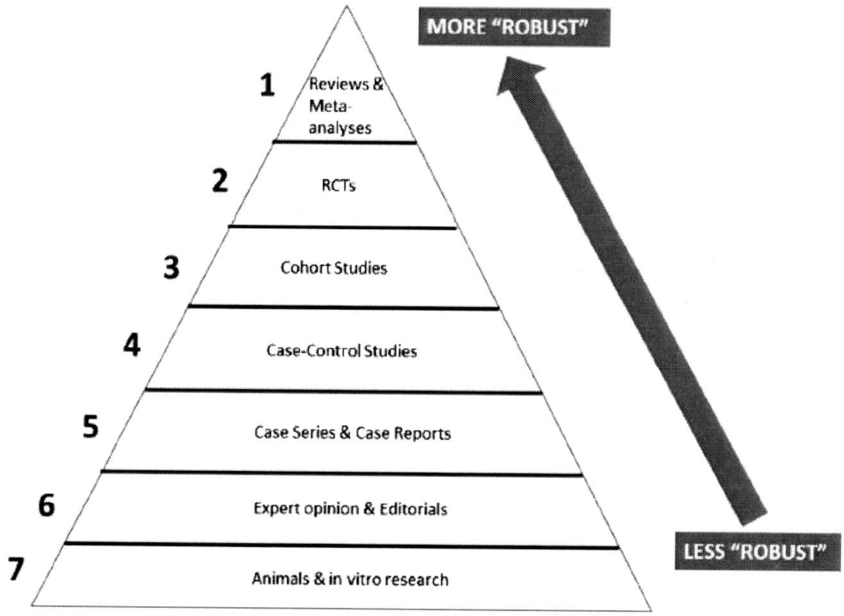

RCTs: Randomized control trials

Figure 2. Hierarchy level of evidence. [9]

Advantages of Application of Evidence-Based Medicine in Clinical Practice

- Allows clinicians and patients access to the most recent clinical knowledge.
- Guides prescribing decisions to get predictable improvement in patient condition.
- Help to sort through misleading drug marketing, and opinions to assess the benefits and risks of various treatments.
- It can enhance healthcare service through the development of common approaches and guidelines
- It can assist in making better use of limited resources by allowing them to evaluate the cost-effectiveness of treatments and services

An example is the use of streptokinase, a thrombolytic agent used in ischemic stroke. It was used to dissolve the clot and restore blood supply to the ischemic part. But three clinical trials (known as MAST-E, MAST-I, and ASK had to stop using it as it contributed to a high mortality rate because of severe bleeding. And it was replaced with alteplase, another thrombolytic agent with fewer adverse events. [10]

The use of hormone replacement therapy (HRT) in postmenopausal women is another example. Without adequate and high-quality evidence, the companies promoted the use of HRT. Only after a large clinical trial revealed that HRT may be dangerous have clinicians stopped.

Take an example of the treatment of eclampsia. Back in 1992, to treat convulsions that may occur during eclampsia diazepam was widely used. Only 2% of physicians prescribed magnesium sulfate which was proven by clinical trials to be more effective and related to decreasing maternal mortality compared to diazepam.

Limitations

Limited applicability of evidence to an individual patient: [11]

Evidence that is most applicable to a patient is the one coming from a study on him alone and the scope of such studies is very limited. Only chronic conditions with repeatable outcomes (unlike MI, stroke, or death) may be suitable for implementation on patients, so we can't generalize the result to all patients and guarantee the same benefits.

Lack of consistent and coherent evidence: This is another big problem. For a wide range of clinical practice-related questions, there is little incoherent evidence or the studies may not answer the question you are searching for.

Need time from clinicians: To conduct EBM it may take a lot of deep searching which requires time and knowledge about certain terminology of which some clinicians are not completely aware of the body of evidence continues to change, which requires a clinician aware of the recent updates to use the best therapeutic option.

Steps of Evidence-Based Medicine

Five key steps (5 As) are involved in the EBM process

1. Ask for the needed information by formulating your clinical question.
2. Acquire the best evidence that answers your question.
3. Assess or appraise the relevance, quality, and importance of the evidence.
4. Apply the evidence-in your practice or to your patient.
5. Access or Evaluate the outcome

Ask for the needed information by formulating your clinical question.

There are four types of questions to be asked as follow: Therapy, Diagnostic test, Prognosis, and Harm.

1. Therapy questions encompass all types of interventions, including medical, surgical, behavioral, psychological, and counseling issues
2. Diagnostic tests use a single or a combination of strategies (clinical, laboratory, imaging, and others) to distinguish between individuals who have and do not have the disease.
3. Prognosis questions, simply seek to predict the future course of patients with specific characteristics, such as stage I breast cancer.
4. Harm questions are concerned with the adverse effects of potentially harmful therapeutic agents on patients.

In patients with a particular clinical presentation.

A well can help to identify what you want to know. There are 4 elements of a good EBM question:

P = Patient or problem being addressed.
I = Intervention or exposure being considered.
C = Comparison intervention or exposure when relevant.
O = Outcome or the clinical outcomes of interest.

This is called the PICO from the initial letters of the four words: Patient, Intervention, Comparison, and Outcome. Most journal articles are based on the PICO research question.

An example: In a patient with a history of chronic smoking, does the administration of varenicline be more bupropion as compared to a nicotine replacement therapy (NRT) be a better therapy in causing long-term abstinence from smoking?

P = chronic smoker.
I = varenicline.
C = nicotine replacement therapy (NRT).
O = long-term abstinence from smoking

Another example: A 50-year-old gentleman with COPD who is bedridden suddenly develops breathlessness and hypertension. You suspect pulmonary embolism and order a ventilation-perfusion (V/Q) scan; however, you do not know and want to know how good the V/Q scan in the diagnosis of pulmonary embolism is. Before searching the literature, you start to formulate the question:

Patients: middle-aged men with COPD, bedridden and suspected to have pulmonary embolism

Intervention: ventilation-perfusion scan
Comparison: gold standard (pulmonary angiography)
Outcome: diagnosis of pulmonary embolism

Acquire (allocate) searching resources that answer your question.

Once your question is well-formulated, the next step is to find the currently available evidence to answer it. To do this efficiently, you may do two things: where to search and how to search or searching strategies.

Searching the PubMed

PubMed is free and probably the most searched system. The system keeps improving regularly and by the time you read this, the system may have added new features. It may be useful to keep in mind:

1. Easy searching: Simply type a word, phrase, or sentence into the search box. When you click 'search,' you will see the results. The word or phrase you choose should be based on your question, and it should be in PICO format. Any order is acceptable, but 'intervention' and 'patients' often produce more relevant results.
2. Related articles and reviews: To the right of the retrieved list of articles, there are some citations of related articles and two options below them: 'reviews' and 'all related articles'. You can expand your search by clicking on them. By using the display button, you can arrange the retrieved articles by 'publication date.'

3. Limits: This option allows you to limit your PubMed retrieval results to publication type (such as meta-analysis), year of publication (such as the last 5 years), language (such as English), age and sex of study subjects, and so on. There are two ways to go about it: directly through a button beneath the search box or in a direct PubMed search, all of these options are displayed on the left panel, and you can select as many as you want to narrow your results.
4. Clinical queries: PubMed has this search tool (you can find it on the lower half of the PubMed homepage where you can enter the term you want to search. using 'clinical queries can easily provide relevant studies as well as systematic reviews on the topic, in addition, it can help you either to 'broad' or 'narrow' search and article types such as 'therapy,' 'diagnosis,' and 'prognostic.'
5. MeSH terms: MeSH is an abbreviation for medical subject heading.
   This is the MEDLINE-controlled vocabulary.
   The use of MeSH terms is beneficial in retrieving information that would otherwise be missed.
6. History and combining terms: One of the choices below the search box is the 'History' tab. By displaying this, you can find search terms used in your most recent search session. They're all numbered.
   You can combine them by entering the numbers after # and selecting the 'AND' or 'OR' Boolean operators.

Searching Strategies

For precise search Boolean operators can be used. Boolean Operators are simple words (AND, OR, NOT) that are used as conjunctions in a search to combine or exclude keywords, yielding more focused and productive results as shown in Table 4.

Table 4. Boolean operators

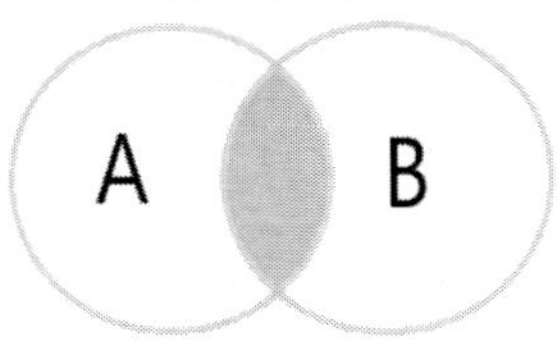 A AND B	Retrieves the articles having concept A and concept B in the same record. Using AND, the number of hits retrieved decreases
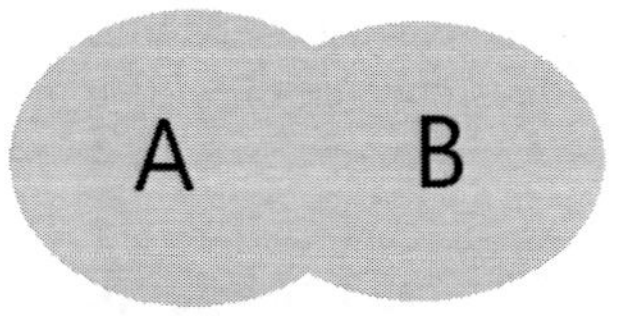 A OR B	Retrieves the articles containing either concept A or concept B. Used usually to connect synonyms or related terms. Using OR, the number of hits retrieved increases.
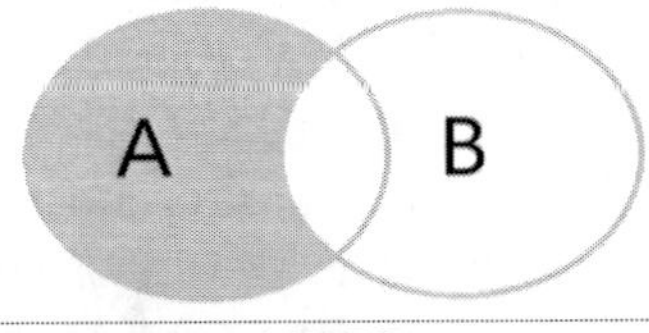 A NOT B	Retrieves the articles containing concept A but not concept B. Use with caution as it might eliminate some relevant records.

AND

Narrow result, as it requires both terms to be in the search result If one term appears in the document but the other does not, the item is not included in the resulting list. example: when we search for diabetes and hypertension, the search result will include articles that talk about both diabetes and hypertension.

OR

Broadens the search. both terms will be in the search result. For example: when we search for diabetes or hypertension, the search result will contain any articles talking about either diabetes or hypertension.

NOT

Narrow the search may be too exclusively the first term is searched, followed by subtracting any records containing the term after the operators from the results. For example, when we search for diabetes, not hypertension, The search result will contain articles talking only about diabetes, and articles about hypertension will be omitted.

Other operators can be used as the following: Truncation (asterisk) (*) can be used to the wide search result to include various word endings and spelling, for example, plan *retrieves plans, plants plan.

Assess or Appraise the Relevance, Quality, and Importance of the Evidence

Once you identified the literature that may answer your question, it needs to be critically appraised to determine if it is worth using. Critical Appraisal includes four issues: Relevance, Validity, Consistency, and results. We will focus on critical Appraisal for a Therapy Paper.

Relevance refers to what extent the research paper meets your information needs. when reading the abstract and comparing the research question in the paper to your clinical question, you will know if this paper is relevant and would answer your question or not. In addition to relevancy, to determine if you can use this paper to answer your question you need to check validity.

Validity refers to the extent to which the results are true and free from bias. There are two types of validity, internal and external validity.

Internal validity is defined as the extent to which the observed results reflect the truth in the population we are studying and are thus not the result of methodological errors. Internal validity should check the following points as explained in detail in Table 5.

1. Presence of a control group with adequate size and statistical power.
2. Appropriate Randomization method of the control group with concealed allocation.
3. Comparable groups at baseline and concealed group allocation.
4. Absence of Co-intervention Bias.
5. Adequate Compliance.
6. Adequate follow-up length.
7. Blind assessment.

Table 5. Internal validity check questions

1. Was There a Control Group?		
1a. Why do we ask this question?	**1b. where do we find the answer to this question?**	**1c. How do we interpret the answer?**
because progress can happen naturally or because of the Hawthorne effect, a placebo effect	In the abstract of the paper.	If the answer is yes, continue to evaluate. If the answer is no, the study cannot be considered conclusive and further search is advocated.
2. Was Control Group Created Through Random Allocation (Randomization)? Was Allocation Concealed?		
2A. Why do we ask this question?	**2b. where do we find the answer to this question?**	**2c. How do we interpret the answer?**
As a follow-up to the first question, we ask this one. If a control group exists, it must be determined whether it is appropriate. How was it made or put together? To avoid biased results. we need to randomize our patients into 2 groups (control or treatment. To do this, the most popular method is like 'coin tossing'. Although computer randomization is ideal and often used in multi-center trials. For randomization to work, patients should be recruited into the study without knowing which group (control or treatment) they will be assigned to (be allocated). This is known as hidden (or blinded) allocation.	The method should tell you how the patients were allocated to groups and whether randomization was concealed or not.	Randomization is considered concealed if: (a) There is an appropriate placebo in a random distribution to which those enrolling patients are blinded. (b) Those enrolling patients must make a call to a center or person who uses a list or computer to assign the patient to one of the study arms. On the other hand, If (a) a list displaying the allocation is being used (b) alternate patients are assigned to one or the other arm (c) odd or even date of birth is used to assign patients to one or the other arm, randomization is not concealed.
3. Were the Groups Balanced (Comparable or Similar) at Baseline?		
3A. Why do we ask this question?	**3b. where do we find the answer to this question?**	**3c. How do we interpret the answer?**
This question is asked to assess whether the difference in outcomes between the two groups can be related to the treatment or not, as well as if the differences observed are likely to be greater (overestimate) or less (underestimate) than the true difference.	A table of "Baseline Characteristics" comparing the randomized groups on several variables that could affect the outcome should be included in the Results.	You concentrate on the critical prognostic factors that you must be aware of from prior research and experience. Compare the percentages of patients in each group who have a prognostic factor. If the percentage of patients is similar you can conclude that prognostic balance exists at baseline.
4. Was There Any Co-intervention Biases?		
4A. Why do we ask this question?	**4b. where do we find the answer to this question?**	**4c. How do we interpret the answer?**
Any intervention that is not being studied is referred to as a co-intervention. If patients in the two groups receive co-interventions unequally and these affect outcomes, they can introduce bias between the groups This is known as co-intervention bias.	The types of interventions provided to the patients in the two arms would be described in the results section in a table comparing the frequency of use of co-interventions while other papers don't mention it.	Consider only those co-interventions that are likely to have an impact on the outcome. Next, consider whether differences in frequency of use would cause (underestimation or overestimation of the effects.
When a drug is in comparison to a placebo, it is apparent that the drug arm may cause adverse effects that need treatments to deal with it.		Then think about the extent to which the direction and degree of distortion may affect the results.

5. Was the Compliance Adequate?		
5A. Why do we ask this question?	**5b. where do we find the answer to this question?**	**5c. How do we interpret the answer?**
Compliance is essential as, in placebo-controlled studies, the effects of the intervention are not seen if study participants do not take the prescribed intervention.	In the result section, the method of measurement and the extent of compliance should be mentioned.	In placebo-controlled studies, if the intervention is found to be superior to a placebo, compliance is not considered a major concern, on the other hand, If the intervention proves ineffective, one probable explanation might be non-compliance.
6. Was the Follow-Up Complete or Adequate?		
6A. Why do we ask this question?	**6b. where do we find the answer to this question?**	**6c. How do we interpret the answer?**
We ask this question because if there is a remarkable loss in patient follow-up, the validity of the results may be adversely affected, and conclusions may be misleading.	Typically, a table in the results section lists the number of patients who were followed up on, as well as their outcomes.	Follow-up losses should be kept to a minimum, preferably less than 20%. However, if only a few patients have the desired outcome, even minor losses to follow-up can bias the results.
7. Measured objective or were the patients and clinicians kept blind to which treatment was being received?		
7A. Why do we ask this question?	**7b. where do we find the answer to this question?**	**7c. How do we interpret the answer?**
It is ideal if the study is 'double-blinded' - that is, both patient and investigator are unaware of treatment allocation to avoid bias in the results.	The paper's Methods section should explain whether the outcome assessment was blinded.	If the outcome is objective eg death then blinding is less critical. If the outcome is subjective (e.g., symptoms or function) then blinding the outcome assessor is critical.

External validity asks, "To which population are the study's findings applicable or generalizable"? External validity is judged by time, place, and person. Can the findings be interpreted to the present or future, to different geographical regions or settings, or patients not included in the study? Is the treatment feasible in my setting? Will the potential benefits of treatment outweigh the potential harm for my patient?

Results

For a therapy paper, results should contain the answer to the following question "How large and precise was the treatment effect". This can be answered by measuring the following items as shown in Table 6:

Table 6. The most important item to check is the result

1. How large was the treatment effect?	
Consider a study in which 20% (0.2) of the control group died and 15% (0.15) of the treatment group died after 2 years of treatment. The result can be expressed as shown below:	
What is the measure?	**What does it mean?**
Relative risk (RR) = Risk of the outcome in the treatment group/Risk of the outcome in the control group. RR = 0.15/0.2 = 0.75 Since RR < 1, it means that the treatment decreases the risk of death.	The relative risk tells us how many times more likely it is that an event will occur in the treatment group relative to the control group. RR of 1 means that there is no difference between the two groups so, the treatment had no effect. An RR <

Table 6. (Continued)

What is the measure?	What does it mean?
	1 means that the treatment decreases the risk of the outcome. An RR>1 means that the treatment increased the risk of the outcome.
Absolute risk reduction (ARR), also known as the absolute risk difference (RD) = Risk of the outcome in the control group- Risk of the outcome in the treatment group. ARR = 0.2-0.15 = 0.05 or 5% So the absolute benefit of treatment is a 5% reduction in death.	The absolute risk reduction tells us the absolute difference in the rates of events between the two groups and indicates the baseline risk and treatment effect.
Relative risk reduction (RRR) = Absolute risk reduction/Risk of the outcome in the control group. Or it can be calculated by subtracting RR from 1. RRR = 1-RR RRR = 0.05/0.2 = 0.25 Or RRR = 1-0.75 = 0.25 So, we can say that the treatment reduces the risk of death by 25% relative to that occurring in the control group.	The relative risk reduction is the complement of the RR It tells us the reduction in the rate of the outcome in the treatment group relative to that in the control group. It is the most reported measure of treatment effects.
The number needed to treat (NNT) = Inverse of absolute risk reduction. (1/ARR). NNT = 1/0.05 = 20. So, we would need to treat 20 patients for 1 year to prevent 1 death.	NNT represents the number of patients we need to treat with experimental therapy to prevent 1 bad outcome and incorporates the duration of treatment.
2. How precise was the estimate of the treatment effect?	
The true risk of the outcome in the population is unknown, and the best we can do is to estimate it based on the trial's sample of patients. This is known as the point estimate. By examining the confidence intervals (CI) for each estimate, we can determine how near this estimate is to the true value. If the confidence interval is narrow, we can be sure that our point estimate accurately reflects the population value. The confidence interval also tells us about the statistical significance of the result. If the value for no effect is outside the 95% confidence interval, the result is statistically significant at the 0.05 level. The results are not statistically significant if the confidence interval includes the value corresponding to no effect.	

Consistency

The degree to which the research results are similar across different analyses in the study and agree with evidence outside the study is referred to as consistency. There are two types of consistency external and internal.

1. Internal consistency examines the various analyses performed in the study. In a therapy paper, for instance, there may be unadjusted and adjusted analyses, analyses for subgroups, sensitivity analyses, and analyses of primary and secondary outcomes. If these analyses produce the same result, say, in favor of the new therapy, the results are said to be internally consistent.
2. External consistency refers to the consistency of study findings with evidence from biology, other studies, and even clinician experience. If the findings do not match one or more of these, the reasons must be investigated

Apply the Evidence in Your Practice or to Your Patient

Once you've determined that the information in the paper is relevant, valid, consistent, and significant, the next question is whether the test or treatment will be beneficial to your patient/practice. You must first evaluate (or best guess) your patient's disease probability or risk of an undesirable outcome, and then consider how these will change as the new test or treatment is applied. Is the risk and cost of the new interventions worth the change? What does your patient think about the advantages and disadvantages of the new test or treatment? These considerations will assist you in deciding whether to apply the paper's findings.

Access or Evaluate the Outcome

The fifth step evaluates the outcomes. Was the new information or procedure application effective? Used effectively? Did the patient experience any side effects?

Should this new information and/or clinical practice technique be applied in day-to-day applications? Has any new data been published in the literature about this information? All these questions should be reviewed to guarantee the optimum application of evidence-based medicine or practice.

Practical Case

Ms. MP, an 86-year-old woman, arrives at the emergency room following a fall at home. A right femur fracture is discovered during the examination. The orthopedic surgeon advises urgent repair and antibiotics before surgery. Ms. MP, her husband for 40 years, has spent her life avoiding medications and relying on natural remedies. Her husband expresses concern about the possibility of diarrhea as a side effect of the antibiotics and inquires whether fermented milk with lactobacillus or another probiotic product would prevent this side effect. Should she start taking a probiotic to avoid this problem?

Application of 5 steps of EBM would be as follows:

Ask a well-built clinical question using the PICO format

P: Hospitalized patient with femur fracture taking antibiotics
I: Use of probiotics
C: Whether to use probiotics or not.
O: Preventing antibiotic-associated diarrhea.

So, the question would be: in an elderly hospitalized patient taking antibiotics, are probiotics helpful in preventing diarrhea?

Acquire the Evidence

Using PubMed Clinical queries, we can search for antibiotics AND diarrhea, AND probiotics. We can limit the search to full-text randomized controlled trials.

Appraise the Evidence

We find the following article and we want to do a critical appraisal to see if it can be used to answer our question.

Beausoleil M. Effect of a Fermented Milk Combining Lactobacillus acidophilus Cl1285 and Lactobacillus Case in the Prevention of Antibiotic-Associated Diarrhea: A Randomized, Double-Blind, Placebo-Controlled Trial. PMCID: PMC2658588 PMID:18026577 [11].

Abstract

Background: Antibiotic-associated diarrhea is an important problem in hospitalized patients. The use of probiotics is gaining interest in the scientific community as a potential measure to prevent this complication. The main objective of the present study was to assess the efficacy and safety of fermented milk containing Lactobacillus acidophilus and Lactobacillus casei which is widely available in Canada, in the prevention of antibiotic-associated diarrhea.

Method: In this double-blind, randomized study, hospitalized patients were randomly assigned to receive either lactobacilli-fermented milk or a placebo daily.

Result: Among 89 randomized patients, antibiotic-associated diarrhea occurred in seven of 44 patients (15.9%) in the lactobacilli group and 16 of 45 patients (35.6%) in the placebo group (OR 0.34,95% CI 0.125 to 0.944; P = 0.05) The median hospitalization duration was eight days in the lactobacilli group, compared with 10 days in the placebo group (P = 0.09). Overall, the lactobacilli-fermented milk was well tolerated.

Conclusion: The daily administration of lactobacilli-fermented milk was safe and effective in the prevention of antibiotic-associated diarrhea in hospitalized patients.

First, we need to check the validity questions as shown in Table 7.

Table 7. Application of validity question to an RCT as a part of critical appraisal

1. Was There a Control Group?	Yes. 89 patients participated in this study 44 patients were assigned to the lactobacillus group (treatment group) and 45 were assigned to placebo (control group).
2. Was Control Group Created Through Random Allocation (Randomization)? Was Allocation Concealed?	Patients were randomly assigned to receive either lactobacilli-fermented milk or a placebo (a lactoserum devoid of microorganisms), administered once daily. Although allocation is not concealed.
3. Were the Groups Balanced (Comparable or Similar) at Baseline?	Participants were well-matched between the two study groups regarding demographic and baseline characteristics.
4. Was There Any Co-intervention Biases?	No, the treatment group receive only lactobacilli-fermented milk.
5. Was the Compliance Adequate?	Yes. All patients who entered the study were accounted for and were compliant with the intervention.
6. Was the Follow-Up Complete or Adequate?	The follow-up period was planned to end 21 days after the last administered antibiotic dose
7. Were measures objective or were the patients and clinicians kept blind to which treatment was being received?	Yes. The study is double-blinded.

Table 8. Application of result parameters to an RCT as a part of critical appraisal

1. How large was the treatment effect?
Experimental (lactobacilli) Event Rate = 7/44 = 15.9% Control (placebo) Event Rate = 16/45 = 35.5%
Absolute Risk Reduction = 35.5%-15.9% = 19.6%
Relative Risk reduction = 19.6%/35.5% = 55.2%
Number Needed To Treat = 1/19.6%=5
2. How precise was the estimate of the treatment effect?
CI 0.125 to 0.944; P = 0.05) so, the result is statistically significant.

Second, we need to check the result parameters as shown in Table 8.

Apply the Information in Your Practice or to Your Patient

The findings of Beausoleil and colleagues are in line with a previous comprehensive study, which showed that probiotics lessen the incidence of diarrhea brought on by antibiotics and hasten their resolution.

Before applying a study's findings to your patient, ask yourself if they fit the study's inclusion criteria. If not, are there any strong arguments against the results applying to your patient? Were all clinically significant outcomes considered? Are the probable treatment advantages worth the risks and expenses involved?

Access or Evaluate the Outcome

After the application of the interventions for this patient (probiotics) we come to the last step is to evaluate the outcome and to see if our intervention has really helped the patient (prevent diarrhea).

Self-Assessment Questions

1. Which of the following is considered one of the advantages of the application of evidence-based medicine in clinical practice?
   a. Allows clinicians and patients access to the most recent clinical knowledge .
   b. Guides prescribing decisions to get predictable improvement in patient condition.
   c. Help to sort through misleading drug marketing, and opinions to assess the benefits and risks of various treatments.
   d. All of the above.

2. According to the hierarchy pyramid of evidence, which of the following is considered the highest degree of evidence
   a. Randomized control trial.
   b. Meta-analysis.
   c. Cohort studies.
   d. Case report.

3. In critical appraisal, which of the following refers to the extent to which the observed results reflect the truth in the study population and are thus not the result of methodological errors?
   a. External validity.
   b. Internal validity.
   c. Relevancy.
   d. Consistency.

4. Which of the following describes the risk of the outcome in the treatment group/Risk of the outcome in the control group?
   a. Relative Risk (RR).
   b. Absolute Risk Reduction (ARR).
   c. Relative Risk Reduction (RRR).
   d. The number needs to treat (NNT).

5. Which of the following is important to check considering internal validity in critical appraisal?
   a. Presence of a control group with adequate size and statistical power.
   b. Appropriate Randomization method of the control group with concealed allocation.
   c. Comparable groups at baseline and concealed group allocation.
   d. Absence of Co-intervention Bias.
   e. All of the above.

References

[1] Association, C. M. (1981). How to read clinical journals: I. Why to read them and how to start reading them critically. *CMAJ*, 124(5), pp. 555-558.

[2] Skelly, A. C., and Chapman, J. (2011). Evidence-based medicine (EBM): origins and modern application to spine care. *Evidence-based spine-care journal*, 2(01), pp. 11-16.

[3] Lewis, S. J., and Orland, B. I. (2004). The importance and impact of Evidence Based Medicine. *Journal of Managed Care Pharmacy*, 10(5 Supp A), pp. S3-S5.

[4] Haynes, R. B. (1996). Transferring evidence from research into practice: 1. The role of clinical care research evidence in clinical decisions. *BMJ Evidence-Based Medicine*, 1(7), p. 196.

[5] Guyatt, G. (2008). The evidence based-medicine working group users' guides to the medical literature. *Essentials of evidence-based clinical practice*.

[6] Sheridan, D. J., and Julian, D. G. (2016). Achievements and limitations of evidence-based medicine. *Journal of the American College of Cardiology*, 68(2), pp. 204-213.

[7] Kang, H. (2016). How to understand and conduct evidence-based medicine. *Korean journal of anesthesiology*, **69**(5), pp. 435-445.

[8] Prasad, K. (2013). *Fundamentals of evidence based medicine*. Springer.

[9] Kromer, J. (2014). *Boolean and Truncation.*

[10] Timm, D. F., Banks, D. E. and McLarty, J. (2012). Critical appraisal process: step-by-step. *South Med J*, 105(3), pp. 144-8.

[11] Beausoleil, M. (2007). Effect of a fermented milk combining Lactobacillus acidophilus Cl1285 and Lactobacillus casei in the prevention of antibiotic-associated diarrhea: a randomized, double-blind, placebo-controlled trial. *Canadian Journal of Gastroenterology*, 21(11), pp. 732-736.

Chapter 7

Pharmacogenomics

Hoda Rabea[1]
Haitham Saeed[1]
Amr Y. Zakaria[2]
Hager Salah[3]
Gehad Hassoub[5]
Ahmed F. Al-Talqani[4]
and Amira B. Kassem[5,*]

[1]Clinical Pharmacy Department, Faculty of Pharmacy, Beni-Suef University, Beni Suef, Egypt
[2]Clinical Pharmacy (Pharmacy Practice) Department, Faculty of Pharmacy, Horus University, Egypt
[3]Pharmaceutical Services Department, King Hamad University Hospital, Bahrain
[4]Department of Clinical Pharmacy, College of Pharmacy, University of Al-Ameed, Iraq
[5]Clinical Pharmacy and Pharmacy Practice Department, Faculty of Pharmacy Damanhour University, Egypt

Learning Objectives

After completing this chapter, the reader would be able to:

- Understanding of the pharmacogenomics concepts
- Recognize the difference between traditional and personalized medicine.
- Prove brief data about the emergence of personalized medicine.
- Highlight the benefit and the limitations of personalized medicine.
- Provide examples of personalized medicine initiatives.
- Know the relationship between pharmacogenetics and personalized medicine
- Be aware of the type of genetic testing used in personalized medicine.

---

* Corresponding Author's Email: Amira.kassem@pharm.dmu.edu.eg.

In: Clinical Pharmacist Tools to Deliver Rational Medication Use
Editor: Mohamed Emam Abdelmobdy Abdelrahim
ISBN: 979-8-88697-857-5

Concepts of Pharmacogenomics

Understanding why individuals respond differently to drug therapy, both in terms of good and bad outcomes, is one of the most difficult research areas in pharmacoepidemiology. The response to pharmacologic drugs varies significantly between individuals. Pharmacogenomics investigates the extent to which genetic variation is responsible for observed differences [1]. When similar effective drug doses are provided to different patients with similar anthropometrics, plasma drug concentrations can vary more than 1,000-fold [2]. Sex, age, disease condition (e.g., renal and hepatic function), drug-drug interactions, drug-food interactions, and pregnancy can influence drug response variability among treated individuals. Despite that, genetics is also expected to control a significant influence, as individual responses to a particular pharmacologic treatment are highly reproducible [3, 4]. Theoretically, identifying genetic variables that affect drug pharmacokinetics (absorption, distribution, metabolism, and elimination) with the pharmacodynamics (the effect on receptor site) could enable customized therapy, potentially improving pharmacological efficacy and minimizing toxicity profiles in a particular population [1, 5-7]. The possibilities for economic savings (through increased therapeutic efficacy) and decreased morbidity and mortality (via increased drug safety and fewer adverse drug reactions [ADRs]) are considerable [8, 9]. Although many ADRs are preventable and are often the results of medication errors, others have unknown etiology and may be related to ethnicity [10].

The terms used below are used to explain aspects that contribute to the effect of a certain drug on a specific individual.

Pharmacogenomics

The role of various components of the genome on drug response is referred to as pharmacogenomics. For genetic sequence variants, structural alterations in chromosomes (e.g., translocations), epigenetic variants (e.g., changes in gene methylation), and variation in gene expression profiles (changes in messenger RNA [mRNA] levels) are among the most commonly investigated (e.g., changes in microRNA). Genetic variation can be inherited from the parents or acquired (e.g., somatic mutation in a tumor). Much pharmacogenomic research has been aided by the advent of high-throughput tools for interrogating the entire genome.

Pharmacogenetics

Pharmacogenetics is a subclass of pharmacogenomics that studies the effect of genetic variation on pharmacological response. In general, pharmacogenetics refers to a single DNA polymorphism or coding variant rather than epigenetic or transcriptomic changes throughout the genome. Pharmacogenetics and pharmacogenomics are frequently used interchangeably in practice.

Pharmacokinetics

Pharmacokinetics (PK) is the study of how a drug travels through the body [11]. The PK of a drug is involved in its absorption, distribution, metabolism, and elimination, all of which affect the drug's effect by changing the concentration of the drug at its site of action.

Pharmacodynamics

Pharmacodynamics (PD) is the therapeutic response of an individual's body to medicine [11]. This is often defined by the drug's affinity and activity at the site of action or receptor.

Genotyping

The process of determining the collection of alleles (variants) at a specific site in the genome is known as genotyping. Single base alterations, insertions, deletions, and tandem repeats are all examples of allele variations.

Genetic Variation

Differences in genetic sequences among individuals in a population are referred to as genetic variation. Single nucleotide polymorphisms (SNPs) are variations in a single base pair that have a population frequency of at least 1%. Insertions, deletions, copy number variants, and short tandem repeats are examples of other types of variation. Mutations are variants that occur at a considerably lower prevalence than one percent of the population. Every form of variation, regardless of frequency, has the potential to influence phenotype, but the impact is dependent on a variety of factors, including the position of the variation within the genome and the functional consequences of the variation.

Epigenetic Changes

Epigenetic alterations are those that affect genes without changing the sequence of the genes. This might happen due to changes in gene methylation or histone modification (methylation, acetylation), both of which can affect transcription rate or gene expression suppression. Modifications in noncoding RNAs and telomere length are examples of other epigenetic changes. These epigenetic modifications can be passed down from parents to children, but they can also be caused by environmental factors. Reduced susceptibility of a tumor to a chemotherapeutic drug due to gene methylation is an example of an epigenetic alteration that influences drug metabolism [12].

Context Historique

Pharmacogenomics originated in the 6th century BC when scientists were supposed to have observed that the beans of fava could lead to illness in some people [13]. Immune-chemist William Boyd observed that native Britons seldom got hemolytic anemia after consuming fava beans, as opposed to Mediterranean ethnicity, and he proposed that this was due to a genetic variation in the early 1940s [13]. It has already been discovered that hemolytic anemia caused by fava bean consumption, which can also be produced by some drugs, is caused by glucose-6-phosphate dehydrogenase insufficiency (G6PD X-linked).

The following ground-breaking discoveries established the present science of pharmacogenetics:

- Recessive traits in non-screened patients with a phenylthiourea phenotype, early interpretation by Snyder in 1932 [14].
- The patients who were born with plasma cholinesterase deficiency had a sustainable paralytic toxic effect to suxamethonium, which was discovered in the 1950s [15].
- Motulsky proposed in mid-1957 that population disparities in drug response and adverse events might be due to genetic variation [16]. Frederich Vogel, a German geneticist, created the phrase "pharmacogenetics" in 1959 [17].
- A series of twin studies undertaken in the early 1960s confirmed the significance of genetics in interindividual variation in drug responsiveness [18, 19]. The research findings confirmed that many medicines' plasma half-lives, particularly warfarin, have closely related pharmacokinetic parameters. Other findings proved significant differences in twins (dizygotic), non-identical siblings, and other people.
- At the end of the 1970s, dual separate investigations linked an autosomal recessive drug metabolic defect to a much greater frequency of adverse effects in specific participants using the antihypertensive debrisoquine [20]. as well as the anti-arrhythmic sparteine [21]. Approximately 10 years later, the metabolism of both medications was caused by locus allelic polymorphisms at the gene of cytochrome P450 2D6 (CYP2D6) [22].

Historically, breakthroughs in the technology of human genetics and good knowledge of the molecular study of drug pharmacokinetics and pharmacodynamics have resulted in the identification of the degree of functional genetic polymorphisms that have the upper hand in drug treatment effects.

Pharmacogenomics: Current and Future Promise

Pharmacogenomics and its forerunner pharmacogenetics investigate the role of genetic variables in inter-individual differences in drug response and safety profile. The main objective of pharmacogenomics is to personalize medications for specific populations depending on the genetic make-up and molecular profile of those populations.

Pharmacogenomics has evolved in tandem with genotyping technology. Despite the completion of the human HapMap project and genome sequencing, the use of pharmacogenomics did not reach its complete clinical application and still had limited use. We offer an outline of recent pharmacogenomics applications in selected individuals, drug dosing, and development, along with illustrated instances of these types. Some of the domain's tribulations besides its prospects will be conferred.

Currently, pharmacogenomics is used to (1) recognize individuals at risk of ADEs; (2) patient inclusion that truly benefits from the treatment; and (3) set the proper doses to assure drug use with safe and effective therapeutic agents, and (4) inform clinical trial design and drug development. These applications will be discussed in the sections that follow.

Who Is at Risk for Pharmacogenomics and ADEs?

Serious adverse drug reactions (SADRs) and toxicity are responsible for a substantial number of extended hospitalizations and fatalities in the United States each year, as well as the exclusion of potential medications from the market and the post-marketing withdrawal of approved drugs [23]. Type A SADRs are predictable occurrences that are dose-related and are based on the drug's pharmacokinetics and pharmacodynamic features. SADRs can also be out of the blue (known as type B idiosyncratically), which is unrelated to dosage, making them much more concerning. Some idiosyncratic SADRs have undergone immuno-allergenic reactions that are still being studied [24]. Pharmacogenomic techniques can identify potential genes associated with ADEs and generate vital biomarkers for screening patients with high risk [25]. The following are some examples of how a genetic marker has been linked to a SADR.

Drug-induced liver injury (DILI), the most prevalent reason for drug withdrawal from the market is DILI. Furthermore, idiosyncratic DILI is responsible for around 13% of acute liver failure in the United States [25]. We can highlight the significance of being capable of identifying patients who are at-risk. The majority of positive genetic-association studies in DILI for particular medications are related to genetic polymorphisms in human leukocyte antigen (HLA) genes or metabolism and transport genes [26, 27]. Flucloxacillin, xilamegatran, and lumiracoxib are examples of drugs that are not available in the United States. Flucloxacillin is an antibiotic used in Europe and Australia to treat staphylococcal infections. In international centers of GWAS, an SNP in the major histo-compatibility complex (MHC), which is nearly related to HLA-B*5701, revealed a highly significant association with flucloxacillin-induced liver failure [27]. Ximelagatran, an inhibitor of thrombin was designed for the curing and chemo-prophylaxis of thromboembolism, which is unsuccessful to meet safety expectations. The retrospective investigation that included both GWAS and large multicentre candidate gene analysis discovered pharmacogenetic relations between increased alanine transaminases and the presence of HLA-DRB1*07 and HLA-DQA1*02 genes [28]. Lumiracoxib, a COX-2 inhibitor (selective), was neither authorized nor withdrawn post-marketing globally due to apprehensions about hepatotoxicity. A GWAS and fine-mapping study has recently discovered a great correlation with the HLA haplotype (HLA-DRB1*1501-HLA-DQB1*0602-HLA-DRB5*0101-HLA-DQA1*0102) which is mostly common [29]. Subsequent studies were performed to reproduce these relationships to "revive the medications," which is demanding. Tribulations may enclose getting well-representative samples from participants experiencing these ADRs in sufficient numbers to allow for GWAS approaches, the involvement of multiple genes, and complicated interactions of gene-environment [30, 31].

In drug causing dermal injury, Abacavir, an anti-human immunodeficiency virus-1 drug, can cause the significant, perhaps deadly type-1 anaphylactic reactions in 5 to 9 percent of treated people. "A double-blind, prospective, randomized multicenter study with 1,956 patients randomly assigned to an HLA-B*5701 prescreening arm or an arm without screening, found that HLA-B*5701T prescreening reduced the risk of hypersensitivity reaction to abacavir." It was considered one of the most valuable pharmacogenetic application in practice. [32]. GWAS studies have recently revealed a link between HLA-A*3101 and carbamazepine-caused potential ADRs in people of Northern European ancestry [33]. Hypersensitivity reactions to allopurinol, which is used in the treatment of hyperuricemia and gout, have also been associated with the HLA-B gene, although with a different allele, HLA-B*5801 [34].

Statin-causing muscular toxicity, Statins treats hyperlipidemia which leads to a variety of myopathies, from minor myalgia to significantly lethal and rare ADRs of rhabdomyolysis. According to a recent GWAS, the SLCO1B1 521T>C SNP is substantially related to myopathy caused by simvastatin [35]. Multiple prospective and retrospective investigations have shown that patients with UGT1A1 reduced function alleles, such as UGT1A1*28, are more likely to develop severe hematological toxicity such as neutropenia. The relation of the UGT1A1 genotype with diarrhea phenotype was not consistent across studies, presumably due to rigorous antidiarrheal medication management [36].

Who Benefits the Most from Efficacy Predictors?

A low percentage of cancer patients can respond to currently known anticancer therapies. Treated patients can also acquire resistance to medication in a short time. Tumor pharmacogenomics exhibit a variety of structural genomic alterations and can be quite diverse. That diversity was seen in patients with similar tumor types as well as within the same cancer patients when different tumor locations are evaluated at the molecular and cellular levels. Oncology pharmacogenomics is a rich prospect of personalizing therapy for certain patients due to this significant variability and the narrow therapeutic index of many anticancer drugs [37, 38]. Tumor types, traditionally separated and classed based on histology, can be also differentiated into molecular subsets. The subgroups can be distinguished through particular genetic abnormalities that "drive" the tumor (the so-called "oncogenic drivers") and be important related to its survival (e.g., point mutations, translocations, amplification). The majority of these genetic changes are acquired or somatic, meaning they are only seen in tumor tissue. With a better understanding of the tumor molecular landscape and signaling, antineoplastic drugs targeting these specific tumor molecular changes (usually in the drug target or related pathway) have been developed. With this technique, impressive response rates have been found in a molecularly defined subset of patients who are positive for the alteration and/or negative for alterations associated with resistance to therapy. This focusing strategy is also believed to have a higher safety profile than most chemotherapy drugs, which are nonselective and designed to fit everyone. Traditional histology, on the other hand, may be broken into smaller and smaller molecular subsets in this situation, adding complexity and challenging drug design. One of the earliest examples is the use of tamoxifen in estrogen receptor-positive metastatic breast cancer. Table 1 summarizes further examples.

Table 1. Examples of targeted oncology drugs and associated tumor molecular changes [39]

Therapeutic agent	Class	Molecular alteration	Tumor type
Tamoxifen	Nonsteroidal antiestrogen	ER expression	Breast
Erlotinib	EGFR TKI	EGFR activating mutation	NSCLC
Lapatinib	EGFR/HER2 TKI	HER2 amplification/overexpression	Breast
Traztuzumab	Monoclonal antibody against HER2	HER2 amplification/overexpression	Breast
Cetuximab/ panitumumab	Monoclonal antibody against EGFR	KRAS mutation a	mCRC
Imatinib	ABL TKI b	BCR-ABL fusion gene by chromosomal translocation	CML
Crizotinib	ALK TKI	ALK rearrangement (e.g., EML4-ALK)	NSCLC
Vemurafenib	BRAF STK inhibitor	BRAF V600E mutation	Melanoma

"*TKI* tyrosine kinase inhibitor, *STK* serine/threonine kinase inhibitor, *mCRC* metastatic colorectal cancer, *NSCLC* non-*small-cell lung cancer, CML chronic myelogenous leukemia.*

Genes: ER(ESR1) estrogen receptor 1; EGFR epidermal growth factor receptor; ERBB2 (HER2) v-erb-b2 erythroblastic leukemia viral oncogene homolog 2, neuro/glioblastoma derived oncogene homolog (avian); KRAS v-Ki-ras2.

Kirsten rat sarcoma viral oncogene homolog; BCR-ABL breakpoint cluster region-Abl tyrosine kinase; EML4-ALK echinoderm microtubule associated protein like 4-anaplastic lymphoma receptor tyrosine kinase; BRAF v-raf murine sarcoma viral oncogene homolog B1.

a. Lack of benefit from therapy in KRAS mutant mCRC.

b. Only relevant target to tumor type was indicated."

Design of Clinical Trials and Drug Development

Pharmacogenomic approaches have been successfully implemented throughout the development phase, from preclinical to phase 3 trials, as well as the post-approval (Figure 1) [40]. In preclinical research, pharmacogenomics could help in the developing of a biological rationale and examine the potential for polymorphic drug kinetics. When the (drug disposition) pathway is known to be polymorphic in early phase clinical trials, pharmacogenomics can be used to exclude patients with lower function alleles (poor metabolizers) or to drive a genotype-guided dosage approach in later phase studies. Furthermore, drug interaction researches can aid in determining the phenotypes' role with impaired normal physiology and biotransformation. The patients' samples gathered for the investigations, on the other hand, were evaluated retrospectively to define the effect of polymorphisms on medication pharmacokinetics and pharmacodynamics [41]. The data gained in these promising studies were helpful to construct phase 3 trials in the future. It can be used to identify individuals who are seeming to be responsive to medication and to exclude those who are at risk of adverse events based on pharmacokinetics or pharmacodynamics. A variety of enrichment strategies based on genetic markers can also be carried out at any stage of the clinical improvement process [40]. Pharmacogenomics also has clinical uses in diseases discovery and risk stratification, diagnosis, disease prognosis expectations, and disease surveillance and drug monitoring as shown in Figure 1 [42].

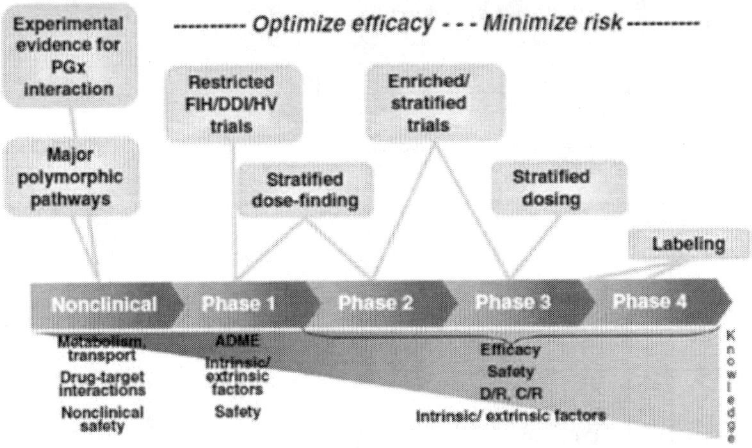

Figure 1. Pharmacogenomic maneuvers in drug development. PGx: Pharmacogenomic, FIH: Frist in human, DDI: Drug-drug interactions, HV: Healthy volunteers, ADME: Absorption, distribution, metabolism, excretion, D/R: Dose-response, C/R: Concentration- response.

Hereafter Prospects

Oncology, psychiatric illnesses, and anticoagulation/thrombosis were the top three therapy areas of pharmacogenetics trials [37]. This snapshot captures the primary driving reasons behind pharmacogenetics and pharmacogenomics approaches, such as efforts to reduce side events and improve successful therapy through specifying the right patient to much correct drug and dose regimen. In psychiatric diseases, therapeutic failure concerning to unspecified therapy may also lead to the employment of pharmacogenetic approaches. It is believed that 40–60% of people must modify their initial prescribed antidepressant. In terms of anticoagulation and thrombosis, the majority of the research described utilized warfarin, which has a limited therapeutic index, significant inter-individual and ethnic heterogeneity related to dose requirements, and a well-known genetic factor attributed with the drug response. What are our plans? GWAS approaches make use of genotype-phenotype associations. One of the rate-limit steps of these methods is the gathering of systematic and specific phenotypes in many studies to study these relations. The problem here is that the current quantity of genomic data has not been matched by large-scale, precise, standardized phenotypic data on individuals—so-called "phenomes." The term "phenomics" was used for describing a rapidly developing "omic" area dedicated to the large-scale study of high-dimensional phenotypes that integrates numerous layers of biology, ranging from molecules to signaling pathways to systems to behavior in health and disease. To provide insights into how genetic variation translates into phenotypes, it is necessary to conduct systematic and thorough acquisition and analysis of phenotypes using diverse methodologies (e.g., omic technologies, clinical, biochemical, imaging) at a high throughput level. The issues of phenomics are similar to those faced by genomics in its early days; how to gather and apply complete (omic; in this case, phenotypic) data. Several phenome projects are currently underway [43]. Steps have also been launched to unify phenotypic criteria for discovery and validation. Phenotypes in major adverse drug reactions, such as drug-induced liver injury, drug-induced skin injury, and drug-induced torsade de pointes, are examples [44]. This purpose of standards and increased phenotype granularity (subtitled "deep phenotyping") may reduce sample heterogeneity and measurement error, resulting in increased study power, improved diagnostics, and, ultimately, a better understanding of genotype-phenotype associations, outcomes, and treatment responses [43, 45, 46]. Following the genomics revolution, phenomics is the next step. It is a vital step to bridge the gap between the laboratory and clinical practice.

Pharmacogenomics Testing and Drug Labeling

Genetic testing can enable targeted actions to prevent or treat disease or its effects. Understanding the limitations and problems of various testing methodologies is critical to improving health and quality of life. The genotype is the DNA blueprint that is associated with the clinical outcomes of a trait or disease (the phenotype). Genetic testing can refer to any form of testing that aids in determining a person's genotype. It can be estimated for germline cells (which give rise to the vast majority of cells in the body) or specific somatic cells such as tumor cells.

In two different settings, the term "genotyping" is used differently:

- Genotype determination
- Guides to the special type of microarray that defines the genotype for a subset of selected nucleotide variants.

According to 2015 advice from the American College of Medical Genetics and Genomics (ACMG) and the Association for Molecular Pathology (AMP), the nomenclature used to describe the results of clinical genetic testing is shifting [47]. This guidance aims to avoid using general, derogatory, or ambiguous terminology like mutation or polymorphism, which refer to genetic variation but do not explain whether the variation is associated with disease.

The term "variant" is used in the ACMG guidance to refer to variance from a reference sequence; variants are categorized into one of five categories for clinical testing [47].

- Benign
- Likely benign
- Pathogenic
- Likely pathogenic (at least 90 percent confidence in pathogenicity)
- Variant of uncertain (or unknown) significance (VUS).

In general, pathogenic or possibly pathogenic variations are regarded as suitable for involvement in clinical care. Pathogenic variations will be referred to as both pathogenic and likely pathogenic variants. These identifications represent the degree of certainty that a mutation is linked to the disease phenotype, but they do not indicate the likelihood of disease development. Factually, the presence of certain genetic variations, as well as other factors such as inheritance type (recessive or dominant), penetrance and expressivity, the individual's age, and other contributory genetic and environmental factors, all influence disease likelihood. The classification of a variant is based on available data, which includes family studies (testing of additional family members, such as parents, can determine if the variant segregates with disease in a family), epidemiologic data, and laboratory testing, which can include functional studies in cells or animals (demonstration of modified protein function) [47].

The term "mutation" is still used in a variety of contexts, including discussions of known mutations, disease pathophysiology, and laboratory procedures.

The phrase single nucleotide polymorphism (SNP) has been used to describe variants found in a significant proportion of the usual, or healthy, population (traditionally defined as >1%). However, as previously stated, when referring to genetic testing, this word might be ambiguous. SNP is also used to describe a sort of panel testing that only looks for a subset of nucleotide alterations (as in "SNP array"). This can be done by DNA testing for the suspected ailment(s)and information on the genetic cause(s) of the condition or presenting features. Selective variations (specific nucleotide substitutions or other alterations) or the complete gene (every coding nucleotide and the nucleotides near the splice sites in the gene's coding region) can be evaluated for each gene. The method employed is determined by the objective of the testing as well as the present state of knowledge about the mutations in that gene that can cause disease. For example: Siblings and offspring of a pathogenic BRCA1 variant carrier can be screened for the familial pathogenic variant rather than all known pathogenic BRCA1 variants. When the majority of cases are caused by a small number of variants, one approach is to genotype for the most common variants first, followed by a reflex to more comprehensive testing of all potential variants (e.g., using sequencing) if the initial testing is negative but the disease is still a concern.

Sequencing is a technique. The more thorough approach to sequencing entails examining all nucleotides across the gene to detect all potentially harmful or likely pathogenic variations. Sequencing has two key advantages: it tests all sites in the gene and it can identify unusual variants that would not be found using genotyping panels.

The copy number variation is in addition to screening for single base-pair alterations, detection of exon or gene deletions or duplications is frequently required as part of a clinical evaluation. In the term, an entire chromosomal analysis is performed. Certain illnesses, such as Down syndrome (trisomy 21), are linked to chromosome aneuploidies. Segmental chromosomal gains and losses, also known as CNVs, chromosome translocations, or other structural rearrangements, can be linked to genetic disorders.

Testing Methods

Genetic testing can refer to any type of testing that helps determine an individual's genotype (The genotype can be defined as the DNA blueprint that is associated with the clinical manifestations of a trait or disease). It can be determined for the germline (cells arising from the germ cells and applicable to most cells in the body) or for selected somatic cells such as tumor cells [71].

There are many methods to detect genetic diseases to personalize a specific treatment option. Direct DNA analysis take two ways:

1. Using microarray analysis to assess the copy number of sections of chromosome.
2. Determining information of DNA sequence [73].

Choosing the appropriate method relies on the presenting feature(s), the availability of tests for the suspected condition(s), and the available genetic information of the condition or presenting feature [73].

Later in this chapter, genetics testing methods and its clinical applications will be explain with more details.

Self-Assessment Questions

1. What is the difference between Pharmacogenomics and Epigenetic?
2. Who is at Risk for Pharmacogenomics and ADEs?
3. Who Benefits the Most from Efficacy Predictors?

Personalized Medicine

Definition of Personalized Medicine

Personalized medicine (PM) also known for precision medicine is based on tailoring a treatment individualized to patient specific disease. PM is based on identifying genetic, epigenomic, and clinical data that will allow us to gain a better understanding of how a person's unique genomic profile makes him susceptible to certain diseases. In addition to the traditional approach (One-Size-Fits-All), PM approach is a complete extension to enhancing our ability to predict the precise diagnosis of the diseases and which medical treatments will be safe and effective for individual patient [48, 49].

Personalized medicine supporters point to its potential for considerable health advantages for patients, practitioners, and society, including: Better medical judgement; Treatments that are adapted to a patient's sequence variations or genotype rather than the general population; Enhanced disease preventive measures, such as lifestyle and behavioral modifications, as well as pharmaco-prevention; Avoidance of ineffective drugs; It can reduce exposure to potentially harmful drugs, which leads to a lower incidence of treatment-related adverse effects and consequences

History Relevant to Personalized Medicine

When talking about history of personalized medicine there had been many initiatives throughout the history. For reasons of brevity, we will only focus the most basic theme behind personalized medicine. In 1902, the first account of recessive inheritance in humans was published.

Sir Archibald Garrod, an Oxford-educated physician, established the first relation between genetic inheritance and inheritance low of Mendel on one hand and susceptibility to various diseases on other hand. [50]. Garrod studied many rare diseases with obvious, visible phenotypic manifestations as alkaptonuria, albinism, cystinuria and pentosuria. Among these conditions, his research on alkaptonuria gained him some popularity when he discovered that some members of families with alkaptonuria had measurably outlying values for some specific basic biochemical assays, such as urine, compared to family members who did not have alkaptonuria. This led him to a conclusion that alkaptonuria developed because 'altered course of metabolism' between affected individuals, which was later proven correct [51]. Although personalized medicine has its origins in genetic studies, it is agreed widely that other factors, such as environmental factors, developmental phenomena and epigenetic modifications, and behaviors, must all be considered when determining the most appropriate treatment for an individual patient [52].

Benefits of Wide Application of Personalized Medicine

Better understanding of the underlying mechanisms by which various diseases occur. Provide treatments that are tailored to a patient's sequence variants rather than the unspecific treatment that fits the general population. Customize disease-prevention strategies, such as lifestyle and behavioral changes, as well as pharmaco-prevention. Avoid prescribing medication with low efficacy. Reduced exposure to potentially toxic medications, resulting in a lower incidence of treatment-related side effects and complications. Identify different genetic mutation that leaded to drug resistance [53]. Several studies have shown that having genetic information available improves patient adherence to behavior modification and other disease prevention strategies as the following examples:

Smoking cessation: Smokers who tested severely AAT deficient were significantly more likely to report a quit attempt (59%) than were those who tested normal (26%).

Alpha-1 antitrypsin (AAT) is an enzyme important for lung function. its deficiency has many implications specially in smokers. In a study of 199 Smokers who tested severely AAT deficient (homozygous for an AAT null allele) were significantly more likely to report a quit attempt (59%) than either mutation carriers (heterozygotes; 34%) or individuals with a normal genotype (26%) [54].

Another example illustrating that having genetic risk factor for a disease may be a motive for patients to take a step toward modifying their behavior toward a positive of their illness. In a study of 261 smokers individuals those who were informed that they had genetic risk factors for heart disease were more likely to report a desire to quit than individuals in a high-risk (but non-genetic) group. A considerable proportion of respondents said their decisions were influenced by the belief that quitting smoking would result in fewer heart attacks [55].

Familial hypercholesteremia: a study involving 781 patients suffering from familial hypercholesterolemia revealed that use cholesterol-lowering medication has increased from 51% to 81%two years after learning genotype status in addition, significant reductions in low-density lipoprotein C levels were noted [56].

Oncology pharmacogenetics, there are numerous therapy protocols for different types of cancer. Guidelines for determining the most appropriate treatment would help in the initiation of successful therapy at the earliest feasible time. Pharmacogenomics can be a useful tool in the selection of appropriate therapy based on individual variations in the drug pathway genes to avoid medication failure [4].

Examples of Personalized Medicine initiatives

There have been a great many examples of interventions tailored to individual patient profiles, virtually all of them based on genetic profiles:

Mutation-Specific Therapies

Rather than developing a drug and then assessing factors that reduce its safety and effectiveness through observational and follow up studies on individuals given the drug, as with warfarin and imatinib, there are now efforts to identify, for example, genetic profiles possessed by patients and then design therapies that uniquely target those profiles [48].

For example, ivacaftor is a drug used for cystic fibrosis treatment, a disease which have a unique gene mutation in CFTR gene. the CFTR gene's encoded protein has many functions one of them is to act as gate like structure that open and close to control the movement of salts in and out of cells. Different mutations in the CFTR gene cause different types of dysfunctions one of which is interfering with the opening and clothing of gate mechanism. the close of the gate causing a build-up of mucus and other material in the lungs. Ivacaftor is designed to open the gate for longer periods of time in the presence of certain mutations that tend to cause the gate to be closed. Therefore, ivacaftor is only useful for the small subset of CF patients whose CFTR mutations lead to this specific gating problem [57].

Personalizing Early Detection Strategies

It is important for an individual to be monitored if he or she has high risk factors for a disease or susceptible to recurrence of a disease. To make claims about evidence or signs of disease or a pathogenic process, it is now believed that such monitoring should be done using 'personal thresholds' rather than 'population thresholds.'

Personal thresholds are based primarily on legacy values of a measure, or a measure collected on an individual over time, which are used to predict how deviant future values of that indicator may be for that individual. Population thresholds are obtained from epidemiologic data and population surveys, for instance, cholesterol levels higher than 200 as a predictor of risk for coronary artery disease, or systolic blood pressure higher than 140 as an indicator of high blood pressure, stroke risk, or heart disease [58].

Drescher et al. [59], for example, investigated the utility of personal thresholds implemented to longitudinal CA125 levels gathered on a group of women, who developed ovarian cancer. The authors discovered that, except for one case, using personal thresholds would have detected the occurrence of ovarian cancer one year earlier than using population thresholds.

Personalizing Disease Prevention

There are many examples of the influence of using genetic information on decreasing the incidence of disease development in addition to minimizing complications from standard treatment.

One of these examples about colorectal cancer, the third leading cause of cancer deaths, despite being a highly preventable illness. In 2012 Liao et al. noticed that taking aspirin postoperatively in colorectal cancer patients with somatic mutation in the PIK3CA gene showed decreased risk for cancer-specific deaths and an improvement in overall survival than patients whose cancers had the wild-type PIK3CA gene [60].

More research was done In 2015, by Nan et al. the study reported that risk of developing colorectal cancer with aspirin use varied according individual's genotype, with individuals possessing different genotypes having either lower, higher or no change in their risk of colorectal cancer development with aspirin use(29). Illustrating that aspirin consumption can have serious consequences including intestinal and intracranial hemorrhage, would be ideal to restrict the use of aspirin to those individuals who are genetically predisposed to have a side effect [61].

As another example, in 2018, Jeon et al. focused on the importance to use expanded risk prediction models for identifying when to start screening for colorectal cancer. Currently the guidelines only use two variables: age and family history. Jeon et al. showed implementing information about individual's environmental exposure and genetic profile, specifically the existence of colorectal cancer associated genetic variants, would shift recommendations for screening time by 12 years for men and 14 years for women. A person's risk of developing colorectal cancer has been studied and explained using area under the curve (AUC), where an AUC of 1.0 would suggest a model with perfect predictive accuracy, AUC was 0.63 for men and 0.62 for women.

Accuracy of relevant predictions about an individual's risk for colorectal cancer has been studied and suggests that the area under the curve (AUC) value for a model including environmental and genetic factors, where an AUC of 1.0 would suggest a model with perfect predictive accuracy, was 0.63 for men and 0.62 for women when taking environmental exposure and genetic profile in consideration. This is compared to an AUC value of 0.53 (men) 0.54 (women) when only family history information was considered [62].

The Relationship between Personalized Medicine and Pharmacogenetics

Personalized medicine is based on pharmacogenetics. Patients with a variety of diseases like cancer routinely undergo genetic testing as part of patient care, enabling physicians to select treatments that improve chances of survival and reduce exposure to adverse effects.

Genetic testing can refer to any type of testing that helps determine an individual's genotype (The genotype can be defined as the DNA blueprint that is associated with the clinical manifestations of a trait or disease). It can be determined for the germline (cells arising from the germ cells and applicable to most cells in the body) or for selected somatic cells such as tumor cells. [63].

American College of Medical Genetics and Genomics (ACMG) uses the term variant, which refers to variation from a reference sequence; for clinical testing, variants are classified into one of five categories Pathogenic: likely pathogenic (at least 90 percent confidence in pathogenicity), variant of uncertain (or unknown) significance (VUS), likely benign and benign [63].

Purpose of Genetic Testing

Diagnostic Genetic Testing

Used to make or confirm the clinical diagnosis of a disorder. For hereditary cancer syndromes, diagnostic testing may be a useful tool for identifying the most appropriate treatment strategies. Examples include more extensive or less extensive cancer surgeries or use of targeted chemotherapy or biologic therapy known to be effective or ineffective in tumors with certain genotypes [64].

Predictive Testing

Used to predict disease risk (pre-symptomatic testing). Predictive testing is a way to assess risk of a disease in patient who has strong hereditary factors. Knowledge of an elevated risk for a specific disease may contribute to risk-reduction interventions. Increased monitoring or prophylactic surgery for variants linked to hereditary cancer syndromes, or additional testing or interventions for variants linked to hypertrophic cardiomyopathy are examples of predictive testing importance [64].

Carrier testing identifies unaffected carriers of an autosomal recessive disorder or of a sex-linked disorder or a balanced chromosomal rearrangement. Carrier analysis can be conducted in families with a family history of a particular genetic condition or in specific populations where pathogenic variants for a specific condition are relatively common, such as Tay Sachs disease in people of Ashkenazi Jewish ancestry [64].

Extent of DNA Analysis

There are many methods to detect genetic diseases to personalize a specific treatment option. Direct DNA analysis take two ways:

1. Using microarray analysis to assess the copy number of sections of chromosome. used to detect chromosomal deletions and duplications.
2. Determining information of DNA sequence. Sequence variants may be sought in a single gene, in a panel of several or many genes, in the exome or in the whole genome.

Choosing the appropriate method relies on the presenting feature(s), the availability of tests for the suspected condition(s), and the available genetic information of the condition or presenting features [65].

Selected Variants

For some diseases analysis of only one or two genetic variants is enough to confirm a diagnosis as: hereditary hemochromatosis is associated with the presence of two variants, p.Cys282Tyr (p.C282Y) and p.His63Asp (p.H63D), so testing for the presence of these variants alone is reasonable and omits extraneous information.

Another example of individual variant genotyping is testing a specific pathogenic BRCA1 variant in high-risk patients whom siblings and first degree relatives are carriers for the same specific variant. Which will be more specific than analyzing all known pathogenic BRCA1 variants [66].

Entire Gene

Analysis of the entire gene is important in some diseases where the disease has many pathogenic variants to which disease gene is highly sensitive and this variants occur at many locations along DNA.

Examples include the breast and ovarian cancer genes, BRCA1 and BRCA2 genes involved in breast and ovarian cancer and CFTR gene responsible for cystic fibrosis [65].

Single-Nucleotide Genotyping Panels

For diagnosis of some diseases testing for the presence of the most common variants is done first, followed by a more detailed comprehensive testing of all potential variants. this is mostly applied when if the initial testing is negative but the patient has a high for the disease. This method is commonly used for cystic fibrosis inspection, where a panel of 25 CFTR gene variants correctly classifies more than 90% of patients of European ancestry. Although, in non-European ancestry, extensive testing should be regarded. as some rarer ethnic variants are not well represented on these panels [67].

Sequencing – is a more comprehensive approach in which all nucleotides across the gene are evaluated to recognize all possible pathogenic or likely pathogenic variants. In addition to genotyping panel, sequencing allows testing all genes' positions, so that rare variants that are difficult to be included on genotyping panels can be easily identified. As in hemophilia B where the initial sequencing of f9 gene is important. Sequencing has two types the first, "gene sequencing panels," can be limited to one gene, to a set of genes involved in a related disease. Another type is "extended genome-wide" or if it is limited to coding regions of all genes, it is called (whole exome sequencing)or (WES). This gene involves in coding and noncoding regions, it is called (whole genome sequencing) or (WGS). Sequencing can be performed using traditional methods (Sanger sequencing) or next generation sequencing (NGS) methods. NGS uses massive parallel sequencing in a high throughput format. consequently, it can produce a huge amount of sequence data (the entire exome or genome) orders of magnitude faster than traditional methods [68].

Entire chromosome – it is called chromosome analysis or karyotyping, in order to detect anomalies, patient chromosomes are evaluated to determine their number and structure. Chromosome analysis is done to help in the diagnosis of many Some disorders as Down syndrome (trisomy 21) caused by the presence of an extra chromosome (21) and chronic myelogenous leukemia caused by a translocation between chromosome number9 and 22 (9;22). Prenatal detection of chromosome abnormalities is now widely used to detect fetal chromosome aberrations early in pregnancy. This method helps parents to seek counseling about the right decision if an abnormality is detected. Noninvasive prenatal screening (NIPS) using cell-free DNA is increasingly being used instead of (or in addition to) invasive testing such as amniocentesis for prenatal detection of chromosome abnormalities [69].

Direct to Consumer Testing (DTC)

Conventional or traditional Genetic testing is a process in which physicians collect clinically necessary samples from patients and send them to a laboratory for genetic analysis. according to the results they discuss the best therapeutic options with patients. On the other hand, Direct-to-consumer (DTC) genetic testing is different. The consumers learn about DTC genetic testing from TV commercials, the internet, or in-store advertising, and request that the tests be conducted by DTC companies of their selection. If conventional genetic testing is a clinician-based test, then DTC genetic testing is a consumer-based one [70]. This included testing for risk variants associated with certain medical conditions as celiac disease, factor XI deficiency, G6PD deficiency, and late-onset Alzheimer disease. as well as ancestry testing (also called genealogy testing. In the Impact of Personal Genomics Study survey, 54 of 961 respondents

(5.6 percent) who had recently undergone DTC testing reported either starting a new medication or changing a medication they were already taking based on the results of DTC tests. Results of DTC testing should not be used to make a new diagnosis or initiate a new treatment without returning to a physician to take the proper treatment action suitable ensures the result applies to the tested individual [71].

Other Personalized Medicine Platforms

The early focus of personalized medicine was the use and the development of genetic-based tests. Other strategies referred as "omic" are established to provide a more complete characterization of risk, including variability in genetic regulation, epigenetics, and cellular metabolism.

Transcriptomics also called Gene expression profiling – is based on analysis of mRNA (of individual genes or panels of gene targets). the whole transcriptome analysis (also known as RNA-Seq) is also possible and can be used for variant interpretation analysis. Expression of gene is vulnerable to many factors as cellular, genetic, and environmental factors, which makes gene expression a particularly a unique target for profiling malignant cells [72].

Microbiomics: is the study of the microbes (typically bacteria) that live in or on an individual. An example is the gut bacteria which may affect the immunity or chance of obesity [73].

Epigenomics is the study of the DNA alteration (often methylation) that influence gene expression. Unlike genomic changes, epigenomic changes are influenced by the environment and can change with age, stress, or exposure to the individual or previous generations [74].

Metabolomics is the large-scale study of small molecules, commonly known as metabolites, within cells, biofluids, tissues or organism. It has a role in detection of disease, such as necrosis, Alzheimer's, and inflammation, evaluation of toxicity (especially liver toxicity) in new drugs it is also an important tool that can identify cancer biomarkers and drivers of tumorigenesis.

Proteomics is the qualitative and quantitative examination of a biological sample's protein composition. These procedures, which are typically performed using modified polyacrylamide gelelectrophoresis (PAGE) or matrix-assisted laser desorption/ionization (MALDI) methodologies, enable measurements of the kinds and quantities of proteins in a biological sample. Certain malignancies are being studied using proteomics tests.

These applications are increasingly being used in clinical practice, and efforts are being made to develop reliable, assays for these platforms. In oncology, for example, gene expression profiling of malignant cells is becoming a major diagnostic and prognostic tool.

One of the earliest example is and implementations of gene expression profiling in oncology focused on single genes, is determining estrogen receptor expression status in breast cancer for informing prognosis and chemotherapeutic options Additionally, whole transcriptome expression profiling techniques have been applied to tumor.0samples with high success rates [75].

Obstacles for Implementation

Despite early successes in the introduction of a limited number of pharmacogenetic analysis, multiple barriers prevent the widespread application of personalized medicine as standard clinical practice across all medical fields. The development of validated biomarkers and genetic assays represents an important obstacle, as does the amount of data resulting from genetic testing and the high cost of most genetic assay. Other ethical and data storage challenges will remain [76].

Limited Predictive Value of Most Tests

PM has only limited examples where genetic testing make a remarkable rule in guiding therapeutic recommendations for healthy individuals, although diagnostic genetic testing may be very effective for recurrence risk estimation. However, in for example oncology field there are an increasing number of variants associated with disease susceptibility and pharmacogenetic variations [76].

Lack of Physician Knowledge

The lack of knowledge about the general concepts of genetic health care member specially the physician. Besides many medical practitioners do not feel they are prepared enough to provide counseling genetic testing [50] and the number of clinical geneticists in North America and in some other countries is considered to be low to meet expected demands [77].

Inadequate Informatics Infrastructure

The record-keeping for clinical laboratory data record for each patient in health care facilities is not adequate to accommodate for NGS data required for sequencing. Although newer approaches that include an easily accessible electronic medical record (EMR) are under development. the majority of those in place would need substantial improvement to accommodate the data storage and processing needs anticipated for genomic data [77].

Presence of Interfering Data

Analysis of the masses of data than can result from next-generation sequencing (NGS) technologies and much of this data can be of no remarkable importance of the target of the test and can be misleading [78].

Information Provenance and Patient Privacy Issues

Many questions arise when considering how personal genomic information should be managed. Who is the responsible for ordering genetic test and how much information should be transferred to other health care team whom patient deals with.

Would the pediatrician be responsible for dealing with data related to a condition of adulthood onset. and should the clinician inform his patients if result of the test tell that the disease has no cure [63].

Reimbursement and Financial Issues

Changes in the reimbursement policies is required needed to enhance personalized medicine initiative to be applied widely in many health care aspects. Several attempts is needed to modify the Medicare clinical laboratory fee schedule to accommodate the reimbursement for complex genetic tests [79].

Genetic Discrimination

Discrimination based on who should have the test or the results of genetic testing or denial of insurance coverage. Many jurisdictions such as the Genetic Insurance Non-discrimination Act (GINA) in the United States have tried to put protections in place. So, no patient can feel uncomfortable to undergo these testing [79].

Societal Issues and Misconceptions

Concern that misconception of the importance of genetic testing may result in a medicalization of society, whereby healthy individuals become preoccupied or obsessed with disease prevention based on their DTC results and undergo unnecessary tests or procedures. One study of individuals who underwent DTC genome profiling found no measurable evidence for increased anxiety, comparing baseline and post-testing anxiety scores.

Genome sequencing may recognize "high-risk" alleles or pathogenic variants in some individuals. With the limited available understanding of risk concepts or penetrance of mutations and risk alleles, this could make patient uncomfortable and lead to incorrect desions.in addition some patient may develop depressed mode when advised of increased risk for sensitive issues, such as oncological disorders or behavioral traits. Acceptance of genetically based treatment recommendations may be low, among certain families. the revelation or failure to reveal genetic information may have an impact on family dynamics [78].

Self-Assessment Questions

1. Purpose of genetic testing involve all the following except:
   a. Diagnostic genetic testing
   b. Predictive genetic testing
   c. Carrier testing
   d. Next generation sequencing

2. Which of the following is considered a limitation of PM?
   a. Reimbursement and financial issues
   b. Lack of physician knowledge
   c. Inadequate informatics infrastructure
   d. All the above

3. Concerning other PM platforms what of the following is based on Analysis of mRNA (individual genes or panels of gene targets)
   a. Epigenomics
   b. Transcriptomics
   c. Metabolomics
   d. Microbiomics

4. A more comprehensive approach in which all nucleotides across the gene are evaluated to recognize all possible pathogenic variants
   a. Single-nucleotide genotyping panels
   b. Sequencing
   c. Selected variants analysis
   d. Non of the above.

Application of Personalized Medicine in Oncology

Oncology is perhaps the most established field of medicine where the application of pharmacogenomics and personalized meet. The primary role of molecular oncology often focusses on somatically mutated genes, germline genetic variation that can affect some cancer treatments.

This chapter provides an overview of some germline or constitutional DNA variants that associated with inter-individual variability in response (either safety or efficacy) in cancer treatment.

Polymorphic variant alleles are frequently found in genes coding for metabolism enzymes, this enzyme can convert a prodrug to its active form or catalyze the elimination of the drug outside the body. One of these enzymes is the cytochrome P450 (CYP450) superfamily, which has a direct impact on the pharmacokinetics of many drugs.

Furthermore, genetic variations in cell surface receptors can alter drug transport, affecting pharmacodynamics as well [80].

Oncology supportive care deals with side effects resulting from chemotherapeutic agents with the target of dealing with them while eradicating cancerous cells. Having certain genetic pathogenic variants can make this adverse effect even worse and makes traditional treatment options ineffective. So, the identification of Germline variation can potentially be very important in the selection and administration of cancer drugs. It has been difficult to demonstrate clinical utility for cancer pharmacogenetic testing, and this is an ongoing area of research.

Clinical tests for a restricted number of genes with clinical validity are currently available. Cancer treatments and associated genes with germline genetic variants that affect patient response will be discussed focusing on examples of higher degree of evidence will be discussed in detail below [81].

Fluoropyrimidines and DPYD Molecular Target

The fluoropyrimidines agent including 5-fluorouracil (5-FU) and its oral inactive prodrugs tegafur and capecitabine, they are indicated for treating many solid tumors as colorectal cancer, breast cancer and other gastrointestinal tract cancers.

The primary mechanism of 5-FU activation is inhibition of the thymidylate synthase enzyme, which is included in the folate homocysteine cycle as well as purine and pyrimidine synthesis. Furthermore, the fluorouridine triphosphate metabolite can be integrated into RNA instead of uridine triphosphate, causing RNA processing and protein synthesis to be disrupted [82]. 5-FU owes a narrow therapeutic index and, in spite of being generally tolerated. However, about 10- 40% of individuals who receive 5-FU develop severe toxicity as nausea, vomiting, neutropenia, severe diarrhea, mucositis, stomatitis, and hand-foot syndrome.

Table 2. CPIC recommended dosing of fluoropyrimidines by DPYD genotype/phenotype

Phenotype (genotype)	Examples of diplotypes	Implication s for phenotypic measures	Dosing recommendations
Homozygous or compound heterozygous variant DPD deficiency, at risk for toxicity with drug exposure (two nonfunctional alleles	*2/*2 *2/*13 *13/*13	drugs Complete DPD deficiency and increased risk for severe or even fatal drug toxicity when treated with fluoropyrimidine drugs	Select another alternative drug
Heterozygous or intermediate activity (one functional allele 1, plus one nonfunction al allele)	*1/*2 *1/*13	Decreased DPD activity (Leukocyte DPD by activity at 30-70% that of the normal population). And increased risk for severe or even fatal drug toxicity when treated with fluoropyrimidine drugs.	Start with at least a 50% reduction in starting dose followed by titration of dose based pharmacokinetic test (if available).
Homozygous wild-type or normal, high DPD activity (two or more functional 1 alleles)	*1/*1	Normal DPD activity and "normal" risk for fluoropyrimidine tox city	Use label - recommended dosage and administration

(DPD) * dihydropyrimidine dehydrogenase enzyme, (CPIC) * Clinical Pharmacogenetics Implementation Consortium.

The rate-limiting step of 5-FU enzyme is dihydropyrimidine dehydrogenase (DPD) converting 5-FU to dihydrofluorouracil [83]. Notably, multiple germline genetic polymorphism in the DPYD gene on chromosome 1p21.3 cause decreased DPD activity and increased drug half-life. Approximately 3–8% of patients, depending on ethnicity, have partial DPYD. deficiency, elevating 5-FU exposure by 1.5 times comparing to normal DPYD activity.

Complete DPYD deficiency is uncommon (prevalence 0.1-0.2%), but it might lead to life threatening toxicities when exposed to regular doses of 5-FU.

Clinical Pharmacogenetics Implementation Consortium (CPIC) set guidelines regarding patients with DPYD variant suggesting a 50% decline in initial dose for heterozygous patients for a nonfunctional DPYD enzyme variant and for those who are homozygous or compound heterozygous for two nonfunctional DPYD variants an alternate therapy should be considered as shown in Table 2 [84].

Genetic Testing

For DPYD, genetic testing can be performed by DNA extraction from blood or from other tissues, which usually entails genotyping the DPYD 2A reduced activity allele [85]. However, other different variant alleles may have been identified. Some labs may offer whole gene DPYD sequencing, which will recognize all known and new sequence variants, although many of which may be clinically insignificant [85].

Limitations of Testing: DPYD

Because targeted DPYD genotyping cannot detect alleles that have not been directly investigated, genotyping with a negative result doesn't really exclude the likelihood that a patient has another DPYD variant. Although complete gene sequencing will identify all DPYD variants, infrequent or new variants will most likely be of unknown clinical relevance. Furthermore, other genes, such as ABCB1, MTHFR, and TYMS (which will not be detected by DPYD genetic testing), could have an impact on responses to 5-FU [86].

Tamoxifen and CYP2D6

Cytochrome (CYP2D6) is one member of P450 metabolizing enzymes. CYP2D6 play a key role in a phase I metabolism. It participates in the metabolism of nearly 25% of all licensed drugs. CYP2D6 is associated with interindividual genetic polymorphism. About 5-10% of the population are called poor metabolizer (PM) as they carry 2 nonfunctional alleles. while 1–30% are ultrarapid metabolizers as they carry duplications of functional alleles [87].

Tamoxifen is a SERMs (selective estrogen receptor modulator). it inhibits cancerous (ER) estrogen receptor positive cells from having the required estrogen for growth. Although, its metabolites also function as aromatase inhibitors, lowering the amount of estrogen in the body [88]. Tamoxifen metabolism is complex, with most of the metabolism mediated via the 4-hydroxylation and N-demethylation pathways, each of which produce the extremely potent secondary metabolite Endoxifen. Endoxifen which is considered the primary metabolite responsible for the efficacy of tamoxifen treatment. Andis is formed from N-desmethyltamoxifen primarily through hydroxylation by cytochrome P450- 2D6 (CYP2D6) [89].

Therapeutic levels of endoxifen are rapidly achieved in for ultrarapid and normal metabolizers in addition, it is recommended to begin with standard dose of (20 mg/d) besides, they should avoid concomitant administration of other drugs moderate/strong CYP2D6 inhibitors [90].

On the other hand, CYP2D6 PMs typically have reduced levels of endoxifen than those who are extensive metabolizers, as a result, reduced efficacy and worse prognosis are expected. consequently, guidelines recommend that PMs take an alternative therapy such as aromatase inhibitors and if it is contraindicated, an increase in tamoxifen is warranted to 40 mg/d [90].

Many studies on the potential pharmacogenetic association between tamoxifen response and CYP2D6 genotype have been conducted based on the highly polymorphic nature of the CYP2D6 gene on chromosome 22q13.2 and the central role that CYP2D6 plays in the metabolism tamoxifen to endoxifen, some of these studies found a link between loss-of-function CYP2D6 alleles and poor prognoses [91].

Others, however, found no link and concluded that clinical CYP2D6 genotyping is unnecessary [92].

These contradictory findings have prompted ongoing debate about the clinical relevance of CYP2D6 in tamoxifen response, in addition to a recent meta-analysis by the International Tamoxifen Pharmacogenomics Consortium (ITPC. The ITPC, clarified the link between CYP2D6 being poor metabolizer and poorer invasive disease-free survival hazard ratio51.25; 95% CI51.06, 1.47; P50.009. Nevertheless, this happened only when post-hoc rigorous inclusion criteria (e.g., dose, duration of treatment, menopausal status, and genotyping quality) were used, as no effect was found when limited or no exclusion criteria were used among the heterogeneous study populations [93]. While much work had been done in the last few years to standardize patient inclusion criteria, in addition to disease and outcome phenotypes, the clinical utility and implementation of CYP2D6 genotyping prior to tamoxifen therapy remains debatable.

Irinotecan and UGT1A1

Molecular Target

Irinotecan is used to treat metastatic colorectal cancer. It is usually given in conjunction with other anticancer medications (e.g., 5-FU, leucovorin). It is also used in advanced small cell lung cancer combined with cisplatin. Irinotecan inhibits activity of topoisomerase I enzyme and thus preventing DNA replication causing cell death. Irinotecan is metabolized to its active SN-38, which is glucoronized to SN-38 glucoronic acid (SN-38G) which enter the liver to be detoxified via conjugation by the uridine diphosphate glucuronosyltransferase (UGT) 1A1 enzyme, this enzyme releases SN-38G into the intestines for elimination.

The most significant variant UGT1A1 allele is the *28 allele, which is a promoter polymorphism with seven thymine-adenine (TA) dinucleotide repeats, whereas the normal allele has six thymine-adenine (TA) dinucleotide repeats. This abnormal allele decreases UGT function by about 70%. The prevalence of the *28 allele is 51% in Africans, while in Caucasians is 29-45%, 16% in Asian populations. the allele which is responsible for reducing UGT1 activity in Asian patients is UGT1A1*6 [94].

Furthermore, UGT1A1*228 heterozygotes show a 25% reduction in enzyme activity, whereas homozygotes have such a 70% decline in enzyme activity and an increased risk of myelosuppression, neutropenia, and diarrhea, due to SN-38 buildup [95].

Clinical Utility: UGT1A1

Although the Evaluation of Genomic Applications in Practice and Prevention (EGAPP) Working Group concluded that there was insufficient evidence to recommend either for or against routine UGT1A1 genotyping in metastatic colorectal cancer patients taking irinotecan [96].

The French National Network of Pharmacogenetics has evaluated irinotecan dosing based on UGT1A1 genotype and suggested no dose change in carriers of the UGT1A1*28 allele when their given dose of irinotecan is 180 mg/m2/wk but proposed a dose reduction of 25-30% in *28/*28 patients when the dose is 180-230 mg/m2 2-3 weekly and contraindicating use when the dose is 240 mg/m2 2-3 weekly. on the other hand, on the other hand, The Dutch Pharmacogenetics Working Group guidelines for UGT1A1 and irinotecan, recommended starting with 70% of the standard initial dose in *28/*28 patients regardless of dose, with no dose modification in heterozygote patients and an increase dose if it was tolerated, dose escalation is guided by neutrophil count monitoring [97].

UGT1A1 genetic testing can be based on extracting DNA from blood or other different tissues, and typically involves testing for the UGT1A1*28 TA repeat polymorphism. The most used assay is a lab-developed test that employs fluorescent PCR amplification. and capillary electrophoresis this assay will detect the five [(TA)5TAA] and eight [(TA)8TAA] repeat alleles. The five TA repeat allele is thought to preserve transcription efficiently, whereas the unusual eight TA repeat allele, like the seven TA repeat allele, indicates irinotecan sensitivity [98].

Limitations of Testing: UGT1A1

Testing for the UGT1A1*28 TA repeat polymorphism will not reveal any other coding UGT1A1 variants that could affect irinotecan metabolism Furthermore, other genes, such as CYP3A4 may influence irinotecan toxicity risk and will not be discovered by UGT1A1 genetic testing [99].

Rasburicase and G6PD Deficiency

Molecular Target

Rasburicase is a drug used in oncology supportive care approved by the FDA as a prophylactic or as a treatment of hyperuricemia occurring during tumor lysis syndrome (TLS). TLS occur when cancer cells are being destroyed extensively releasing many cellular components in the blood including uric acid. Rasburicase is a urate oxidase enzyme that act on uric acid converting it to hydrogen peroxide and allantoin which is easily eliminated from the body by the kidneys [100].

Rasburicase is contraindicated in glucose-6-phosphate dehydrogenase deffecient patients. G6PD gene is located on the X chromosome at Xq28.73,74. G6PD enzyme is the rate-limiting enzyme in pentose phosphate pathway (PPP). it plays an important role by converting glucose-6-phosphate to 6-phosphogluconolactone. this step concomitantly reduces nicotinamide adenine dinucleotide phosphate (NADP+) to NADPH which is required to maintain cellular levels of reduced glutathione. reduced glutathione protects cells from oxidative stress by neutralizing reactive oxygen species. Oxidative stress is defined as an increase in the level of reactive oxygen species (ROS) that can lead to cell damage. ROS are chemically reactive species containing oxygen such as superoxide and hydrogen peroxide [101].

Sharp increases in ROS, on the other hand, overwhelm cellular antioxidant defences, including glutathione-mediated reduction, and erythrocytes are especially vulnerable to oxidative stress because of their function as oxygen carriers and reliance on G6PD. Infections, foodstuffs (for example, fava beans in favism), and specific drugs, such as primaquine, nitrofurantoin, and rasburicase, can all cause oxidative stress [102].

Rasburicase's oxidation of uric acid to allantoin can result in oxidative stress due to the production of hydrogen peroxide. Rasburicase is associated with hemolytic anemia and in rare cases methaemoglobinaemia in patients with G6PD deficiency, which is caused by oxidation of haemoglobin iron, resulting in methaemoglobin and hypoxia. the main medicinal treatment in this case is methylene blue, which is contraindicated due to the risk of exacerbating oxidative stress, making management challenging. Restricting it to high flow oxygen, ascorbic acid and blood transfusions. So, it is vital to identify G6PD genetic variants to avoid such consequences [103].

The World Health Organization categorizes G6PD variants into five groups as shown in Table 3.

Table 3. The World Health Organization categorizes G6PD variants into five group

WHO class	Enzyme activity	Associated phenotype	Variant example
I	Severe deficiency	Congenital non- spherocytic hemolytic (CNSHA)	Tondela, Palermo
II	<10% severely deficient	Risk of acute hemolytic anemia	Mediterranean, Canton, Chatham
III	10-60% moderate deficiency	Risk of acute hemolytic anemia	deficiency A- Haplotype, Asahi, Orissa, Kalyan-Kerala
IV	60-150% normal activity	No clinical manifestations	B (wildtype), A, Mira d'Aire, Sao Borja
V	150% enhanced activity		Hektoen

Class I variants are extremely rare, linked with G6PD activity 10% of normal and occur in symptomatic patients with chronic no spherocytic hemolytic anemia (CNSHA); classes II and III have G6PD activities 10% and 10-60%, respectively, and are not related to CNSHA and thus individuals are asymptomatic the majority of the time; class IV variants have normal activity, and class V is confined with variants with higher activity [104].

The two most well-known variants are the Mediterranean (G6PDMed, class II) and African American (G6PDA-, class III). G6PD deficiency seems to affect approximately 400 million people worldwide, with a higher prevalence in Africa, Southeast Asia, the Mediterranean, and the Middle East. The prevalence of G6PD deficiency is related with the global distribution of malaria, suggesting that G6PD deficiency developed and is maintained because of selection pressure exerted by Plasmodium parasites [101].

Molecular Testing

G6PD genetic testing can be done using DNA extracted from whole blood or other tissues, and typically includes targeted genotyping of a panel of G6PD-deficient alleles. G6PD deficiency occurs in male more than females as it is X-linked and so only 1 class I, II, or III variant is required (hemizygosity). Females, on the other hand, are rarely homozygous or compound heterozygous for G6PD deficiency [105].

Table 4. The CPIC guidelines recommendation among G6PD deficient patients

Phenotype	Examples of diplotypes	Implications for phenotypic measures	Dosing recommendations for rasburicase
Normal. A male carrying a non-deficient allele or a female carrying to non-deficient (class IV alleles	Male B, Sao Boria. Female B/B, B/Sao Boria	Low or reduced risk for hemolytic anemia.	No reason to hold rasburicase based on G6PD status.
Variable. A female carrying one nondeficient (class IV) and one deficient (class I-III) allele.	B/A-, B/ Mediterranean, B/ Bangkak	Unknown risk of hemoktc anemia	To assertion that G6PD status is normal, enzyme activity must be measured; alternatives include allopurinol
Deficient with CNSHA. A Male, male carrying a class I, II or III allele or a female carrying two deficient class I-III alleles.	A Male A-, Orissa, Kalyan-Kerala, Mediterranean, Canten, Chatham, Bangkok,		Deficient with CNSHA. A Male, male carrying a class I, II or III allele or a female carrying two deficient class I-III alleles.

(CNSHA)* Congenital non- spherocytic hemolytic, (G6PD)* glucose-6-phosphate dehydrogenase deficiency patients.

When specific variants of known functional consequence are detected in G6PD, genotyping can be sufficient to establish the diagnosis of G6PD deficiency. The absence of specific variants, however, does not rule out G6PD deficiency due to the presence of untested or unrecognized variants, and thus G6PD phenotyping is frequently required to establish G6PD deficiency.

Regardless of the absence of a prospective randomized clinical trial effectively evaluating the benefit of G6PD genotype directed rasburicase therapy, the available evidence was used to notify the CPIC guidelines, which suggest an alternative therapy to rasburicase in G6PDdeficient patients as shown in Table 4 [84].

Limitations of Testing: G6PD

Because targeted G6PD genotyping cannot detect alleles that have not been directly interrogated, a negative genotyping result does not exclude the possibility that a patient possesses another G6PD variant. Furthermore, other genes may affect rasburicase responses that are not detected by G6PD genetic testing. G6PD genotyping alternatives that directly assess

G6PD enzyme activity are available and may be utilized to confirm a diagnosis of G6PD deficiency [81].

Thiopurines and Thiopurine Methyl Transferase

Molecular Target

Thiopurines (azathioprine, mercaptopurine, and thioguanine) are used for the treatment of acute lymphoblastic leukemia and in autoimmune diseases treatment. Specifically, mercaptopurine for lymphoid malignancies, and thioguanine for myeloid leukemias.

Thiopurines are prodrugs that are metabolized by hypoxanthine guanine phosphoribosyl transferase to active potentially toxic, thioguanine nucleotides (TGNs), which are inactivated by thiopurine methyltransferase (TPMT). These drugs are analogs of the nucleic acid guanine and are incorporated into RNA and DNA causing cell death.

Variant alleles of TPMT are linked to lower enzyme activity and, as a result, greater TGN levels, leading to significant pharmacological effects. Individuals who inherit two loss-of-function alleles are significantly more likely to develop life-threatening myelosuppression leading to excessive TGN exposure [106].

The TPMT gene on chromosome 6p22.3 has 31 variant alleles, many of them have missense mutations associated with decreased in vitro activity [107].

TPMT*2, *3A, *3B, and *3C are the most studied and tested variant alleles. TPMT 3A, which contains two missense variants in cis, p.Ala154Thr and p.Tyr240Cys. and is the most common variant allele associated with low TPMT activity in Caucasians. Many heterozygous patients have moderate to severe myelosuppression, whereas homozygous wild-type patients have lower TGN metabolite levels and a lower risk of myelosuppression [108]. Taken together these data prompted CPIC practice guidelines recommending dose reductions and/or alternate therapies among loss- of-function TPMT allele carriers as seen in Table 5.

More recently, NUDT15 variant has been identified by genome-wide association and it was found to have a strong influence thiopurine intolerance in ALL patients. NUDT15 encodes a nucleoside diphosphatase that catalyzes the cytotoxic thioguanine triphosphate (TGTP) metabolite's conversion to thioguanine monophosphate which is less toxic. TGTP binds to DNA, forming DNA-TG, an antileukemic metabolite. 47 Impaired NUDT15-mediated catabolism lead to high levels of TGTP and, later, DNA-TG, increasing the risk of myelosuppression [109].

The first NUDT15 SNP linked with thiopurine toxicity was rs116855232 (c.415C > T), resulting in substitution in p. R139C amino acid leading to in vitro complete losing of protein stability enzymatic activity. Carriers of this allele show an elevation of levels and subsequently severe myelosuppression.

in ALL patients following the standard maintenance doses of mercaptopurine, the risk of developing myelosuppression is 14.5-fold higher in carriers of the p. R139C variants than in wild-type individuals.49 in addition, in a pediatric ALL cohort study, Individuals homozygous for p.R139C tolerated only 8% of the standard dose. The p.R139C allele in NUDT15 has received the most attention and thus has the greatest evidence for clinical application. However, the NUDT15 contains many other variants with varying frequencies, many of them have no data on functional activity [110].

Table 5. CPIC practice guidelines recommending dose modifications among loss- of-function TPMT allele carriers

Examples of Phenotype	Example of diplotypes	Implications for pharmacologic measures	Dosing recommendation for thioguanine
Heterozygote or intermediate activity (one functional allele *1, plus one nonfunctional allele.)	*1/*2, *1/*3A, *1/*3B, *1/*3C, *1/*4	Extremely high concentrations of TNG metabolites, fetal toxicity without dose decrease.	Start with drastically reduced doses (reduce daily dose by 10-fold and dose thrice weekly instead of daily) and adjust doses of thioguanine based on degree of myelosuppression and disease-specific guidelines. Allow 4-6 weeks to reach steady state after each dose adjustment. In setting of myelosuppression, emphasis should be on reducing thioguanine over other agents. For nonmalignant conditions, consider alternative nonthiopurine immunosuppressant therapy
Homozygous or compound heterozygote variant, mutant, low, or deficient activity (two nonfunctional alleles)	*3A/*3A *2/*3A, *3C/*3A, *3C/*4,*3C/*2, *3A/*4	Moderate to high concentrations of TGN metabolites but note that TNG after thioguanine 5-10 xhigher than TNG after mercaptopurine or azathioprine.	Start with reduced doses (reduce by 30-50%) and adjust doses of thioguanine based on degree of myelosuppression and disease specific guidelines. Allow 2-4 weeks to reach steady state after each dose adjustment. In setting of myelosuppression, and depending on other therapy, emphasis should be on reducing thioguanine over other agents
Homozygous wild-type or normal, high activity (Two functional *1 alleles	*1/*1	Lower concentrations of TGN metabolites but note that TNG after thioguanine 5-10 xhigher than TNG after mercaptopurine or azathioprine.	Start with normal starting dose. Adjust doses of thioguanine and of other myelosuppressive therapy without any special emphasis on thioguanine. Allow 2 weeks to reach steady state after each dose adjustment

(TGN)* thioguanine nucleotides.

A recent study was conducted to overcome this limitation. using saturation mutagenesis to recognize 54 residues where variants resulted in protein instability. Variants in 17 residues altered NUDT15 activity without influencing protein stability. As more patients undergo whole-genome sequencing, the information obtained by Yang and colleagues50 will become more useful when determining all potential variants that may impact enzyme activity and the need to tailor dose.

While inherited TPMT dysfunction appears to have a greater impact on the risk of thiopurine-induced intolerance in people of European or African ancestry, NUDT15 risk alleles appear to be more relevant in individuals of Asian and Hispanic ancestry. As a result, in the future, when individualizing 6-mercaptopurine dose, both genes should be investigated regardless of ethnicity, as emphasized by the latest CPIC guideline [111].

Genetic Testing

TPMT testing can be done using DNA extraction from either blood or other tissues, and I targeted genotyping is done for of the TPMT2, 3A, 3B, and 3C allele. In the Caucasian, African-

American, and Asian populations, PCR-based assays that investigate the three common variants detect 80-95% of people who have low and intermediate enzyme activity [112].

Limitations of Testing: TPMT

Because targeted TPMT genotyping cannot detect alleles that are not investigated directly, a genotyping negative result does not exclude the possibility that a patient has another TPMT allele causing myelosuppression .Although complete gene sequencing will detect all TPMT variants, rare or novel variants are likely to be of uncertain clinical significance. Furthermore, other genes, such as ITPA may affect thiopurine responses and will not be identified by TPMT genetic testing [81].

Other Examples of Lower Evidence

ABCB1 and Chemotherapy Toxicity

The adenosine triphosphate (ATP)-binding cassette (ABC) subfamily B (MDR/TAP) member 1 (ABCB1) gene encodes for P-glycoprotein 1 (P-gp), which is a widely expressed membrane-associated ATP dependent efflux pump with broad substrate specificity. Oncology drug substrates for P-gp include doxorubicin, docetaxel, paclitaxel, and vincristine; doxorubicin and vincristine both induce P-gp.

Multi drug resistance (MDR) is a leading cause of chemotherapeutic drugs failure in metastatic cancer patients. Although it is a complex and poorly understood phenomenon, basal and drug-induced P-gp overexpression in cancer cells has been linked to treatment failure in several types of cancer [113].

ABCB1 shows high level of genetic polymorphism, but most studies have focused on one or more of three common ABCB1 variants and/or haplotypes: c.1236C > T (rs1128503, a synonymous variant), c.2677G > T/A (rs2032582, a missense variant), and c.3435C > T (rs1045642, a synonymous variant). Furthermore, ABCB1 c.1199G > A (a missense variant) has also been demonstrated to improve in vitro efflux transport of the tyrosine kinase inhibitors imatinib, dasatinib, and nilotinib.

In some studies, genetic variation in ABCB1 is related to cancer ADRs such as anthracycline-induced cardiotoxicity, paclitaxel-medicated peripheral neuropathy and neutropenia, and vincristine neurotoxicity. Small sample sizes and interethnic variability may account for some of this variation. However, there is currently insufficient evidence to support ABCB1 genotyping [114].

CYP3A7 and CYP3A-Metabolised Chemotherapeutics

CYP3A4, 3A5, 3A7, and 3A43 are members of the human CYP3A subfamily. The primary fetal hepatic CYP is CYP3A7.116 After birth CYP3A7 expression decreases while CYP3A4 expression increases. CYP3A7 mRNA expression varies greatly, and CYP3A7 is detectable in 10% of adult livers, accounting for 9-36% of total CYP3A protein [115].

The allele, CYP3A7*1C, is caused by the replacement of 60 bp of its promoter region by the corresponding region of the CYP3A4 adult promoter and is linked to increased hepatic and intestinal CYP3A7 expression. Surprisingly, a borderline significant interaction (P interaction =.06) was discovered between carrying CYP3A7*1C, treatment with a CYP3A-substrate chemotherapeutic on one hand and increased mortality in breast or lung cancer and disease progression in chronic lymphocytic leukemia on the other hand. These findings are particularly remarkable because CYP3A metabolism roughly 30% of clinically used drugs [116].

SLCO1B1 and Methotrexate

Methotrexate is mentioned before is a chemotherapeutic agent involved in the treatment of ALL. The solute carrier organic anion transporter family member 1B1 (SLCO1B1) gene encodes the hepatic xenobiotic influx transporter, organic anion transporter polypeptide 1B1 (OATP1B1).

Paediatric ALL, candidate gene studies and a GWAS27 identified genetic variants in SLCO1B1 that are linked to decreased methotrexate clearance.

The major variant probably the reduced function SLCO1B1 SNP, rs4149056 (c.521T > C, p.V174A), because s many other recognised SLCO1B1 variants (e.g., rs4149081, rs11045879, rs11045821125,126) are in linkage disequilibrium with rs41490566 [117]. Remarkably, an interaction (SNP-SNP) has been discovered between gain-of-function rs2306283 (c.388A > G, p.N130D) and methotrexate clearance rs4149056, which identify the most common SLCO1B1 haplotypes (*1a, *1b, *5, *15). The rs2306283 ancestral A allele is related with even reduced methotrexate clearance within each rs4149056 genotype group.

70-90% of methotrexate is eliminated in urine. The SLCO1B1 rs4149056 and rs2306283 variants alter many specific metabolites in urine significantly. Furthermore, these metabolites are considered substrates for renal organic anion transporters (OATs) like methotrexate, and half of them were linked to methotrexate toxicity. This implies that clearance and toxicity of methotrexate may be influenced by complex transporter-transporter interactions mediated by endogenous substrates [118].

Self-Assessment Questions

1. Multiple germline genetic variants in the DPYD gene on chromosome 1p21.3 in patient receiving 5-FU can lead to which of the following
   a. Decreased DPYD activity and increase drug half life
   b. Increase DPYD activity and increase drug half life
   c. Increased drug clearance
   d. None of the above

2. UGT1A1*228 homozygote who has an approximate 70% reduction in UGT1A1 enzyme activity possess an increased risk for which of the following
   a. Myelosuppression
   b. diarrhea,
   c. neutropenia
   d. All the following

3. Thiopurines are prodrugs that are metabolized by hypoxanthine guanine phosphoribosyl transferase to active potentially toxic, thioguanine nucleotides (TGNs), which are inactivated by
   a. DPYD
   b. TPMT
   c. G6P
   d. ABCB1

Applications of Pharmacogenetics in Cardiovascular Drug Therapy

Genetics and medication metabolism are the most overlapping that can affect pharmacotherapy [119]. The metabolism affecting the drug, and convert it either to a more or less active form consequently will affect patient response for the medication. An inherited enzyme deficiency can render prodrugs that needs activation as clopidogrel, ineffective due to reduce transformation into the active metabolite that give the required drug's effects. When drugs like warfarin are given in their active form, a deficit in an enzyme might result in increased drug exposure, which can cause dangerous adverse effects. The Clinical Pharmacogenetics Implementation Consortium (CPIC) provides guidelines for gene–drug links that have important evidences to enhance the use of pharmacogenomics in clinical decisions to make pharmacogenetic testing easier in practice [120]. The Dutch Pharmacogenetics Working Group (DPWG), the Canadian Pharmacogenomics Network for Drug Safety (CPNDS), as well as societies offer similar advice point [121, 122]. Clopidogrel, warfarin, and simvastatin are three medicines that are addressed in three guidelines. The DPWG also offers advice on how to take these medications.

In clinical practice, pharmacogenetics is used to assist patients. deciding on prescriptions. Here We talk about the potential example for cardiovascular pharmacogenetics to grow.

Clopidogrel

After percutaneous coronary intervention (PCI), dual antiplatelet medication plus acetylsalicylic acid and a P2Y purinoceptor 12 (P2Y12 receptor) inhibitor clopidogrel, ticagrelor, or prasugrel is the drug of choice to minimize the risk of adverse cardiovascular events [123].

Guidelines recommend that prasugrel or ticagrelor are superior to clopidogrel in individuals with acute coronary syndrome (ACS) because of their greater efficacy in clinical trials [124, 125]. Despite the fact that the usage of these newer medicines is growing, they are associated with increased costs and bleeding risks [124-126]. Clinical trials failed to demonstrate the variations in patients with ACS, and mainly 30% of those patients has lack in the cytochrome P450 (CYP) 2C19 enzyme, which definitely reduces the efficiency of clopidogrel. Clopidogrel is as efficacious as an alternate medication following the PCI with whom enzymes are fully active, according to data from a 2019 study [127].

Pharmacogenetics

Clopidogrel is a medication that goes through metabolism in mainly two phases to be converted in its active metabolite, which blocks platelet activation permanently [128]. Clopidogrel is activated by many of CYP enzymes. CYP2C19, on the other hand, is implicated in both processes and has effect in the bioactivation of clopidogrel [129].

The CYP2C19 gene has a high degree of polymorphism, *with alleles *1* signifying alleles associated with normal activity and alleles *2 and *3 were associated with no activities, respectively (Table 6) [130, 131]. patients who have two non-functional alleles (also known as loss-of-function) (as *2/*2) are called poor metabolizers (PMs) they mainly lost the function. Intermediate metabolizers (IMs) are characterized by one nonfunctional allele (as the *1/*2) which reduces the activity of enzymes. Where The *17 allele, on the other hand, is related with higher enzyme function and grants the phenotypes of rapid metabolizer (RM; *1/*17 genotype) and ultra-rapid metabolizer (UM; *17/*17 genotype) (Table 7). Mainly 30% of people are PMs or IMs, with the remaining 30% being RMs or UM.

Although other less prevalent no-function alleles have been identified, the US Association of Molecular Pathology considers the *2, *3 and *17 alleles to be the only ones that are required for testing.

Table 6. CYP2C19 alleles and functional activity

CYP2C19 alleles	Function
*1	Normal function
*2,*3 ⇨ more common in patients	No function
4, 5,*6,*7,*8	No function
*17	Increase the function

Table 7. CYP2C19 genotypes and phenotypes

Phenotype	Genotype	Example
Ultra rapid (UM)	Two alleles that increase function	*17/*17
Rapid metabolizer (RM)	One normal function allele plus one alleles that increase function	*1/*17
Normal metabolizer (NM)	Two normal function allele	*1/*1
Intermediate metabolizer (IM)	One normal function allele plus one No function allele OR One No function allele plus one alleles that increase function	*1/*3 Or *3/*17

Exposure to CYP2C19 and clopidogrel Compared to normal function alleles (NM) phenotype (that is, *1/*1 genotype), the CYP2C19 PM and IM are linked with decreased exposure to the bioactive clopidogrel derivative and enhanced platelet reactivity during therapy [132, 134]. Higher clopidogrel doses have been studied as a way to compensate for the lower antiplatelet effects seen in IMs and PMs. In IMs, increasing the dose to 225 mg per day produces platelet inhibition comparable to a 75mg per day dose in NMs, however in PMs, a dose which is high as 300mg per day won't be effective [134-136]. Because the CYP2C19 genotype has no effect on the pharmacokinetics or pharmacodynamics of prasugrel or ticagrelor, without contraindications, these medicines are preferred over clopidogrel dosage increase in IMs and PMs (as increase the risk of bleeding [137-139].

Its unclear how the *17 allele affects clopidogrel responsiveness. This variant improved platelet aggregation inhibition and enhance the chance of bleeding with clopidogrel, according to an early study 35, but study did not account for the *2 allele. Because the *2 and *17 alleles are merely found on the same haplotype, it's questionable if the observed effects were caused by the inclusion or exclusion of the *17 allele or the *2 allele.

Clinical Practice

In 2010, the FDA authorized a label update for clopidogrel that includes a boxed warning indicating reduced clopidogrel efficacy in PMs (but not IMs), for whom alternative P2Y12 inhibitors are advised 51. same statement on the clopidogrel label has been approved by the European Medicines Agency, the Japanese Pharmaceutical and Medical Devices Agency, and other regulatory organizations. In their list of gene–drug combinations where the findings justify therapeutic management suggestions [140], The FDA is in charge of both IMs and PMs. The CPIC clopidogrel recommendations cover both IMs and PMs, with an emphasis on patients with an ACS and PCI who have considerable data, whereas the DPWG extends counseling to patients with stroke [141]. With no existence of a contraindication, the recommendations recommend prasugrel or ticagrelor in CYP2C19 IMs or PMs, but they do not recommend genetic testing. The American College of Cardiology (ACC) and the American Heart Association (AHA) produced joint PCI recommendations in 2016 that advise against routine genotyping for all PCI participants, citing a lack of randomized trial (RCT) information at the point [123]. Both institutions, though, propose that screening be explored in greater risk individuals, and for individuals with a no-function variant, either prasugrel or ticagrelor is indicated, same to CPIC.

One of the most common examples of a no-function allele is CYP2C19 testing to recommend the usage of antiplatelet treatment after PCI. In clinical practice, pharmacogenetic testing is used [119, 142]. As per ACC/AHA recommendations, some institutions retain screening for patients who are at high risk of cardiovascular events based on clinical manifestation, while some other sites genotype the bulk of PCI patients [142].

Most institutions use clinical counseling notes or automated decision assistance to offer alternate P2Y12 inhibitor medication for both IMs and PMs.

Oral Anticoagulants

The direct-acting oral anticoagulants (DOACs) apixaban, dabigatran, edoxaban, and rivaroxaban, as well as the vitamin K antagonist warfarin, Thrombotic disorders are treated and avoided with these drugs.

The therapeutic index of warfarin is somewhat narrow, which necessitates multiple INR monitoring to provide optimum anticoagulation, which is defined as an INR of 2–3 for most applications. Patients' required dosages of warfarin to obtain an INR of 2–3 from 1mg to >10mg per day88. Although genotype has a significant role in dosage variability in medical care, however, it is poorly studied. Instead, all patients are usually started on the same dose of warfarin (for example, 5 milligrams per day). For the first 1–3 days of treatment, loading dosage (for illustration, 10 mg) are often used, with later dose modifications based on an INR result [143, 144], especially in Europe. However, in people with bleeding disorders, these 'fixed-dose' techniques can lead to excessive anticoagulation. Genotypes linked to decreased warfarin metabolism or higher susceptibility to the drug. In patients with warfarin-resistance genes, however, delays in achieving therapeutic anticoagulation might occur, particularly when there isn't a load dose.

Pharmacogenetics

When compared to warfarin, DOACs have a broader therapeutic index and don't need to be monitored often, as well as are linked to lower risk of cerebrovascular embolism and other thrombotic events, as well as a lower risk of cerebral hemorrhage [145, 146]. Whereas gene mutations with in CES1 gene have been linked to dabigatran serum concentrations and hemorrhage incidence, there seems to be no definitive proof of genetic links to DOAC efficacy [147]. Because of its superior profile to warfarin, DOAC use has elevated during the last ten years. DOACs represented for much more than 30% of orally anticoagulant in the U.s by 2015, and 50% of atrial fibrillation orders in Norway [148, 149]. Nevertheless, because DOACs are more expensive, have lesser compliance rates, and lesser indications than warfarin, and the price of reversal agents for DOACs in the event of over-anticoagulation, warfarin is still usually recommended, especially in older patient populations and those with significant comorbid conditions
[150, 151].

Clinical Practice

Genetic relationships in pharmacogenetics. CYP2C9 and VKORC1 are the main genes that affect warfarin response, with CYP4F2 playing a modest role). S-warfarin (the more active enantiomer) clearance is reduced by the CYP2C9*2, *3, *5, *6, *8, and *11 alleles, lowering patient dose requirements [152-154]. The *2, *8, and *11 alleles were associated to weekly dose drops of 5–7 mg, with the *3 and *5 alleles showing up to 14 mg per week decreases [155, 156].

These variations are also linked to an elevated risk of bleeding and over-anticoagulation, with a significant likelihood of hemorrhage remaining throughout warfarin treatment [157, 158].

In people of European ancestry, the *2 and *3 alleles are the most prevalent, whereas the *5, *6, *8, and *11 alleles are mainly found in people of African heritage.

The protein target of warfarin is vitamin K epoxide reductase complex 1 (VKORC1), and uncommon mutations leads to warfarin tolerance and the urge for escalation for doses (e.g., 20 mg per day) to maintain effective anticoagulation effect [159]. VKORC1 expression is lowered and warfarin dose requirements are reduced when there is variation, c.1639G > A (rs9923231), in the regulatory region of VKORC1 is present [159, 160]. Asians have a higher prevalence of the −1639 AA (very sensitive) genotype than Europeans, while Africans have a higher prevalence of the −1639 GG (lower sensitivity) genotype. This difference explains why Asians receive lower dosages and Africans receive larger amounts than Europeans [161].

Vitamin K1 is converted to hydroxyl-vitamin K1 by the CYP4F2 enzyme. In the presence of the *3 allele (rs2108622), CYP4F2 activity is lowered, as a consequence, more vitamin K1 is available for decrease to vitamin K hydroquinone and coagulation factors stimulation [162]. In European and Asian populations [163], the *3 allele is linked to increased warfarin dose requirements than the *1 variant. In groups with African heritage, however, no association has been found [164-166].

VKORC1 and CYP2C9 are the major genetic determinants to warfarin dose required in people of European or Asian ancestry, according to GWAS [165-167]. A GWAS in an African-American sample found rs12777823, a novel variance in the CYP2C locus on chromosome 10 associated to lower warfarin dose requirements (50). While this single-nucleotide polymorphism (SNP) is distributed throughout the genome, its connection with warfarin reaction corresponds to those of African ancestry [168]. As a basis, rather than being a functional polymorphism, rs12777823 is more likely to be in genetic linkage with a functional polymorphism (or variants) seen in African heritage populations. Following that, a GWAS revealed a mutation on chromosome 6 upstream of EPHA7 associated to the risk of serious bleeding in African Americans using warfarin with an INR of 4.

This mutation is only found in people of African descent, with an allele frequency of 7%, and its link with bleed incidence reached genome-wide importance when the detection and replication cohorts were integrated. The SNP appears to improve bleeding risk prediction when included in the HAS-BLED score, but this finding has to be verified [169].

Algorithms for Dosing

The International Warfarin Pharmacogenetics Consortium (IWPC) [170] and Gage and colleagues [171] have created dosage procedures that take into account genotype (VKORC1 1639G > A, CYP2C9*2 and CYP2C9*3 alleles) as well as patient characteristics that affect warfarin response (such as age, BMI, and administration of CYP2C9 inhibitors) to aid in calculating starting warfarin dosages (both accessible at The IWPC algorithm) For individuals receiving CYP2C9 inducers (such as phenytoin or rifampin), algorithms produce identical dose estimations. The CYP2C9*5, *6, *8, *11, or rs12777823 variant is not included in either documented algorithm; however, the *5 and *6 alleles, as well as the CYP4F2*3 allele, are included in the online version of warfarin dosing algorithm [172].

Application of Pharmacogenetics in Antibiotics Drug Therapy

Aminoglycosides

They're normally provided intravenous or intramuscularly to manage Gram-negative pathogenic bacteria, or as a combination therapy for Gram-positive pathogenic bacteria,

Therapeutic dosage monitoring (TDM) is needed since kinetics fluctuate between patients and excessive concentrations in blood are linked to increased risk. Sensorineural hearing loss (cochleotoxicity) and vestibulotoxicity are two ototoxic adverse effects of aminoglycoside medications. These toxicities are usually depending on dose and occur in people who take large doses of aminoglycosides for a long time. However, significant bilateral sensorineural hearing loss happened from case reports, imply that some people are prone to aminoglycoside-induced hearing loss (AIHL) [173].

Pharmacogenetics

And unlike other actionable pharmacogenetic factors that modify drug metabolism and thus drug response, mutations in the gene under analysis here candidates tend to severe AIHL after exposure to current standard aminoglycoside dosages.

Based on the patient's diplotype, no metabolizer status can be determined. Instead, the presence of a pathogenic MT-RNR1 variant in a person can be considered a risk factor for AIHL [174].

This CPIC recommendation assume that genetic screening has been performed and that an MT-RNR1 variant has been detected, irrespective of the testing procedures used. The existence of an MT-RNR1 alteration known to cause AIHL is enough to determine a phenotypic category, while lack of a variant does not exclude out AIHL [175].

Clinical Practice

Numerous studies investigating the link connecting MT-RNR1 mutations and AIHL contain serious limitations. Many of clinical studies that demonstrate the link of having MT-RNR1 variants and AIHL [176-179]. The entirety of these investigations are small cohort studies wherein authors found people with a high occurrence of AIHL and genotyped MT-RNR1 (Table 8).

Prescriptions for Treatment

If the patient has an MT-RNR1 mutation that impels to AIHL, the essential pharmacogenetics advice is to exclude aminoglycoside antibiotics if only the higher risk of AIHL is balanced by the intensity of infection and with no other options of treatments. (Table 9).

No enough studies demonstrated the fact that some aminoglycosides cause more severe adverse medication reactions than others. As a result, this recommendation applies to all aminoglycosides class for Individuals with MT-RNR1 mutations that make them liable to AIHL, avoidance of aminoglycosides is a must and used only if the danger of infection without effective and safe alternatives outweighs the risk of permanent hearing. We suggest using an aminoglycoside for the shortest time possible if there is no effective alternative, consulting an infectious disease Physician for different regimens, therapeutic drug monitoring (TDM), and regular AIHL evaluation, either within or following the treatment, in discussion with an audio vesicular health care professional [180-182].

People who have no noticeable MT-RNR1 variants or who have MT-RNR1 variants that believed to be non-attributing to AIHL (standard). AIHL is commonly associated with various risks, such as preterm birth, renal failure, severe immune reaction, long duration, and high serum level [183, 184]. Therefore, irrespective of if the MT-RNR1 mutation tends to lead to AIHL or not, it is important to take cautions such as assessing the renal function of the patient, assessing therapeutic medication, and administering the lowest effective dose possible. In conclusion, even if a patient with a potentially active MT-RNR1 variation has been treated with aminoglycosides in the past and has not developed AIHL as a result of those treatments, this does not decrease the chance that they could do so with subsequent dosages.

Table 8. MT-RNR1 phenotype based on genotype

Likely phenotype	Genotypes
MT-RNR1 increased risk of AIHL	Patients are linked to high risk of AIHL
MT-RNR1 normal risk of AIHL	Patients are linked to normal risk of AIHL
MT-RNR1 uncertain risk of AIHL	Patients are linked uncertain risk of AIHL.

Adapted from the Clinical Pharmacogenetics Implementation Consortium Guideline for the Use of Aminoglycosides Based on MT-RNR1 Genotype.

Table 9. Advisable use aminoglycoside in adult and children with the MT-RNR1 phenotype

Phenotype Therapeutic recommendations	Significance for phenotypic Characteristics	Therapeutic suggestions	Classification of recommendations	Considerations
MT-RNR1 increased risk of AIHL	Very high risk	Avoid unless risk of hearing loss is overweighed infection	Strong	If aminoglycoside is the only choice, evaluate for the incidence of hearing loss and use lowest effective dose and shortest duration, monitor other parameters
MT-RNR1 normal risk of AIHL	Normal risk	Use at well established doses for short period with monitoring.	Strong	Patients who do not have MT-RNR1 aminoglycoside-induced hearing loss variants, the aminoglycoside-related hearing loss is at high chance particularly at high doses or long-term use.
MT-RNR1 uncertain risk of AIHL	Minimal or no risk	aminoglycoside may be at well established doses for short period with monitoring.	Optional	Patients who do not have MT-RNR1 aminoglycoside-induced hearing loss variants, the aminoglycoside-associated hearing loss is at high, particularly with high doses or long term use.

Adapted from Clinical Pharmacogenetics Implementation Consortium Guideline for the Use of Aminoglycosides Based on MT-RNR1 Genotype.

Self-Assessment Questions

1. A 78-year-old man is seen for a hypertension follow-up. he takes, lisinopril 20 mg daily, and nifedipine 20 mg daily. For his acute coronary syndrome, he is taking aspirin 325 mg, atorvastatin 20 mg, and clinic blood pressure readings have been 150–154/75–70 mm Hg, heart rate 100 bpm Pharmacogenetics CYP 2C19 was prescribed, if the patient is CYP 2C19 2*/3* what is the best antiplatelet to be added to aspirin?
   a. clopidogrel
   b. ticagrelor

   c. prasugrel
   d. (b or c)
2. Regarding CYP2C19 genotypes and phenotypes, *1/*3 alleles
   a. Two alleles that increase function
   b. Two normal function allele
   c. One normal function allele plus one No function allele
   d. None of the above

3. Based on MT-RNR1 Genotype, using gentamycin in patients with uncertain risk of AIHL
   a. can be used for a short period
   b. Avoid use unless benefit overweight risk
   c. Use at normal doses for the required period
   d. Switch to another class

Important Websites in Pharmacogenomic

1. Pharmacogene Variation (PharmVar)
   https://www.pharmvar.org/

The Pharmacogene Variation (PharmVar) Consortium is the new home for PGx gene nomenclature serving as a centralized 'Next-Generation' Pharmacogene Variation data repository. The major focus of PharmVar is to catalogue allelic variation of genes impacting drug metabolism, disposition and response and provide a unifying designation system (nomenclature) for the global pharmacogenetic/genomic community.

2. Pharmacogenomics Global Research Network (PGRN)
   https://www.pgrn.org/

The mission of the Pharmacogenomics Global Research Network is to catalyse and lead research in precision medicine for the discovery and translation of genomic variation influencing therapeutic and adverse drug effects.

3. *Clinical Pharmacogenetics Implementation Consortium* (*CPIC*)
   https://cpicpgx.org/

International consortium which is interested in facilitating use of pharmacogenetic tests for patient care. CPIC's goal is to address the barrier to clinical implementation of pharmacogenetic tests by creating, curating, and posting freely available, peer-reviewed, evidence-based, updatable, and detailed gene/drug clinical practice guidelines. CPIC guidelines follow standardized formats, include systematic grading of evidence and clinical recommendations, use standardized terminology, are peer-reviewed, and are published in a leading journal with simultaneous posting to cpicpgx.org, where they are regularly updated.

4. Pharmacogenetics and Pharmacogenomics Knowledge Base (PharmGKB)
   https://www.pharmgkb.org/

The PharmGKB is a pharmacogenomics knowledge source that includes clinical information including clinical guidelines and drug labels, potentially clinically actionable gene-drug associations and genotype-phenotype relationships. PharmGKB collects, curates and distributes knowledge about the impact of human genetic variation on drug responses through the following activities:

- Annotate genetic variants and gene-drug-disease relationships via literature review
- Summarize important pharmacogenomic genes, associations between genetic variants and drugs, and drug pathways
- Curate FDA drug labels containing pharmacogenomic information
- Enable consortia examining important questions in pharmacogenomics
- Curate and participate in writing pharmacogenomic-based drug dosing guidelines
- Contribute to clinical implementation projects for pharmacogenomics through collaborations
- Publish pharmacogenomic-based drug dosing guidelines, very important pharmacogene summaries and drug-centered pathways
- Display all information on the website and provide comprehensive downloads.

References

[1] Maitland-van der Zee, A. H., A. de Boer, and H. G. Leufkens, The interface between pharmacoepidemiology and pharmacogenetics. *European journal of pharmacology*, 2000. 410(2-3): p. 121-130.

[2] Ingelman-Sundberg, M., Pharmacogenetics: an opportunity for a safer and more efficient pharmacotherapy. *Journal of internal medicine*, 2001. 250(3): p. 186-200.

[3] Drazen, J. M., E. K. Silverman, and T. H. Lee, Heterogeneity of therapeutic responses in asthma. *British medical bulletin*, 2000. 56(4): p. 1054-1070.

[4] Evans, W. E. and H. L. McLeod, Pharmacogenomics—drug disposition, drug targets, and side effects. *New England Journal of Medicine*, 2003. 348(6): p. 538-549.

[5] Vesell, E. S., Therapeutic lessons from pharmacogenetics. *Annals of internal medicine*, 1997. 126(8): p. 653-655.

[6] Wang, L., H. L. McLeod, and R. M. Weinshilboum, Genomics and drug response. *New England Journal of Medicine*, 2011. 364(12): p. 1144-1153.

[7] Zakaria, A.. Effect of Genetic Variations on Pharmacokinetics and Pharmacodynamics of High Dose of Methotrexate in Pediatric Osteosarcoma. in *Pediatric Blood & Cancer*. 2020. Wiley 111 River St, Hoboken 07030-5774, NJ USA.

[8] Lazarou, J., B. H. Pomeranz, and P. N. Corey, Incidence of adverse drug reactions in hospitalized patients: a meta-analysis of prospective studies. *JAMA*, 1998. 279(15): p. 1200-1205.

[9] Kongkaew, C., P. R. Noyce, and D. M. Ashcroft, Hospital admissions associated with adverse drug reactions: a systematic review of prospective observational studies. *Annals of Pharmacotherapy*, 2008. 42(7-8): p. 1017-1025.

[10] Classen, D. C. Adverse drug events in hospitalized patients: excess length of stay, extra costs, and attributable mortality. *JAMA*, 1997. 277(4): p. 301-306.

[11] Preskorn, S. H. and C. R. Hatt, How pharmacogenomics (PG) are changing practice: implications for prescribers, their patients, and the healthcare system (PG series part I). *Journal of Psychiatric Practice®*, 2013. 19(2): p. 142-149.

[12] Li, D. Integrative approaches for studying the role of noncoding RNAs in influencing drug efficacy and toxicity. *Expert Opinion on Drug Metabolism & Toxicology*, 2022: p. 1-13.

[13] Tantisira, K. and S. T. Weiss, Overview of pharmacogenomics. *UpToDate*. MA, USA, 2013.

[14] Snyder, L. H., Studies in human inheritance. IX. The inheritance of taste deficiency in man. *Ohio J Sci*, 1932. 32(5): p. 436-40.

[15] Kalow, W., Familial incidence of low pseudocholinesterase level. *The Lancet,* 1956. 268(6942): p. 576-577.

[16] Motulsky, A. G., Drug reactions, enzymes, and biochemical genetics. *Journal of the American Medical Association*, 1957. 165(7): p. 835-837.

[17] Vogel, F., Moderne probleme der humangenetik, in *Ergebnisse der inneren medizin und kinderheilkunde*. 1959, Springer. p. 52-125.

[18] Vesell, E. S. and J. G. Page, Genetic control of drug levels in man: phenylbutazone. *Science*, 1968. 159(3822): p. 1479-1480.

[19] Lee, S., *Automating the Interpretation of Pharmacogenetic Data*, 2019.

[20] Mahgoub, A. Polymorphic hydroxylation of debrisoquine in man. *The Lancet,* 1977. 310(8038): p. 584-586.

[21] Eichelbaum, M. Defective N-oxidation of sparteine in man: a new pharmacogenetic defect. *European journal of clinical pharmacology*, 1979. 16(3): p. 183-187.

[22] Gonzalez, F. J. Characterization of the common genetic defect in humans deficient in debrisoquine metabolism. *Nature*, 1988. 331(6155): p. 442-446.

[23] Becquemont, L., Pharmacogenomics of adverse drug reactions: practical applications and perspectives. *Pharmacogenomics*, 2009. 10(6): p. 961-969.

[24] Wu, X., J. Gu, and M. R. Spitz, Strategies to identify pharmacogenomic biomarkers: candidate gene, pathway-based, and genome-wide approaches, in *Genomics and Pharmacogenomics in Anticancer Drug Development and Clinical Response.* 2008, Springer. p. 353-370.

[25] Ma, Q. and A. Y. Lu, Pharmacogenetics, pharmacogenomics, and individualized medicine. *Pharmacological reviews*, 2011. 63(2): p. 437-459.

[26] Andrade, R. J. Drug-induced liver injury: insights from genetic studies. *Pharmacogenomics*, 2009. 10(9): p. 1467-1487.

[27] Huang, Y. S., Tailored drug therapy for mitigating drug-induced liver injury: is this the era of genetic screening? *Personalized Medicine*, 2010. 7(1): p. 5-8.

[28] Kindmark, A. Genome-wide pharmacogenetic investigation of a hepatic adverse event without clinical signs of immunopathology suggests an underlying immune pathogenesis. *The pharmacogenomics journal*, 2008. 8(3): p. 186-195.

[29] Singer, J. B. A genome-wide study identifies HLA alleles associated with lumiracoxib-related liver injury. *Nature genetics*, 2010. 42(8): p. 711-714.

[30] Tujios, S. and R. J. Fontana, Mechanisms of drug-induced liver injury: from bedside to bench. *Nature reviews Gastroenterology & hepatology*, 2011. 8(4): p. 202-211.

[31] Pirmohamed, M., Pharmacogenetics of idiosyncratic adverse drug reactions. *Adverse Drug Reactions*, 2010: p. 477-491.

[32] Mallal, S. HLA-B* 5701 screening for hypersensitivity to abacavir. *New England Journal of Medicine*, 2008. 358(6): p. 568-579.

[33] McCormack, M. HLA-A* 3101 and carbamazepine-induced hypersensitivity reactions in Europeans. *New England Journal of Medicine*, 2011. 364(12): p. 1134-1143.

[34] Somkrua, R. Association of HLA-B* 5801 allele and allopurinol-induced Stevens Johnson syndrome and toxic epidermal necrolysis: a systematic review and meta-analysis. *BMC medical genetics*, 2011. 12(1): p. 1-10.

[35] Link, E. SLCO1B1 variants and statin-induced myopathy--a genomewide study. *The New England journal of medicine*, 2008. 359(8): p. 789-799.

[36] Walko, C. M. and H. McLeod, Pharmacogenomic progress in individualized dosing of key drugs for cancer patients. *Nature Reviews Clinical Oncology*, 2009. 6(3): p. 153-162.

[37] Carlquist, J. F. and J. L. Anderson, Pharmacogenetic mechanisms underlying unanticipated drug responses. *Discovery Medicine*, 2011. 11(60): p. 469-478.

[38] Lovly, C. M. and D. P. Carbone, One size does not fit all. *Nature Reviews Clinical Oncology*, 2011. 8(2): p. 68-70.

[39] Jänne, P. A., N. Gray, and J. Settleman, Factors underlying sensitivity of cancers to small-molecule kinase inhibitors. *Nature reviews Drug discovery*, 2009. 8(9): p. 709-723.

[40] Zineh, I. and M. A. Pacanowski, Pharmacogenomics in the assessment of therapeutic risks versus benefits: inside the United States Food and Drug Administration. *Pharmacotherapy: The Journal of Human Pharmacology and Drug Therapy*, 2011. 31(8): p. 729-735.

[41] Stingl, J. and J. Brockmöller, Why, when, and how should pharmacogenetics be applied in clinical studies?: current and future approaches to study designs. *Clinical Pharmacology & Therapeutics*, 2011. 89(2): p. 198-209.

[42] Diamandis, M., N. White, and G. M. Yousef, Personalized Medicine: Marking a New Epoch in Cancer Patient ManagementPersonalized Medicine in Cancer Management. *Molecular Cancer Research*, 2010. 8(9): p. 1175-1187.

[43] Houle, D., D. R. Govindaraju, and S. Omholt, Phenomics: the next challenge. *Nature reviews genetics*, 2010. 11(12): p. 855-866.

[44] Pirmohamed, M. The phenotype standardization project: improving pharmacogenetic studies of serious adverse drug reactions. *Clinical Pharmacology & Therapeutics*, 2011. 89(6): p. 784-785.

[45] Lanktree, M. B. Phenomics: expanding the role of clinical evaluation in genomic studies. *Journal of Investigative Medicine*, 2010. 58(5): p. 700-706.

[46] Tracy, R. P., 'Deep phenotyping': characterizing populations in the era of genomics and systems biology. *Current opinion in lipidology*, 2008. 19(2): p. 151-157.

[47] Richards, S. Standards and guidelines for the interpretation of sequence variants: a joint consensus recommendation of the American College of Medical Genetics and Genomics and the Association for Molecular Pathology. *Genetics in medicine*, 2015. 17(5): p. 405-423.

[48] Goetz, L. H. and N. J. Schork, Personalized medicine: motivation, challenges, and progress. *Fertility and sterility*, 2018. 109(6): p. 952-963.

[49] Mathur, S. and J. Sutton, Personalized medicine could transform healthcare. *Biomedical reports*, 2017. 7(1): p. 3-5.

[50] Jørgensen, J. T., Twenty years with personalized medicine: past, present, and future of individualized pharmacotherapy. *The oncologist*, 2019. 24(7): p. e432-e440.

[51] Garrod, A., The incidence of alkaptonuria: a study in chemical individuality. The *Lancet*, 1902. 160(4137): p. 1616-1620.

[52] Carlsten, C. Genes, the environment and personalized medicine: we need to harness both environmental and genetic data to maximize personal and population health. *EMBO reports*, 2014. 15(7): p. 736-739.

[53] du Puch, C. B. M. Benefits of functional assays in personalized cancer medicine: More than just a proof-of-concept. *Theranostics*, 2021. 11(19): p. 9538.

[54] Ashenhurst, J. R. Prevalence of alpha-1 antitrypsin deficiency, self-reported behavior change, and health care engagement among direct-to-consumer recipients of a personalized genetic risk report. *Chest*, 2022. 161(2): p. 373-381.

[55] Sanderson, S. C. and S. Michie, Genetic testing for heart disease susceptibility: potential impact on motivation to quit smoking. *Clinical genetics*, 2007. 71(6): p. 501-510.

[56] Huijgen, R. Two years after molecular diagnosis of familial hypercholesterolemia: majority on cholesterol-lowering treatment but a minority reaches treatment goal. *PLoS One,* 2010. 5(2): p. e9220.

[57] Davis, P. B., U. Yasothan, and P. Kirkpatrick, Ivacaftor. *Nature reviews Drug discovery*, 2012. 11(5): p. 349-351.

[58] Schork, N. J. and L. H. Goetz, Single subject (n-of-1) studies in translational nutrition research. *Annual review of nutrition*, 2017. 37: p. 395.

[59] Drescher, C. W. Longitudinal screening algorithm that incorporates change over time in CA125 levels identifies ovarian cancer earlier than a single-threshold rule. *Journal of clinical oncology*, 2013. 31(3): p. 387.

[60] Liao, X. Aspirin use, tumor PIK3CA mutation, and colorectal-cancer survival. *New England Journal of Medicine*, 2012. 367(17): p. 1596-1606.

[61] Nan, H. Association of aspirin and NSAID use with risk of colorectal cancer according to genetic variants. *JAMA*, 2015. 313(11): p. 1133-1142.

[62] Jeon, J. Determining risk of colorectal cancer and starting age of screening based on lifestyle, environmental, and genetic factors. *Gastroenterology*, 2018. 154(8): p. 2152-2164. e19.

[63] Franceschini, N., A. Frick, and J. B. Kopp, Genetic testing in clinical settings. *American Journal of Kidney Diseases*, 2018. 72(4): p. 569-581.

[64] Hewitt, A. C. a. M., *Genetics and dysmorphology*. 2022: Elsevier.

[65] Benjamin A Raby, M., MPH, Wendy Kohlmann, MS, CGC, Deborah Hartzfeld, MS, CGC, *Genetic testing*. 2021, UpToDate, Waltham, MA.

[66] Carlos A Bacino, M., FACMG, *Genomic disorders: An overview*, ed. T. W. Post. Jun 22, 2022., UpToDate in Waltham, MA.

[67] Das, S., G. R. Abecasis, and B. L. Browning, Genotype imputation from large reference panels. *Annu Rev Genomics Hum Genet*, 2018. 19(1): p. 73-96.

[68] Peter J Hulick, M., MMSc, FACMG, *Next-generation DNA sequencing (NGS): Principles and clinical applications*, ed. T. W. Post. 2022: UpToDate, Waltham, MA,.

[69] Glenn E Palomaki, P., P. Geralyn M Messerlian, and M. Jacquelyn V Halliday, *Prenatal screening for common aneuploidies using cell-free DNA*, ed. T. E. Post. Jul 2022.: UpToDate, Waltham, MA.

[70] Oh, B., Direct-to-consumer genetic testing: advantages and pitfalls. *Genomics & informatics*, 2019. 17(3).

[71] Majumder, M. A., C. J. Guerrini, and A. L. McGuire, Direct-to-consumer genetic testing: value and risk. *Annual Review of Medicine*, 2021. 72: p. 151-166.

[72] Katrina Steiling, M., MSc and M. *Stephanie Christenson, MAS, Tools for genetics and genomics: Gene expression profiling*, ed. Ted. W. Post. 2022: UpToDate, Waltham, MA.

[73] Cynthia L Sears, M., *Anaerobic bacteria: History and role in normal human flora*, ed. Ted. W. Post. 2019: UpToDate, Waltham, MA.

[74] Maria E Figueroa, M., *Principles of epigenetics*, ed. Ted. W. Post. 2022: UpToDate, Waltham, MA.

[75] Holmes, E., I. D. Wilson, and J. K. Nicholson, Metabolic phenotyping in health and disease. *Cell*, 2008. 134(5): p. 714-717.

[76] Tiberi, D. Limitations of personalized medicine and gene assays for breast cancer. *Cureus*, 2017. 9(3).

[77] Walt, D. R. Lessons learned from the introduction of personalized genotyping into a medical school curriculum. *Genetics in Medicine*, 2011. 13(1): p. 63-66.

[78] Brothers, K. B. and M. A. Rothstein, Ethical, legal and social implications of incorporating personalized medicine into healthcare. *Personalized medicine*, 2015. 12(1): p. 43-51.

[79] Overby, C. L. and P. Tarczy-Hornoch, Personalized medicine: challenges and opportunities for translational bioinformatics. *Personalized medicine*, 2013. 10(5): p. 453-462.

[80] Carr, D. F., R. M. Turner, and M. Pirmohamed, Pharmacogenomics of anticancer drugs: Personalising the choice and dose to manage drug response. *Br J Clin Pharmacol*, 2021. 87(2): p. 237-255.

[81] William B. Coleman, G. J. T., Personalized Medicine in Cancer Treatment, in *Diagnostic Molecular Pathology: A Guide to Applied Molecular Testing*. 2016, Academic Press. p. 582.

[82] Thorn, C. F. PharmGKB summary: fluoropyrimidine pathways. *Pharmacogenetics and Genomics*, 2011. 21(4): p. 237-242.

[83] Froehlich, T. K. Clinical importance of risk variants in the dihydropyrimidine dehydrogenase gene for the prediction of early-onset fluoropyrimidine toxicity. *International journal of cancer*, 2015. 136(3): p. 730-739.

[84] Caudle, K. Clinical Pharmacogenetics Implementation Consortium guidelines for dihydropyrimidine dehydrogenase genotype and fluoropyrimidine dosing. *Clinical Pharmacology & Therapeutics*, 2013. 94(6): p. 640-645.

[85] Saif, M. DPYD* 2A mutation: the most common mutation associated with DPD deficiency. *Cancer chemotherapy and pharmacology*, 2007. 60(4): p. 503-507.

[86] Schwab, M. Role of genetic and nongenetic factors for fluorouracil treatment-related severe toxicity: a prospective clinical trial by the German 5-FU Toxicity Study Group. *Journal of clinical oncology*, 2008. 26(13): p. 2131-2138.

[87] Cascorbi, I., Pharmacogenetics of cytochrome p4502D6: genetic background and clinical implication. *European Journal of Clinical Investigation*, 2003. 33: p. 17-22.

[88] Wu, X. The tamoxifen metabolite, endoxifen, is a potent antiestrogen that targets estrogen receptor α for degradation in breast cancer cells. *Cancer research*, 2009. 69(5): p. 1722-1727.

[89] Klein, D. J. PharmGKB summary: tamoxifen pathway, pharmacokinetics. *Pharmacogenetics and genomics*, 2013. 23(11): p. 643.

[90] Goetz, M. P. Clinical Pharmacogenetics Implementation Consortium (CPIC) guideline for CYP2D6 and tamoxifen therapy. *Clinical Pharmacology & Therapeutics*, 2018. 103(5): p. 770-777.

[91] Goetz, M. P. The impact of cytochrome P450 2D6 metabolism in women receiving adjuvant tamoxifen. *Breast cancer research and treatment*, 2007. 101(1): p. 113-121.

[92] Regan, M. M. CYP2D6 genotype and tamoxifen response in postmenopausal women with endocrine-responsive breast cancer: the breast international group 1-98 trial. *Journal of the National Cancer Institute*, 2012. 104(6): p. 441-451.

[93] Province, M. A. CYP2D6 genotype and adjuvant tamoxifen: meta-analysis of heterogeneous study populations. *Clinical Pharmacology & Therapeutics*, 2014. 95(2): p. 216-227.

[94] Perera, M. A., F. Innocenti, and M. J. Ratain, Pharmacogenetic testing for uridine diphosphate glucuronosyltransferase 1A1 polymorphisms: are we there yet? *Pharmacotherapy: The Journal of Human Pharmacology and Drug Therapy*, 2008. 28(6): p. 755-768.

[95] Zhang, D. Characterization of the UDP glucuronosyltransferase activity of human liver microsomes genotyped for the UGT1A1* 28 polymorphism. *Drug metabolism and disposition*, 2007. 35(12): p. 2270-2280.

[96] Palomaki, G. E. Can UGT1A1 genotyping reduce morbidity and mortality in patients with metastatic colorectal cancer treated with irinotecan? An evidence-based review. *Genetics in Medicine*, 2009. 11(1): p. 21-34.

[97] Swen, J. Pharmacogenetics: from bench to byte—an update of guidelines. *Clinical Pharmacology & Therapeutics*, 2011. 89(5): p. 662-673.

[98] Rubinstein, W. S. The NIH genetic testing registry: a new, centralized database of genetic tests to enable access to comprehensive information and improve transparency. *Nucleic acids research*, 2012. 41(D1): p. D925-D935.

[99] van der Bol, J. M. A CYP3A4 Phenotype–Based Dosing Algorithm for Individualized Treatment of IrinotecanCYP3A4 Phenotype–Based Dosing of Irinotecan. *Clinical Cancer Research*, 2010. 16(2): p. 736-742.

[100] Sundy, J. S. Efficacy and tolerability of pegloticase for the treatment of chronic gout in patients refractory to conventional treatment: two randomized controlled trials. *JAMA*, 2011. 306(7): p. 711-720.

[101] Belfield, K. D. and E. M. Tichy, Review and drug therapy implications of glucose-6-phosphate dehydrogenase deficiency. *The Bulletin of the American Society of Hospital Pharmacists*, 2018. 75(3): p. 97-104.

[102] Bubp, J., M. Jen, and K. Matuszewski, Caring for glucose-6-phosphate dehydrogenase (G6PD)–deficient patients: implications for pharmacy. *Pharmacy and Therapeutics*, 2015. 40(9): p. 572.

[103] Sonbol, M. B. Methemoglobinemia and hemolysis in a patient with G6PD deficiency treated with rasburicase. *American journal of hematology*, 2013. 88(2): p. 152-154.

[104] Group, W. H. O. W., Glucose-6-phosphate dehydrogenase deficiency. *Bull World Health Organ*, 1989. 67(6): p. 601-11.

[105] van den Broek, L., E. Heylen, and M. van den Akker, Glucose-6-phosphate dehydrogenase deficiency: not exclusively in males. *Clinical case reports*, 2016. 4(12): p. 1135.

[106] Relling, M. Clinical Pharmacogenetics Implementation Consortium guidelines for thiopurine methyltransferase genotype and thiopurine dosing. *Clinical Pharmacology & Therapeutics*, 2011. 89(3): p. 387-391.

[107] Appell, M. L. Nomenclature for alleles of the thiopurine methyltransferase gene. *Pharmacogenetics and genomics*, 2013. 23(4): p. 242.

[108] Relling, M. V. Mercaptopurine therapy intolerance and heterozygosity at the thiopurine S-methyltransferase gene locus. *Journal of the National Cancer Institute*, 1999. 91(23): p. 2001-2008.

[109] Yang, J. J. Inherited NUDT15 variant is a genetic determinant of mercaptopurine intolerance in children with acute lymphoblastic leukemia. *Journal of clinical oncology*, 2015. 33(11): p. 1235.

[110] Chiengthong, K. NUDT15 c. 415C> T increases risk of 6-mercaptopurine induced myelosuppression during maintenance therapy in children with acute lymphoblastic leukemia. *Haematologica*, 2016. 101(1): p. e24.
[111] Relling, M. V. Clinical pharmacogenetics implementation consortium guideline for thiopurine dosing based on TPMT and NUDT 15 genotypes: 2018 update. *Clinical Pharmacology & Therapeutics*, 2019. 105(5): p. 1095-1105.
[112] Zhou, S., Clinical pharmacogenomics of thiopurine S-methyltransferase. *Current Clinical Pharmacology,* 2006. 1(1): p. 119-128.
[113] Waghray, D. and Q. Zhang, Inhibit or evade multidrug resistance P-glycoprotein in cancer treatment: Miniperspective. *Journal of medicinal chemistry*, 2017. 61(12): p. 5108-5121.
[114] Ceppi, F. Polymorphisms of the vincristine pathway and response to treatment in children with childhood acute lymphoblastic leukemia. *Pharmacogenomics*, 2014. 15(8): p. 1105-1116.
[115] Sim, S. C. CYP3A7 protein expression is high in a fraction of adult human livers and partially associated with the CYP3A7* 1C allele. *Pharmacogenetics and genomics*, 2005. 15(9): p. 625-631.
[116] Zanger, U. M. and M. Schwab, Cytochrome P450 enzymes in drug metabolism: regulation of gene expression, enzyme activities, and impact of genetic variation. *Pharmacology & therapeutics*, 2013. 138(1): p. 103-141.
[117] Ramsey, L. B. Genome-wide study of methotrexate clearance replicates SLCO1B1. *Blood, The Journal of the American Society of Hematology*, 2013. 121(6): p. 898-904.
[118] Martinez, D. Endogenous metabolites-mediated communication between OAT1/OAT3 and OATP1B1 may explain the association between SLCO1B1 SNPs and methotrexate toxicity. *Clinical Pharmacology & Therapeutics*, 2018. 104(4): p. 687-698.
[119] Volpi S, Bult CJ, Chisholm RL, Deverka PA, Ginsburg GS, Jacob HJ. Research directions in the clinicaRelling, M. V and Klein, T. E. (2011) 'CPIC: clinical pharmacogenetics implementation consortium of the pharmacogenomics research network,' Clinical Pharmacology & Therapeutics, 89(3), pp. 464–467.l implementation of phar. *Clin Pharmacol Ther.* 2018;103(5):778–86.
[120] Relling M V, Klein TE. CPIC: clinical pharmacogenetics implementation consortium of the pharmacogenomics research network. *Clin Pharmacol Ther.* 2011;89(3):464–7.
[121] Ross CJD, Visscher H, Sistonen J, Brunham LR, Pussegoda K, Loo TT. The Canadian Pharmacogenomics Network for Drug Safety: a model for safety pharmacology. *Thyroid.* 2010;20(7):681–7.
[122] Swen JJ, Nijenhuis M, de Boer A, Grandia L, Maitland-van der Zee A-H, Mulder H. Pharmacogenetics: from bench to byte—an update of guidelines. *Clin Pharmacol Ther.* 2011;89(5):662–73.
[123] Levine GN, Bates ER, Bittl JA, Brindis RG, Fihn SD, Fleisher LA. 2016 ACC/AHA guideline focused update on duration of dual antiplatelet therapy in patients with coronary artery disease: a report of the American College of Cardiology/American Heart Association Task Force on Clinical Practice Guidelines. *J Am Coll Cardiol.* 2016;68(10):1082–115.
[124] Wallentin L, Becker RC, Budaj A, Cannon CP, Emanuelsson H, Held C. Ticagrelor versus clopidogrel in patiets with acute coronary syndromesn. *N Engl J Med.* 2009;361(11):1045–57.
[125] Wiviott SD, Braunwald E, McCabe CH, Montalescot G, Ruzyllo W, Gottlieb S. Prasugrel versus clopidogrel in patients with acute coronary syndromes. *N Engl J Med.* 2007;357(20):2001–15.
[126] Dayoub EJ, Seigerman M, Tuteja S, Kobayashi T, Kolansky DM, Giri J. Trends in platelet adenosine diphosphate P2Y12 receptor inhibitor use and adherence among antiplatelet-naive patients after percutaneous coronary intervention, 2008-2016. *JAMA Intern Med.* 2018;178(7):943–50.
[127] Claassens DMF, Vos GJA, Bergmeijer TO, Hermanides RS, Van't Hof AWJ, Van Der Harst P. A genotype-guided strategy for oral P2Y12 inhibitors in primary PCI. *N Engl J Med.* 2019;381(17):1621–31.
[128] Kazui M, Nishiya Y, Ishizuka T, Hagihara K, Farid NA, Okazaki O. Identification of the human cytochrome P450 enzymes involved in the two oxidative steps in the bioactivation of clopidogrel to its pharmacologically active metabolite. *Drug Metab Dispos.* 2010;38(1):92–9.
[129] Sangkuhl K, Klein TE, Altman RB. Clopidogrel pathway. *Pharmacogenet Genomics.* 2010;20(7):463.

[130] Caudle KE, Dunnenberger HM, Freimuth RR, Peterson JF, Burlison JD, Whirl-Carrillo M. Standardizing terms for clinical pharmacogenetic test results: consensus terms from the Clinical Pharmacogenetics Implementation Consortium (CPIC). *Genet Med.* 2017;19(2):215–23.

[131] Gaedigk A, Ingelman-Sundberg M, Miller NA, Leeder JS, Whirl-Carrillo M, Klein TE. The Pharmacogene Variation (PharmVar) Consortium: incorporation of the human cytochrome P450 (CYP) allele nomenclature database. *Clin Pharmacol Ther.* 2018;103(3):399–401.

[132] Mega JL, Close SL, Wiviott SD, Shen L, Walker JR, Simon T. Genetic variants in ABCB1 and CYP2C19 and cardiovascular outcomes after treatment with clopidogrel and prasugrel in the TRITON–TIMI 38 trial: a pharmacogenetic analysis. *Lancet.* 2010;376(9749):1312–9.

[133] Umemura K, Furuta T, Kondo K. The common gene variants of CYP2C19 affect pharmacokinetics and pharmacodynamics in an active metabolite of clopidogrel in healthy subjects. *J Thromb Haemost.* 2008;6(8):1439–41.

[134] Varenhorst C, James S, Erlinge D, Brandt JT, Braun OÖ, Man M. Genetic variation of CYP2C19 affects both pharmacokinetic and pharmacodynamic responses to clopidogrel but not prasugrel in aspirin-treated patients with coronary artery disease. *Eur Heart J.* 2009;30(14):1744–52.

[135] Carreras ET, Hochholzer W, Frelinger III AL, Nordio F, O'Donoghue ML, Wiviott SD. Diabetes mellitus, CYP2C19 genotype, and response to escalating doses of clopidogrel. *Thromb Haemost.* 2016;116(07):69–77.

[136] Mega JL, Hochholzer W, Frelinger AL, Kluk MJ, Angiolillo DJ, Kereiakes DJ. Dosing clopidogrel based on CYP2C19 genotype and the effect on platelet reactivity in patients with stable cardiovascular disease. *JAMA.* 2011; 306(20):2221–8.

[137] Price MJ, Murray SS, Angiolillo DJ, Lillie E, Smith EN, Tisch RL. of genetic polymorphisms on the effect of high-and standard-dose clopidogrel after percutaneous coronary intervention: the GIFT (Genotype Information and Functional Testing) sInfluencetudy. *J Am Coll Cardiol.* 2012;59(22):1928–37.

[138] Mega JL, Close SL, Wiviott SD, Shen L, Hockett RD, Brandt JT. Cytochrome P450 genetic polymorphisms and the response to prasugrel: relationship to pharmacokinetic, pharmacodynamic, and clinical outcomes. *Circulation.* 2009;119(19):2553–60.

[139] Wallentin L, James S, Storey RF, Armstrong M, Barratt BJ, Horrow J. Effect of CYP2C19 and ABCB1 single nucleotide polymorphisms on outcomes of treatment with ticagrelor versus clopidogrel for acute coronary syndromes: a genetic substudy of the PLATO trial. *Lancet.* 2010;376(9749):1320–8.

[140] Mullard A. FDA tackles gene-drug interactions. *Nat Rev Drug Discov.* 2020;19(4):226–7.

[141] Scott SA, Sangkuhl K, Stein CM, Hulot J, Mega JL, Roden DM. Clinical Pharmacogenetics Implementation Consortium guidelines for CYP2C19 genotype and clopidogrel therapy: 2013 update. *Clin Pharmacol Ther.* 2013;94(3):317–23.

[142] Empey PE, Stevenson JM, Tuteja S, Weitzel KW, Angiolillo DJ, Beitelshees AL. Multisite investigation of strategies for the implementation of CYP2C19 genotype-guided antiplatelet therapy. *Clin Pharmacol Ther.* 2018;104(4):664–74.

[143] Pirmohamed M, Burnside G, Eriksson N, Jorgensen AL, Toh CH, Nicholson T. A randomized trial of genotype-guided dosing of warfarin. *N Engl J Med.* 2013;369:2294–303.

[144] Stewart A, Ganguli A, FitzGerald R, Pirmohamed M. Variation in warfarin prescribing and dosing in the UK: a national survey of anticoagulation clinics. *J Clin Pharm Ther.* 2015;40(4):466–71.

[145] Proietti M, Romanazzi I, Romiti GF, Farcomeni A, Lip GYH. Real-world use of apixaban for stroke prevention in atrial fibrillation: a systematic review and meta-analysis. *Stroke.* 2018;49(1):98–106.

[146] Ntaios G, Papavasileiou V, Makaritsis K, Vemmos K, Michel P, Lip GYH. Real-world setting comparison of nonvitamin-K antagonist oral anticoagulants versus vitamin-K antagonists for stroke prevention in atrial fibrillation: a systematic review and meta-analysis. *Stroke.* 2017;48(9):2494–503.

[147] Paré G, Eriksson N, Lehr T, Connolly S, Eikelboom J, Ezekowitz MD. Genetic determinants of dabigatran plasma levels and their relation to bleeding. *Circulation.* 2013;127(13):1404–12.

[148] Ziakas PD, Kourbeti IS, Poulou LS, Vlachogeorgos GS, Mylonakis E. Medicare part D prescribing for direct oral anticoagulants in the United States: cost, use and the "rubber effect." *PLoS One.* 2018;13(6):e0198674.

[149] Kjerpeseth LJ, Ellekjaer H, Selmer R, Ariansen I, Furu K, Skovlund E. Trends in use of warfarin and direct oral anticoagulants in atrial fibrillation in Norway, 2010 to 2015. *Eur J Clin Pharmacol.* 2017;73(11):1417–25.

[150] Ho KH, van Hove M, Leng G. Trends in anticoagulant prescribing: a review of local policies in English primary care. *BMC Health Serv Res.* 2020;20(1):1–8.

[151] Zhu J, Alexander GC, Nazarian S, Segal JB, Wu AW. Trends and variation in oral anticoagulant choice in patients with atrial fibrillation, 2010–2017. *Pharmacother J Hum Pharmacol Drug Ther.* 2018;38(9):907–20.

[152] Allabi AC, Gala J, Horsmans Y, Babaoglu MO, Bozkurt A, Heusterspreute M. Functional impact of CYP2C9* 5, CYP2C9* 6, CYP2C9* 8, and CYP2C9* 11 in vivo among black Africans. *Clin Pharmacol Ther.* 2004;76(2):113–8.

[153] Dickmann LJ, Rettie AE, Kneller MB, Kim RB, Wood AJJ, Stein CM. Identification and functional characterization of a new CYP2C9 variant (CYP2C9* 5) expressed among African Americans. *Mol Pharmacol.* 2001;60(2):382–7.

[154] Scordo MG, Pengo V, Spina E, Dahl ML, Gusella M, Padrini R. Influence of CYP2C9 and CYP2C19 genetic polymorphisms on warfarin maintenance dose and metabolic clearance. *Clin Pharmacol Ther.* 2002;72(6):702–10.

[155] Asiimwe IG, Zhang EJ, Osanlou R, Krause A, Dillon C, Suarez-Kurtz G. Genetic factors influencing warfarin dose in Black-African patients: a systematic review and meta-analysis. *Clin Pharmacol Ther.* 2020;107(6):1420–33.

[156] Cavallari LH, Langaee TY, Momary KM, Shapiro NL, Nutescu EA, Coty WA. Genetic and clinical predictors of warfarin dose requirements in African Americans. *Clin Pharmacol Ther.* 2010;87(4):459–64.

[157] Higashi MK, Veenstra DL, Kondo LM, Wittkowsky AK, Srinouanprachanh SL, Farin FM. Association between CYP2C9 genetic variants and anticoagulation-related outcomes during warfarin therapy. *JAMA.* 2002;287(13):1690–8.

[158] Limdi NA, McGwin G, Goldstein JA, Beasley TM, Arnett DK, Adler BK. Influence of CYP2C9 and VKORC1 1173C/T genotype on the risk of hemorrhagic complications in African-American and European-American patients on warfarin. *Clin Pharmacol Ther.* 2008;83(2):312–21.

[159] Rost S, Fregin A, Ivaskevicius V, Conzelmann E, Hörtnagel K, Pelz H-J. Mutations in VKORC1 cause warfarin resistance and multiple coagulation factor deficiency type 2. *Nature.* 2004;427(6974):537–41.

[160] Johnson JA, Caudle KE, Gong L, Whirl-Carrillo M, Stein CM, Scott SA. Clinical Pharmacogenetics Implementation Consortium (CPIC) guideline for pharmacogenetics-guided warfarin dosing: 2017 update. *Clin Pharmacol Ther.* 2017;102(3):397–404.

[161] Limdi NA, Wadelius M, Cavallari L, Eriksson N, Crawford DC, Lee M-TM. Warfarin pharmacogenetics: a single VKORC1 polymorphism is predictive of dose across 3 racial groups. *Blood, J Am Soc Hematol.* 2010;115(18):3827–34.

[162] McDonald MG, Rieder MJ, Nakano M, Hsia CK, Rettie AE. CYP4F2 is a vitamin K1 oxidase: an explanation for altered warfarin dose in carriers of the V433M variant. *Mol Pharmacol.* 2009;75(6):1337–46.

[163] Danese E, Raimondi S, Montagnana M, Tagetti A, Langaee T, Borgiani P. Effect of CYP 4F2, VKORC 1, and CYP 2C9 in Influencing Coumarin Dose: A Single-Patient Data Meta-Analysis in More Than 15,000 Individuals. *Clin Pharmacol Ther.* 2019;105(6):1477–91.

[164] Bress A, Patel SR, Perera MA, Campbell RT, Kittles RA, Cavallari LH. Effect of NQO1 and CYP4F2 genotypes on warfarin dose requirements in Hispanic–Americans and African–Americans. *Pharmacogenomics.* 2012;13(16):1925–35.

[165] Cooper GM, Johnson JA, Langaee TY, Feng H, Stanaway IB, Schwarz UI. A gen warfarin maintenance dosenome-wide scan for common genetic variants with a large influence o. *Blood, J Am Soc Hematol.* 2008;112(4):1022–7.

[166] Takeuchi F, McGinnis R, Bourgeois S, Barnes C, Eriksson N, Soranzo N. A genome-wide association study confirms VKORC1, CYP2C9, and CYP4F2 as principal genetic determinants of warfarin dose. *PLoS Genet.* 2009;5(3):e1000433.

[167] Cha P-C, Mushiroda T, Takahashi A, Kubo M, Minami S, Kamatani N. Genome-wide association study identifies genetic determinants of warfarin responsiveness for Japanese. *Hum Mol Genet.* 2010;19(23):4735–44.

[168] Perera MA, Cavallari LH, Limdi NA, Gamazon ER, Konkashbaev A, Daneshjou R. Genetic variants associated with warfarin dose in African-American individuals: a genome-wide association study. *Lancet.* 2013;382(9894):790–6.

[169] De T, Alarcon C, Hernandez W, Liko I, Cavallari LH, Duarte JD. Association of genetic variants with warfarin-associated bleeding among patients of African descent. *JAMA.* 2018;320(16):1670–7.

[170] Consortium IWP. nicEstimation of the warfarin dose with clial and pharmacogenetic data. *N Engl J Med.* 2009;360(8):753–64.

[171] Gage BF, Eby C, Johnson JA, Deych E, Rieder MJ, Ridker PM. Use of pharmacogenetic and clinical factors to predict the therapeutic dose of warfarin. *Clin Pharmacol Ther.* 2008;84(3):326–31.

[172] Finkelman BS, Gage BF, Johnson JA, Brensinger CM, Kimmel SE. Genetic warfarin dosing: tables versus aorithmslg. *J Am Coll Cardiol.* 2011;57(5):612–8.

[173] Tian X, Zhang C, Qin Z, Wang D, Yang J, Zhang X. Impact of CYP2C19 Phenotype and Drug-Drug Interactions on Voriconazole Concentration in Pediatric Patients. *Antimicrob Agents Chemother.* 2021;65(9):e00207-21.

[174] McDermott JH, Wolf J, Hoshitsuki K, Huddart R, Caudle KE, Whirl-Carrillo M. Clinical Pharmacogenetics Implementation Consortium Guideline for the Use of Aminoglycosides Based on MT-RNR1 Genotype. *Clin Pharmacol Ther.* 2022;111(2):366–72.

[175] Barbarino JM, Whirl-Carrillo M, Altman RB, Klein TE. PharmGKB: A worldwide resource for pharmacogenomic information. *Wiley Interdiscip Rev Syst Biol Med.* 2018;10(4):e1417.

[176] Fischel-Ghodsian N, Prezant TR, Chaltraw WE, Wendt KA, Nelson RA, Arnos KS. Mitochondrial gene mutation is a significant predisposing factor in aminoglycoside ototoxicity. *Am J Otolaryngol.* 1997;18(3):173–8.

[177] Usami S, Abe S, Kasai M, Shinkawa H, Moeller B, Kenyon JB. ng loss associated withennGarieetic and clinical features of sensoriural he the 1555 mitochondrial mutation. *Laryngoscope.* 1997;107(4):483–90.

[178] Usami S, Abe S, Akita J, Namba A, Shinkawa H, Ishii M. Prevalence of mitochondrial gene mutations among hearing impaired patients. *J Med Genet.* 2000;37(1):38–40.

[179] Li Z, Li R, Chen J, Liao Z, Zhu Y, Qian Y. Mutational analysis of the mitochondrial 12S rRNA gene in Chinese pediatric subjects with aminoglycoside-induced and non-syndromic hearing loss. *Hum Gene*t. 2005;117(1):9–15.

[180] Shen Z, Zheng J, Chen B, Peng G, Zhang T, Gong S. Frequency and spectrum of mitochondrial 12S rRNA variants in 440 Han Chinese hearing impaired pediatric subjects from two otology clinics. *J Transl Med.* 2011;9(1):1–11.

[181] MacArthur DG, Manolio TA, Dimmock DP, Rehm HL, Shendure J, Abecasis GR. Guidelines for investigating causality of sequence variants in human disease. *Nature.* 2014;508(7497):469–76.

[182] McCormick EM, Lott MT, Dulik MC, Shen L, Attimonelli M, Vitale O. Specifications of the ACMG/AMP standards and guidelines for mitochondrial DNA variant interpretation. *Hum Mutat.* 2020;41(12):2028–57.

[183] Göpel W, Berkowski S, Preuss M, Ziegler A, Küster H, Felderhoff-Müser U. Mitochondrial mutation m. 1555A> G as a risk factor for failed newborn hearing screening in a large cohort of preterm infants. *BMC Pediatr.* 2014;14(1):1–5.

[184] Koo J-W, Quintanilla-Dieck L, Jiang M, Liu J, Urdang ZD, Allensworth JJ. Endotoxemia-mediated inflammation potentiates aminoglycoside-induced ototoxicity. *Sci Transl Med.* 2015;7(298):298ra118-298ra118.

Chapter 8

Pharmacoeconomics

Zahraa Hassan Shehata*

Pharmacoeconomics Unit, Egyptian Drug Authority, Cairo, Egypt

Learning Objectives

After completing this chapter, the reader would be able to:

- Define Pharmacoeconomics, and identify its importance and relationship to other disciplines.
- Differentiate between the four most common types of Pharmacoeconomics studies and when to use them appropriately.
- Categorize cost categories and determine the perspective of the study.
- Select the most appropriate outcome measure for each study.
- Calculate the incremental cost-effectiveness ratio (ICER) and make a decision upon it.
- Interpret the cost-effectiveness plane.
- Recognize the value of modeling in Pharmacoeconomics.

What Is Pharmacoeconomics? Why Is It Important?

Pharmacoeconomics is the science that measures and compares the costs and consequences of pharmaceutical products and services. Pharmacoeconomics helps healthcare decision-makers answer two important questions concerning drug development and drug use.

The first question is related to the development and pricing of new drugs. Recently, there is a clear trend toward using new technologies to produce targeted and personalized medicines. Due to these advancements, the cost of drug development is rapidly increasing, leading to highly expensive medications. Decision-makers need to find a *balanced pricing policy* that provides a rewarding incentive for pharmaceutical manufacturers to continue innovating while ensuring the affordability and accessibility of these new therapies.

* Corresponding Author's Email: zahraa.hassan.shehata@gmail.com.

In: Clinical Pharmacist Tools to Deliver Rational Medication Use
Editor: Mohamed Emam Abdelmobdy Abdelrahim
ISBN: 979-8-88697-857-5

To achieve this, the price of new drugs should be linked to the added drug value (safety, effectiveness, and use) compared to the current treatments. This approach is called *"value-based pricing"* and is applied with the help of Pharmacoeconomics as shown in Figure 1.

Moving to the second question, from the perspective of governments, payers, and health insurance systems, the rapid introduction of many new and expensive treatments adds a high burden on healthcare systems that have limited budgets. Therefore, decision-makers are often concerned with how to make the best use of the *finite* resources available. They also have to decide which new interventions are considered the most efficient use of the *fixed budget.*

For example, as shown in Figure 2, if a new costly drug has been introduced to treat a serious disease that was previously untreated, the amount of money spent on purchasing this drug will be reduced from the budget available for other healthcare services (e.g., dialysis sessions). These missed opportunities are called *"the opportunity cost."* So, decision-makers must decide, which of these investments yields the *highest health benefits* for the population using the same budget. Pharmacoeconomics helps answer this question.

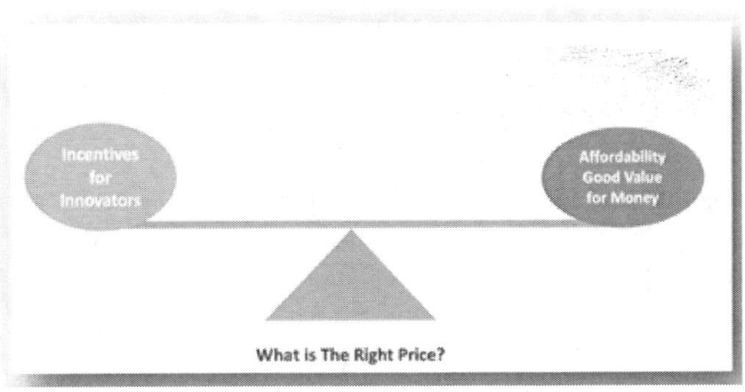

Figure 1. Important factors for appropriate pricing of pharmaceuticals.

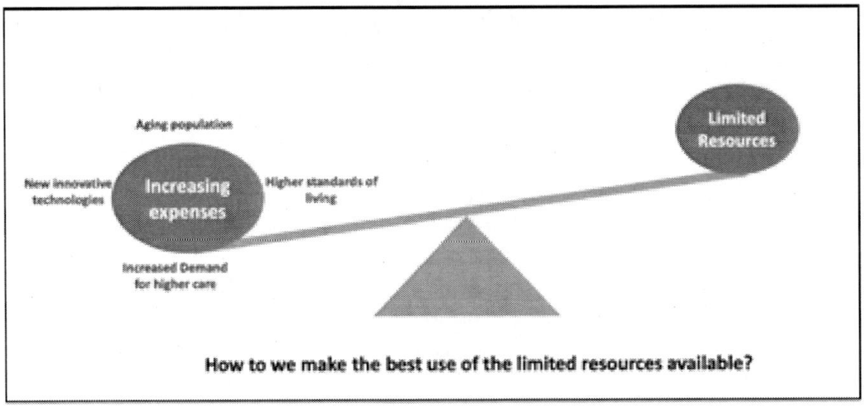

Figure 2. The need for efficient use of limited resource to meet the increasing costs of healthcare.

Pharmacoeconomics is also of high importance when comparing two alternative treatments for the same indication (e.g., a new expensive oncology drug vs. chemotherapy). Despite the higher price of the new drug, it can save money that is spent to administer the chemotherapy in the hospital, treat the adverse events, and prevent future complications from the disease. Pharmacoeconomics allows assessing whether the extra benefits of the new drug are worth the extra cost (after taking into consideration all these future savings).

To conclude, the science of pharmacoeconomics attempts to answer the following two questions:

1- What is the fair price for newly developed drugs?
2- Which drugs are good value for money and should be added to the formulary?

Relation between Pharmacoeconomics and Other Related Disciplines?

After understanding the definition and importance of pharmacoeconomics, it is important to define familiar with other closely related terms. Some of these concepts include: "Health Economics," "Health Technology Assessment," "Economic Evaluation" and others.

As mentioned, pharmacoeconomics is the science that identifies, measures, and compares the costs and consequences of pharmaceutical products and services. According to this definition, pharmacoeconomics focuses primarily on pharmaceuticals (mostly drugs) and tries to evaluate the costs and outcomes of these drugs.

The outcome of a drug includes, for example, patients' health and quality of life. The costs include the drug price as well as all the required resources, such as co-medications, hospitalizations, and management of adverse events. Pharmacoeconomics is sometimes considered a subdiscipline of health economics.

Health Economics

Health economics is the application of the concepts of economics to health care. Economics itself is concerned with the allocation of scarce resources. Therefore, health economics is concerned with the allocation of scarce resources to improve health [1].

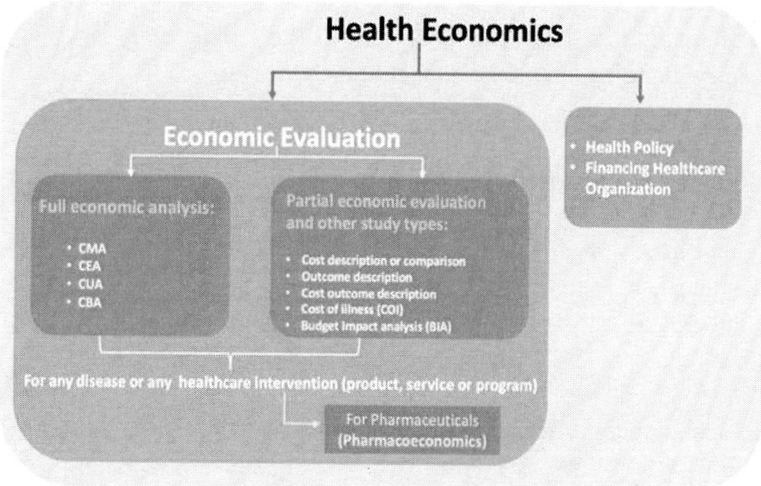

CMA = Cost-Minimization Analysis, CEA = Cost-Effectiveness Analysis, CBA = Cost-Benefit Analysis, CUA = Cost-Utility Analysis.

Figure 3. Different topics included within the concept of health economics and the relation between health economics and Pharmacoeconomics.

According to this definition, health economics is broader than pharmacoeconomics as it *is not concerned with pharmaceutical products only* but includes all types of health-related interventions. Besides, it also includes the broader principles related to *health policy*. For example, it is concerned with how to generate funds for health and how to distribute these funds among different services and different segments of the population through health insurance programs (Figure 3).

As illustrated in Figure 3, health economics includes both health policy aspects and economic evaluations. When the economic evaluation is concerned specifically with pharmaceutical products (including drugs), this is pharmacoeconomics [2].

Economic evaluations include either:

- *Full economic evaluation* which compares both costs and consequences (health outcomes) of two or more interventions and includes four study types that will be discussed later in details. [2]
- *Partial economic evaluations* either consider only one aspect (costs or outcomes) or it does not compare two interventions but can describe only a single intervention. This category includes: [2]
  - *Cost description* when only the costs of one intervention are analyzed.
  - *Cost comparison* is when the costs of two or more interventions are compared.
  - *Outcomes description* when only the outcomes of one intervention are analyzed.
  - *Cost outcome description* when both the costs and outcomes of one intervention are analyzed.
- *Other types of health economic studies include:*
  - *Cost of illness studies (COI).* This type is sometimes considered a type of partial economic analysis in some references. These studies are not concerned with a particular healthcare intervention, but instead, attempt to estimate the economic burden of a specific disease on society [2, 3].
  - *Budget Impact Analysis (BIA).* This analysis is concerned only with the affordability of healthcare interventions (i.e., what will be the impact of adopting a new intervention on the budget of the payer) [4].

Health Technology Assessment (HTA) [5]

Health technology assessment (HTA) is another key concept that is increasingly used nowadays in different healthcare systems. HTA can be defined as a "multidisciplinary process intended to support healthcare decision making by assessing properties and effects of one or more new or existing health technologies in comparison with a current standard in a systematic, transparent, and robust manner.

The assessment process covers 8 core aspects:

1. Health problem and alternatives that are currently used
2. Technical characteristics of the new health technology
3. Safety
4. Clinical effectiveness

5. *Costs and economic evaluation*
6. Ethical aspects
7. Organisational aspects
8. Patient and social aspects
9. Legal aspects

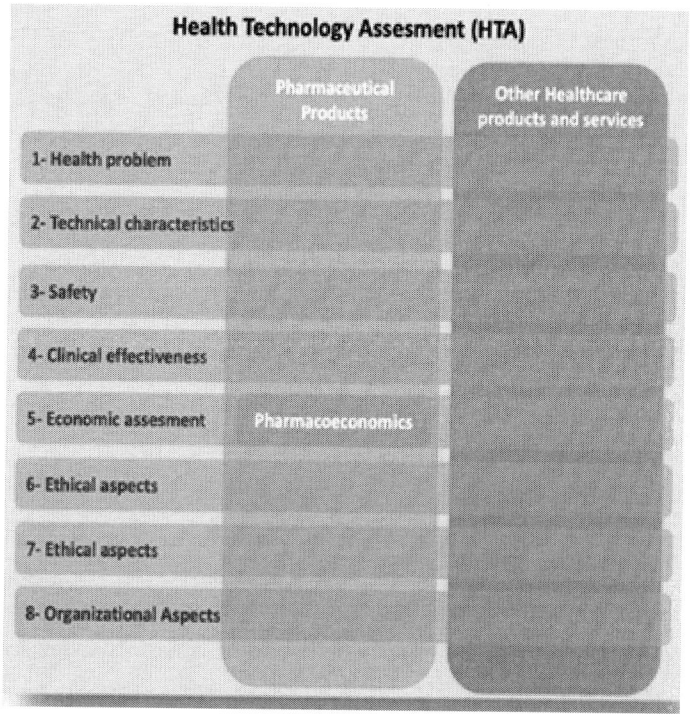

Figure 4. Relation between Health Technology Assessment (HTA) and pharmacoeconomics.

According to this definition (and as illustrated in Figure 4), HTA uses pharmacoeconomics studies as one of its tools to assess the economic aspects of health technology. The term health technology here refers to a variety of products besides drugs, such as medical devices, surgeries, mobile applications, and nonpharmacological interventions.

Starting from here till the end of the chapter, all the concepts that will be discussed apply to all types of interventions or health technologies. However, because this chapter is concentrated on pharmacoeconomics, all examples will be on pharmaceutical products (especially drugs).

What Are the Different Types of Pharmacoeconomic Studies?

Although there are different types of health economic (and pharmacoeconomic studies) as illustrated in Figure 3, the focus of this chapter is only on the most important category of studies which is "Full Economic Analysis". In these types of studies, value for money of drugs are assessed through answering the following questions:

- How much will be paid and what benefits will be gained from using the new drug compared with the current alternatives?
- Is this extra cost worth the extra benefits that will be gained?

Under this category there are four types of studies: [6]

- Cost-Minimization Analysis (CMA)
- Cost-Effectiveness Analysis (CEA)
- Cost-Benefit Analysis (CBA)
- Cost-Utility Analysis (CUA).

In all these four types the aim is to measure the costs and health outcomes of the drug (or any product/service) in comparison with other product/service. In all types, costs are expressed in monetary units (e.g., dollars, euros, EGPs, etc.). The only difference between them is how the outcomes are measured and presented.

Cost-Minimization Analysis (CMA)

CMA is the only type of economic studies in which only costs are measured and compared among alternatives. The reason for this is that the comparison is between two alternatives that have similar (equivalent) efficacy and safety (same outcomes). As both drugs are assumed to have similar outcomes, the aim of the study is only to find the least costly drug.

When conducting this type of analysis, it is essential to find good evidence that both options actually have similar efficacy. This assumption is often hard to prove, which limits the applicability of this method.

A simple example of CMA is comparing two drugs from the same therapeutic class with the same efficacy and safety. However, each drug has a different mode and frequency of administration, resulting in different costs.

Cost-Effectiveness Analysis (CEA)

In CEA, the outcomes are expressed in terms of natural health units, e.g., the number of cases cured, the number of stroke events prevented, the number of life-years gained due to increased patients' survival, etc.

According to this definition, all drugs compared in this type of analysis must be used for the same disease. For example, it is not possible to compare an antidiabetic drug with an anticancer drug using the same health outcomes. There is another limitation of this study type, is that only one health outcome can be assessed at a time. For example, if both drugs have different effects on patients' mortality and morbidity, and they also cause different side effects, all these outcomes cannot be taken into consideration in the same study. The aim of this analysis is to identify the intervention that is considered a good use of the available resources.

Cost-Utility Analysis (CUA)

Cost-utility analysis overcomes the limitations of CEA. To do so, outcomes should be measured using a generic tool that can be used in any disease area and it should also be able to combine all different types of outcomes into one single measure. This tool is called "QALYs" (Quality Adjusted Life Years).

But what is a QALY? A QALY is a way to measure people's health from two dimensions; the number of years they may live (survival) and how well they live (utility). Using this tool, whatever the disease under study and whatever the types of drug effects of interest, they can all be converted into a QALY.

Accordingly, cost-utility analysis compares costs and outcomes among two or more interventions, while outcomes are expressed in terms of QALYs. Both CEA and CUA are the most commonly used types of studies.

Cost-Benefit Analysis (CBA)

What if a government is deciding whether to spend a certain part of the budget on a disease screening program, an educational program, or a water cleaning program? i.e., the comparison is among alternative economic decisions that are not all within the healthcare sector? In this case, outcomes must be converted to a more generic measure. This generic measure is "monetary units."

In cost-benefit analysis, both costs and outcomes are measured in monetary units. Using this approach, it is possible to assess the cost-benefit ratio of certain interventions with (or without) comparison with other alternatives. For example, CUA can answer the question, "For every dollar spent on program X, how many dollars will be saved (or gained)?" This is called the benefit-cost ratio. In other words, it is called "the return on investment."

Benefit-cost ratio = Benefits (B) /Costs (C)

Another way to ask the question is whether this program will result in more money gain than the money that will be invested in its implementation? This is called "the net benefit" which equals benefits minus costs.

Net monetary benefit = Benefits (B) - Costs (C)

The difficult part here is how to convert outcomes to money (how to value the outcomes). Some of the outcomes are easy to measure in terms of money. For example, if the program will save other costs or if it helps people be more productive at work. However, there are benefits that are neither saved resources nor increased productivity. For example, improved health and quality of life. This type of benefit is converted to money using a special tool called the willingness-to-pay threshold which will be discussed later. This type of analysis is not common in the evaluation of pharmaceuticals but is very common in evaluating public health programs as shown in Table 1.

Table 1. Comparison between different types of pharmacoeconomic studies

Type of study	Measurement of costs	Measurement of outcomes	Applications	Limitations
Cost-minimization analysis (CMA)	$	Assumed to be similar	• Compare two drugs (interventions) with similar health outcomes used for the same disease	• It is hard to prove that both drugs have similar health outcomes.
Cost-effectiveness analysis (CEA)	$	Natural units e.g., (life years, prevented attacks, cured cases, etc)	• Compare two drugs (interventions) used for the same disease.	• Cannot compare drugs used for different diseases. • Assess only one type of health outcomes in each study.
Cost-utility analysis (CUA)	$	Quality-adjusted life years (QALYs)	• Compare two drugs (interventions) used for the same or different diseases.	• Measurement of QALYs is challenging. • Cannot compare programs/services outside the health sector.
Cost-benefit analysis (CBA)	$	$	• Assess the return on investment for any product or program. • Compare health program with non-health program. • Commonly used for evaluating public health programs.	• It is difficult to give a monetary value for health and other outcomes as psychological and social benefits.

How Are Costs Measured in Pharmacoeconomic Studies?

Costs are one of the two main pillars in the economic comparison between any two drugs. Costs are usually classified into four categories: direct medical costs, direct non-medical costs, indirect costs, and intangible costs.

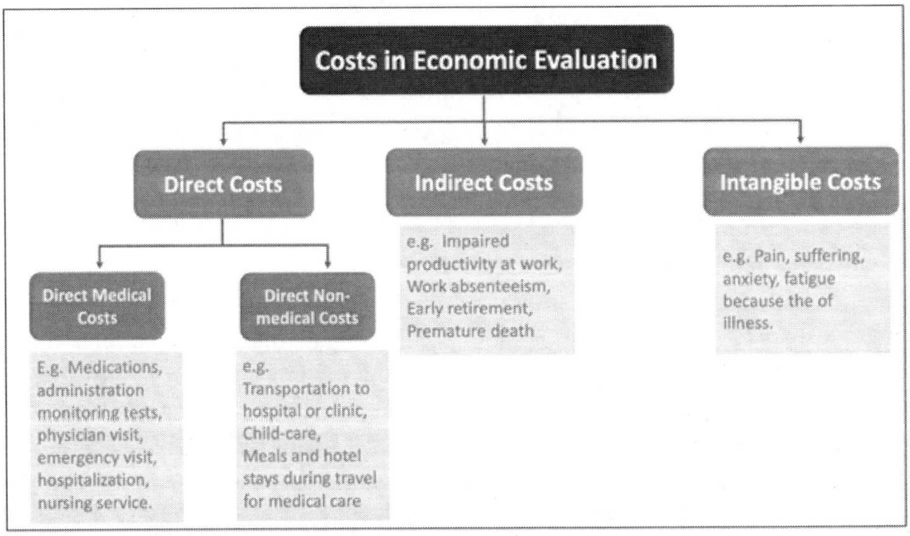

Figure 5. Types of costs included in pharmacoeconomic studies.

In general, direct costs represent actual expenditures incurred because of the disease or the drug use. While indirect costs represent the loss of earnings or productivity. For example, if a patient spent $ 100 to buy a medicine, this is a direct cost. However, if the patient couldn't work for one week because of his illness and lost $100 from his income, this is an indirect cost. Direct costs are further classified into medical and non-medical medical costs as shown in Figure 5 [7].

- *Direct Medical Costs* are easy to measure and usually included in all economic evaluations. They are expenditures related to medical care such as the costs of medications, medication administration, diagnostic tests, physician visits, pharmacist visits, emergency department visits, and hospitalizations.
- *Direct Non-medical Costs* are costs to patients and their families as a result of the disease or the treatment but not involved in the purchasing of medical services. Examples of direct nonmedical costs include the cost of transportation to and from the clinic or the hospital; childcare services for the children of a patient, and cost of hotel stays and meals for the patients and their families to receive treatment in other cities.
- *Indirect costs,* sometimes referred to as "productivity losses." It represents loss of earnings or productivity that affects the patient, his family, or the society from stopping or reducing work because of the disease. These include the productivity losses due to early retirement, sick leaves (absence from work) or impaired productivity at work (for example inability to work effectively because of pain). Indirect costs also include the costs of premature mortality.
- *Intangible Costs* include the costs of pain, suffering, anxiety, or fatigue that occur because of an illness or the treatment. It is difficult to measure or place a monetary value on these types of costs. In cost-utility analysis, intangible costs are included as an outcome within the calculation of utility scores as it will be discussed in the next section.

Perspective of the Study

The perspective is the point of view adopted when deciding which costs and health benefits to be included in the pharmacoeconomic study. In other words, who (what) is the person (or the organization) that is interested to know if the drug is of good value for money or not. Is it the patient himself? The hospital? The insurance company? or the whole society?

The perspective used in the study help determine the following:

- *Which cost categories should be included?* e.g., should non-medical and indirect costs be included in the study or not?
- *Within each category, what resource items should be included?* e.g., should all medical costs be included or some of them? Assume that the drug causes headache as a side effect which requires buying an OTC analgesic from the pharmacy. And study is conducted from the perspective of the third-party payer (health insurance company) who does not cover the cost of buying the analgesic in this case. For this study, the cost of the OTC analgesic should not be included.

- *Which unit cost will be used? (Note that "price" does not necessarily equal the "cost.*
  - For example, if the actual "cost" to perform a surgery is $ 1000.
  - The "price" of this surgery (after adding the hospital profit is $ 2000.
  - If the patient is insured, and the insurance company covers $1600 (80%) while the patient co-payment is $ 400 (20%).
  - In this example, the cost included in the study can be $ 1000, $1600, or $400 according to the study perspective (hospital, insurance company, or patient).

There are several types of study perspectives, the most commonly used ones include:

- *Societal perspective:* here the aim is to measure all costs that affect the society including costs to the insurance company, costs to the patient, costs to the provider/institution, and others. Although this may be the most appropriate and comprehensive perspective, it is difficult and time-consuming and therefore is rarely adopted in economic studies.
- *Payer perspective* (governmental or private insurance system). As mentioned above, in this case, only the amount of the price that is reimbursed (paid by the insurance) should be used in estimating costs. In addition, only medical services covered in the insurance plan are included.
- From the patient perspective, only the patient's out-of- pocket expenses, e.g., co-payments, lost income, and transportation costs should be included as shown in Table 2.

Table 2. Example on common perspectives used in pharmacoeconomic studies

Perspective	Direct Medical costs	Direct non-medical costs	Indirect costs
Patient perspective	Out-of-pocket costs only	Included	Effects on family income
Third-party payer (health-insurance) perspective	Covered costs only	Not included	costs covered by the health-insurance only
Societal perspective	All costs	Included	All costs

Steps in Cost Assessment

Assessing the costs in an economic evaluation involves 3 steps:

1. Identify the relevant resources used.
2. Value these resources (translate to monetary values).
3. Adjust valuations to account for the different timings.

Step 1: Resource Identification [3]

Used resources include for example medications used, number of days in hospital admission, number of visits to the physician, laboratory tests, etc. In an economic evaluation, only relevant resources are included. Relevant resource means those that are related to the disease, the administration of the treatment, or the consequence of the treatment such as treating as an adverse event from the drug.

As pharmacoeconomic researchers are usually comparing two alternatives, they are not interested in the overall costs of each alternative; instead, they are interested in the differences in costs between them. For example, if two drugs require the same monitoring tests with the same frequency and for the same duration, the costs of these tests are not relevant, as they are identical for both alternatives.

Usually, to know which resources are associated with a treatment, there are two possible sources:

- Costs measured during the clinical trial for each patient through record keeping and patient logs.
- Alternatively, costs that are collected retrospectively from medical records or reimbursement claims data. This source better reflects the "real-world" practice.

Step 2: Resource Valuation [3]

To obtain the total cost, the quantity of the resource units used is multiplied by their unit cost or price (according to the perspective). For example, if the patient needs to perform a special monitoring test every 2 weeks i.e., twice a month (quantity) and the cost of this test is $200 (unit cost).

Therefore, in one month the cost of this testing will be 200*2 = $ 400 per month.

Medical costs = Quantity of the Resources used * Unit price

Step 3: Time Adjustments for Costs [7]

Adjusting Past Costs to the Present value

Costs change over time because of inflation. For example, a drug that costs $15 in 2010 may cost $25 in 2020. For this reason, when costs are estimated from information collected more than 1 year ago, an adjustment of costs is needed. This is also referred to as standardization of costs. To do so, either use unit costs of the current year or adjust old costs using inflation rates.

Expressing Future Costs in Today's Value (Discounting)

If costs are estimated based on dollars that will be spent (or saved) in future years, another type of modification is needed called "discounting." People (and businesses) prefer to receive money today rather than later. Therefore, money received today is worth more than the same amount of money received next year or after 5 years. Modifications for this time value are calculated using a discount rate. The discount rate generally accepted for health care interventions is between 3% and 5%.

For example, suppose a new drug will save $ 10,000 for the payer after 5 years. Although this is a good saving, they are still promised to occur after 5 years. Because the payer prefers instant savings, this $ 10,000 equals only about $8500 in today's value (people prefer to receive money today not later). Similarly, if the payer will pay $ 10,000 but after 5 years, this is considered like paying only about $8500 today (people prefer to spend money later not now) as shown in Figure 6.

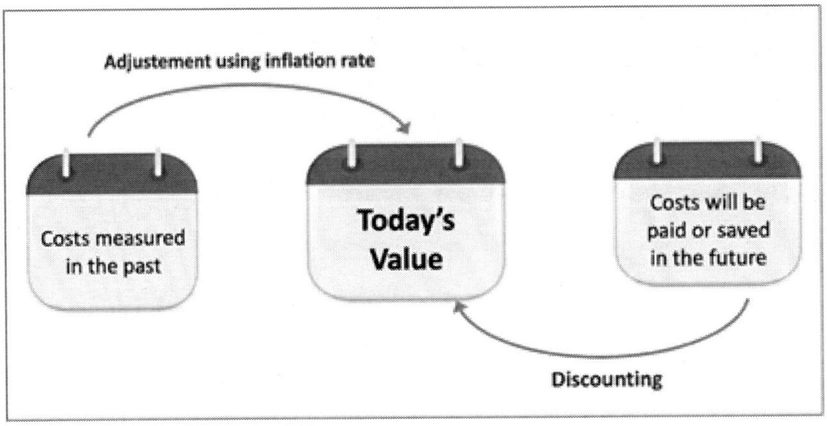

Figure 6. Types of time adjustments used for costs.

How Are Outcomes Measured?

The second component of any economic analysis is the outcome to be measured, that is defined as the expected benefits from an intervention (efficacy). It is worth noting that when the drug effect is measured in a clinical trial under ideal conditions, it is called "efficacy." When the effect of the drug is measured through observational studies or in real-world settings, it is called "effectiveness."

Outcomes also include risks of the products such as adverse events (safety). Therefore, outcomes include both positive and negative outcomes.

Traditionally, pharmacoeconomic references are used to classify outcomes as economic, clinical, and humanistic outcomes (abbreviated as ECHO). Economic outcomes represent for example the money saved money due to reduced occurrence of certain complications or side effects or because the drug administration requires fewer resources compared to the comparator drug or as it allows patients to be more productive at work, etc. All these outcomes are actually no more than the consequences of the clinical outcomes and are measured under the costs as in the previous section. To avoid confusion, the focus of this section is only on clinical outcomes and their effect on the humanistic aspects of the patients.

Types of Outcome Measures

The benefits derived from an intervention can be measured in either natural units or utility units.

1. *Natural units:* As mentioned previously, natural units are used in cost-effectiveness analyses. These are the clinical outcomes that are typically assessed by the clinicians in routine clinical practice or in clinical trials. This type of outcome occurs because of the drug effects on the mortality or the morbidity of the disease.
   - *Mortality (or survival):* Survival is expressed in the economic study as the number of life years. These life years are calculated form the clinical trial which reports

for example the number of patients alive after five years, or median time to death, etc.

- *Morbidity:* The effect of the drug on morbidity can be measured in one of two ways:
  - *Physiological measures (or surrogate endpoints)* such as blood pressure, cholesterol level, or bone mineral density. These are *intermediate outcomes* that are linked with the final clinical events. For example, previous studies have shown that there is an association or link between increased blood pressure and the occurrence of stroke events. Also, between bone mineral density and hip fracture.
  - *Final outcomes* are the clinical events of interest such as stroke or hip fractures.

2. *Utility units:* Utility scores are used to calculate Quality-adjusted life years (QALYs) which are the outcome used in cost-utility analysis.

   It represents the *humanistic* outcome of the drug. In fact, this outcome is also the result of the morbidity (clinical outcome). However, the effect on morbidity here is seen through the eyes of the patient and how it affects his quality of his life.

There are several characteristics and advantages of using utility units in economic studies rather than clinical events:

1. In this method, the effect of the disease and drug are reported by the patient themselves and not by the clinician or anyone else. It is therefore one of the patient reported outcomes (PROs). Some events might not seem serious or important from the perspective of the physician while they have a great impact on the patients' life for example a non-serious diarrhea or rash, etc.
2. Utility is calculated from health-related quality of life (HRQoL). HRQoL incorporates the physical, social, and emotional aspects of the patient's well-being (not only the physical effects). For example, a skin reaction in the face that causes no physical harm to the patient may have serious social and emotional effects in the patient's life that cannot be expressed in clinical terms.
3. As described previously, utility scores provide a generic unit that can be used in any disease area and therefore can be a common measure to compare between interventions used in different diseases.
4. It takes into account different effects of the drug in one measure for example if the drug has high efficacy but also causes many side effects. Both the drug's efficacy and side effects can be presented together in this single value.
5. Utility values are also incorporated with survival to calculate QALYs. In this way, there is one measure that expresses all the effects of the drug on patients' mortality and morbidity i.e., both quality and quantity of life.
6. Finally, utility scores not only represent patients' quality of life but also people's preferences. For example, a person may prefer to live 4 years in full health than living ten years with blindness. This reflects how people value their health and what they prefer as shown in Figure 7.

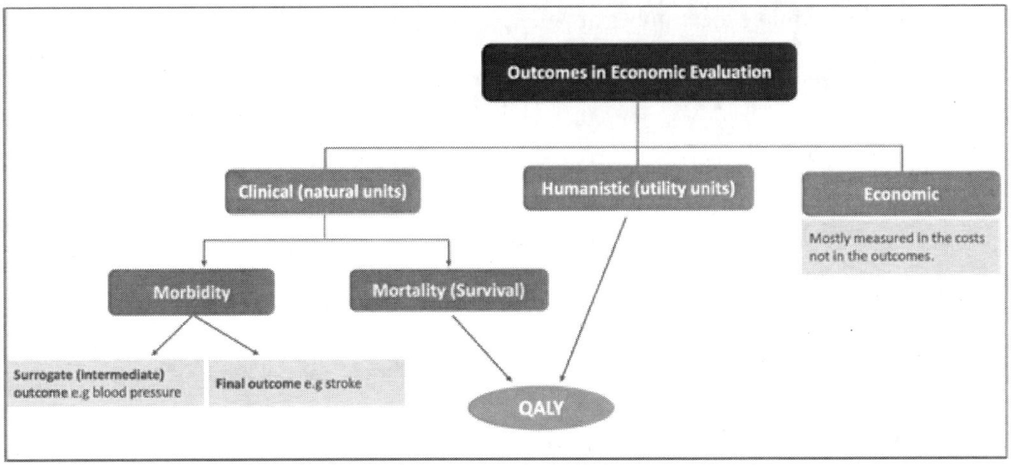

Figure 7. Types of outcome measures used in pharmacoeconomic studies.

HRQoL, Utility and QALYs. What Is the Difference?

In the previous section, three distinctive but closely related terms were mentioned. It is important to define each one of them separately and understand how it is calculated.

1. *Health-related quality of life (HRQoL)*
   This is just a way to describe the health state of the patient from all the dimensions (physical, social, and emotional). It is measured using questionnaires that allow patients to describe their health state. An example of such questionnaires is the EQ-5D questionnaire. The result is only descriptive. For example, the patient's state can be described as follows: some pain, big problems in mobility and no anxiety or depression. HRQoL are always multidimensional and not a single score or number.
2. *Utility values [4]*
   In utility, the health state is not just described, but there is also an interest in how people value their health and what they prefer. In addition, there is a need for one single number that incorporates all dimensions of health.

Utility always takes a value between 0 and 1:

- Zero means people see there is no difference between death and living in this state.
- One means perfect health.
- Sometimes, in very severe morbidity, utility can take a negative value. This means that people prefer dying to living with such morbidity.

There are two ways to generate utility scores:

- *Direct methods:* in these methods, patients with the disease are asked to estimate a utility value that represents their health state using a specific type of questionnaires (outside the scope of this chapter).

- *Indirect methods:* here patients are only describing their health state using HRQoL questionnaires. Then a sample of individuals from the general population are asked to give weights or values for these health states to translate them into a utility value (Figure 8).

  In a simplified example, if a patient with a certain disease described his health (using the HRQoL questionnaire) as follows:

  - no pain
  - serious problems in mobility
  - some problems in self-care
  - serious problems in doing his usual activities
  - severe anxiety or depression.

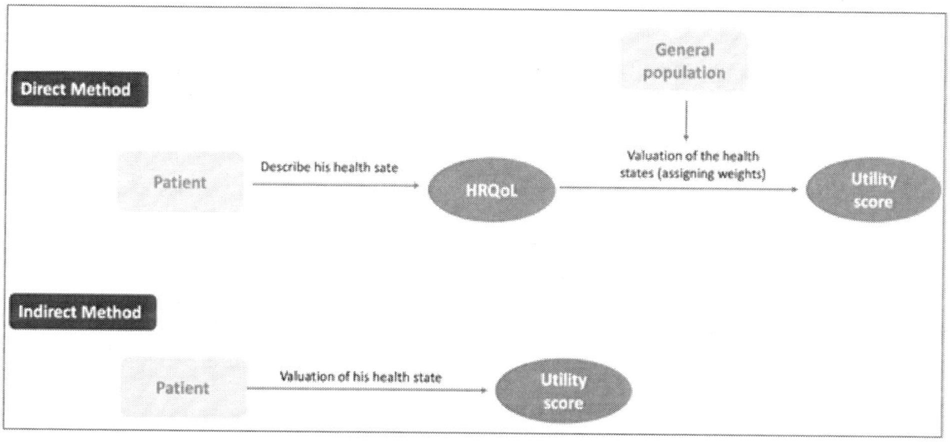

Figure 8. Direct vs indirect methods for generating utility scores.

Then a very large sample of individuals was asked about their preference of living with perfect health for short time or living with in this health state for a longer time. According to this questionnaire, a utility of 0.5 was given for this health state. This means people think there is no difference between living 10 years with this disease or living only 5 years in perfect health.

3. *Quality-adjusted life-years (QALYs) [4]*

This is the final form that is used in the economic study. The QALY combine the effects of the drug on both mortality and morbidity into a single index (combines quantity and quality of life).

QALYs are calculated simply by multiplying the duration of time spent in a given health state by the utility score of this health state. For example, if being blind has a utility of 0.3, spending 10 years as a blind person would give 3 QALYs, which is equivalent to spending 3 years in full health (Figure 9).

QALYs = Life years X Utility score

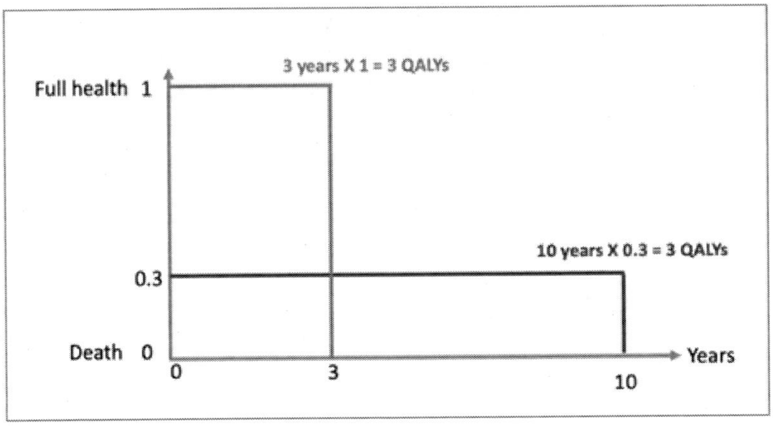

Figure 9. Example on calculating Quality adjusted life years (QALYs).

Presenting the Results and Making Decisions

After calculating all relevant costs and outcomes for both the new drug and the comparator, there are four possible scenarios:

1. The new drug has *higher benefits and lower costs* than the comparator. In this case, the new drug is with no doubt a better choice. No more calculations are required, and the decision is obvious which is to accept the new drug. In this scenario, the new drug is called *"Dominant."*
2. On the opposite side, if the new drug has higher costs and lower benefits than the alternative. Here, it is worse, and the decision is also clear, the new drug should be rejected. In this case, the drug under-study is called *"Dominated."*
3. The new drug can have lower costs and lower benefits than the alternative. This situation rarely occurs.
4. The new drug has higher costs and higher benefits than the alternative. This is the most common scenario when conducting pharmacoeconomic studies. As more efficacious technologies generally come at a higher cost.

In both the last two scenarios there is a need to do further calculations to make the right decision of whether or not to accept the new drug. The focus of this chapter is on the fourth scenario mostly.

There are several ways used to summarize and compare the costs and benefits of both alternatives. Only the incremental cost-effectiveness ratio (ICER) will be discussed here as it is the most commonly used method.

Costs, benefits, and the calculated ICER can be also represented graphically using and cost-effectiveness plane which will be also explained.

In all the examples used in this section, QALY will be used as the outcome measure. However, the exact same methods are used with any other type of outcome measure e.g., life years, cases of stroke, …etc.

Incremental Cost-Effectiveness Ratio (ICER)

Usually, the objective of any pharmacoeconomic study is to decide whether or not to replace a currently used drug with another that is more effective but is also more expensive. In such cases, an estimate of the additional costs spent to obtain the additional benefit is calculated. This is done by calculating the incremental cost-effectiveness ratio (ICER) using the following formula:

$$\text{Incremental cost effectiveness ratio} = \text{Cost}_{\text{New}} - \text{Cost}_{\text{Old}} / \text{Effectiveness}_{\text{New}} - \text{Effectiveness}_{\text{Old}}$$

ICER is the difference in costs (incremental cost) between both drugs divided by the difference in outcomes (incremental effect). In other words, ICER is the extra cost spent to get one extra unit of health (e.g., one QALY, one life year, one cured case…etc). A simplified numerical example on how ICER is calculated is presented in Table 3.

$$\text{Incremental cost effectiveness ratio (ICER)} = \frac{\text{Difference in costs}}{\text{Difference in outcomes}}$$

Table 3. Numerical example on ICER calculation

	Total Costs	Total outcomes
New Drug	$ 100,000	4 QALYs
Old Drug	$ 70,000	2 QALYs
Difference (New – Old)	= 100,000 - 70,000 = $ 30,000	= 4 – 2 = 2 QALYs
ICER	= 30,000/2 = $15,000 per QALY (an additional $ 15,000 should be spent for each one extra QALY)	

What Does a QALY Worth?

In the above example, an ICER of $ 15,000 per QALY was calculated which means that an additional $15,000 should be spent for each one QALY gained using the new drug. The question now is; is $15,000 acceptable or it is too high? Shall the decision-makers accept the new drug with this price, or it is too expensive with respect to the benefits that will be gained.

To answer these questions decision makers (payers) in each country should specify a maximum value they are willing to pay for each one unit of additional health.

- Assume the threshold is $20,000/QALY, in the above example the price per QALY (ICER) is lower than what they are willing to pay (threshold), so they can accept the new drug (the new drug is cost-effective).
- On the other hand, if the threshold is $10,000/QALY, in the above example, the ICER is higher than the threshold and the new drug should be rejected (not cost-effective).

There are different ways to decide the appropriate threshold for each country, but the details of these methods are outside the scope of this chapter.

> Cost-effectiveness Threshold (Willingness to pay threshold)
>
> It is the maximum amount of money the decision maker is willing to pay to gain one unit of health benefit.

Cost-Effectiveness Plane

Differences in costs, differences in effects, ICER and threshold all can be represented graphically using a cost-effectiveness plane. In this graph, the point where the x and y axes cross, indicates the costs and effectiveness for the comparator (old drug). For the new drug, differences in costs are placed on the Y-axis and differences in the effects on the X- axis (Figure 10).

Both axes go from negative to positive values. Because each point on the axis represents the value (costs or effects) of the new drug minus the old drug, when the point is positive it means the new drug is higher (in costs or effects) than the old one.

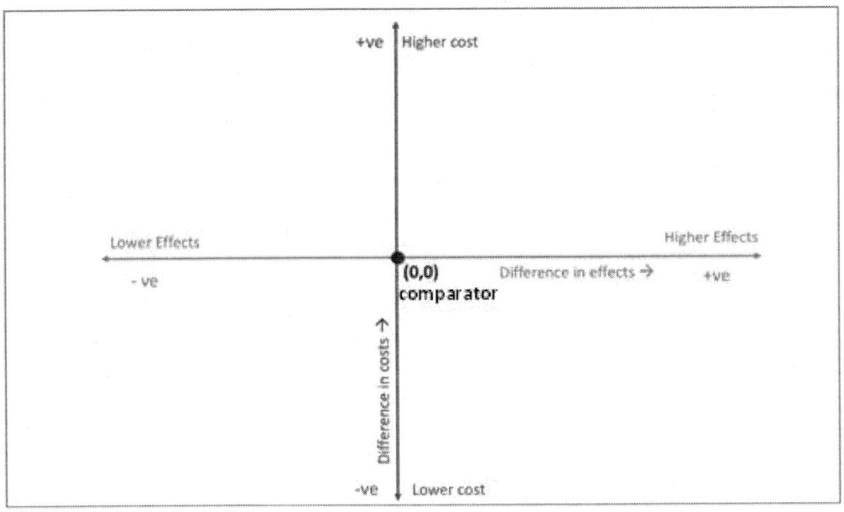

Figure 10. Overview of the cost-effectiveness plane.

As mentioned previously, there are 4 scenarios for the new drug:

1. The new drug is higher benefits and lower costs than the comparator "i.e., dominant". Graphically it lies in the bottom right quadrant on the CE plane. (Point A) in Figure 11.
2. The new drug has higher costs and lower benefits than the alternative "i.e., dominated". Graphically it lies in the top left quadrant on the CE plane. (Point B).
3. The new drug may have lower costs and lower benefits than the alternative. In this case it lies in the bottom left quadrant on the CE plane. (Point C).

4. The new drug has higher costs and higher benefits than the alternative. In this case it lies in the bottom left quadrant on the CE plane. (Point D). And this is the most common scenario in economic studies.

For both the bottom left and top right quadrants (points C and D), neither alternative dominates. In these cases, ICERs should be calculated. In these cases, the ICER is the slope of the line that goes from the origin (0,0) to point C or D (Figure 12).

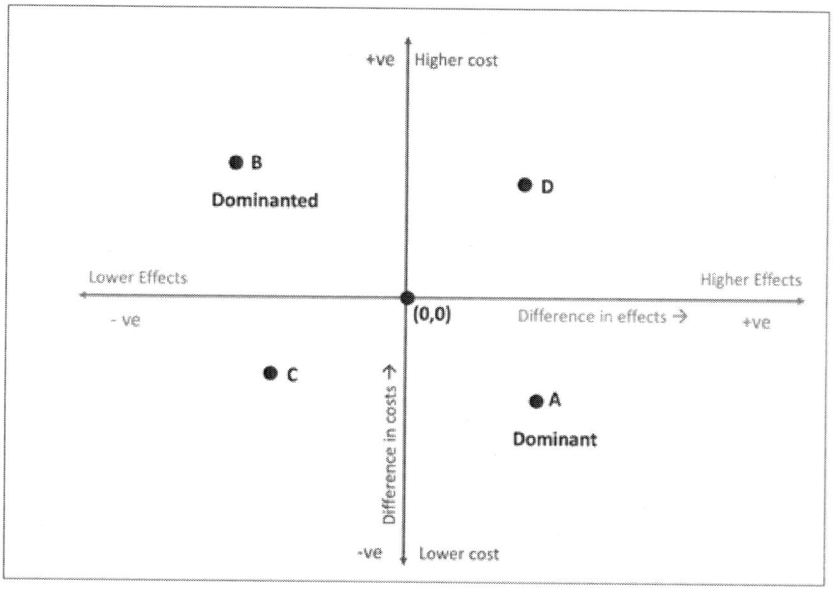

Figure 11. Indication of each quadrant on the cost-effectiveness plane.

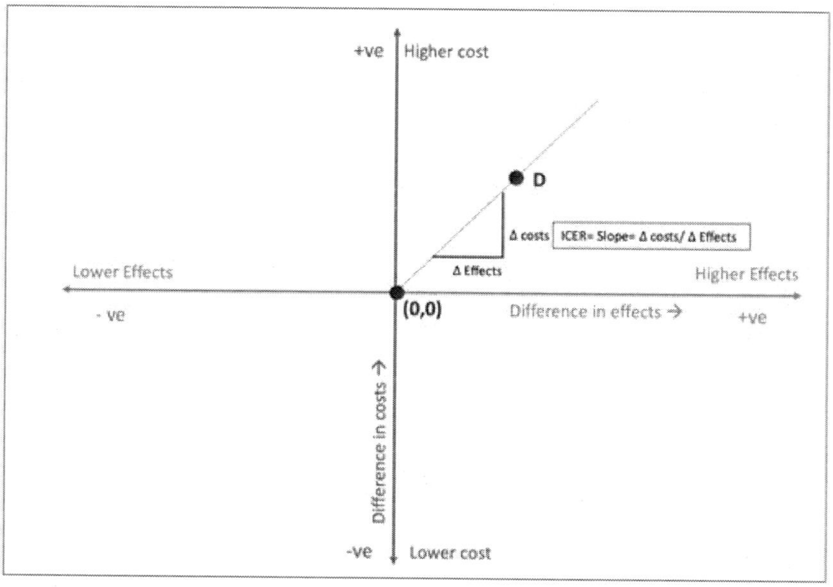

Figure 12. Calculations of the cost-effectiveness threshold represented on the cost-effectiveness plane.

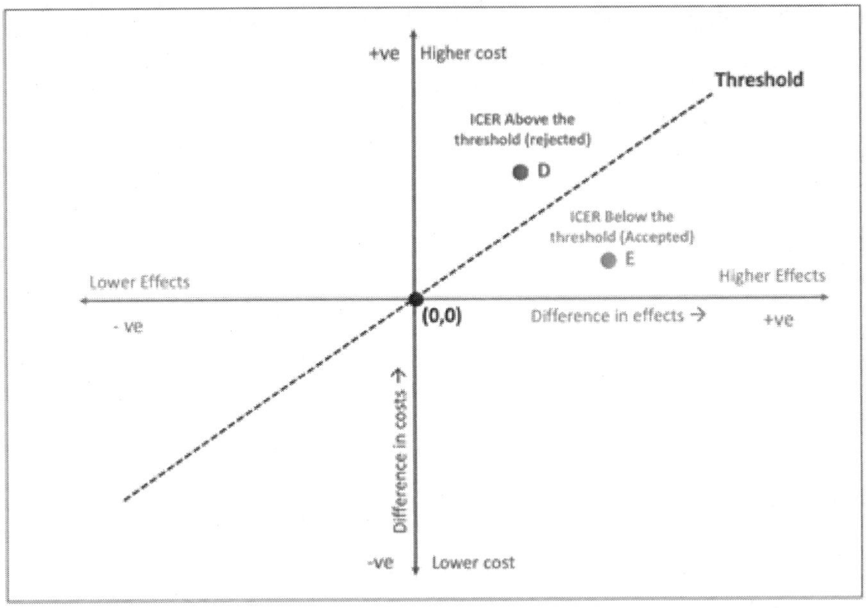

Figure 13. Representation of drugs with ICER above or below the threshold on the cost effectiveness plane.

The cost-effectiveness threshold can be also represented on the cost-effectiveness plane using a line with a slope equal to the threshold (Figure 13). Any point above the line indicates that the ICER is higher than the threshold and the drug is not cost-effective compared to the alternative and should be rejected (Point D). While any point below the line indicates that the ICER is lower than the threshold and the drug is not effective compared to the alternative and can be accepted (Point E).

Modeling in Pharmacoeconomic Studies

As mentioned before, all costs and outcomes that occur as a consequence of using the new drug vs. the alternative should be included in the study. For example, the use of the drug may delay disease progression which in turn delays further complications and finally death. The drug may also cause adverse events which lead to other complications…, etc. Each one of these consequences has its associated costs and outcomes.

These events do not occur in all patients, and if occurred, they do not occur at the same time. For example, only a proportion of patients may develop a certain complication or side effect while others not. This can happen after a month, a year, or ten years.

So how all these data can be analyzed to calculate the results? In principle, the most straightforward way is to measure both costs and outcomes in randomized clinical trials. In this case, costs and outcomes for each patient in the trial are just recorded and summed up. The advantage of this method is retaining the high internal validity of the clinical trial and ensuring that both costs and outcomes are measured in the same setting.

What Are the Limitations of Using Data Only from Clinical Trials?

The abovementioned approach is rarely used in economic studies for several reasons. Among them are:

- Clinical trials usually do not enroll enough patients for a long enough period to collect data about costs.
- Costs in clinical trials do not reflect costs in routine clinical practice. For example, a special test may be done in a trial but rarely done in the real world.
- Clinical trials include patients from different countries, and this cannot provide reliable information about resources and costs in a specific country.
- Clinical trials do not include all types of patients. For example, elderly patients and patients with comorbidities are usually excluded.
- In most cases, clinical trials are done against a placebo while in the economic study the interest is to compare the new drug with another alternative drug. Or there might be an interest to compare the new drug with different alternatives other than the one in the clinical trial.
- Finally, clinical trials are mostly of short duration so they don't capture all consequences of the drug. For example, trials may only measure an intermediate outcome as blood pressure changes but do not last for 10 or 20 years to collect data about the occurrence of stroke and death which are the most relevant outcomes in economic studies.

To overcome all of these limitations, economic studies are done using modeling techniques.

What Is Modelling? [8]

Modeling (also called decision analysis modeling) is a general concept used in pharmacoeconomics and in many other fields, including economics, healthcare, marketing, law, and engineering.

This approach helps in making decisions when there is a need to compare different alternatives that cause different consequences in a systematic way. Modeling is very useful specially when the decision is complex and when researchers are uncertain about some of the available data. It enables complex problems and processes to be broken down into component parts, each of which can be analyzed individually in detail before they are recombined.

In pharmacoeconomic studies, as it is hard to rely on a single clinical trial to estimate costs and outcomes associated with each drug, usually different types of data (epidemiological, clinical, economic) from multiple sources are combined using models. Models are considered a simplified representation of real-world situations.

In these models, mathematical relationships are used to define a series of possible consequences that occur from using alternative drugs.

Types of Models Used in Pharmacoeconomic Studies

There are a number of model types used in pharmacoeconomic studies. The most common ones are decision trees and Markov models.

Decision Tree [3, 4]

A decision analysis tree estimates the consequences of two or more options. It is represented by a tree diagram as in Figure 14.

- Branches of the tree represent all the interventions to be compared (Antibiotic A and Antibiotic B in this example).
- A series of possible consequences are coming out from these branches (Clinical success, failure, and adverse events)
- The likelihoods of the occurrence of the consequences are called 'transition probabilities.'

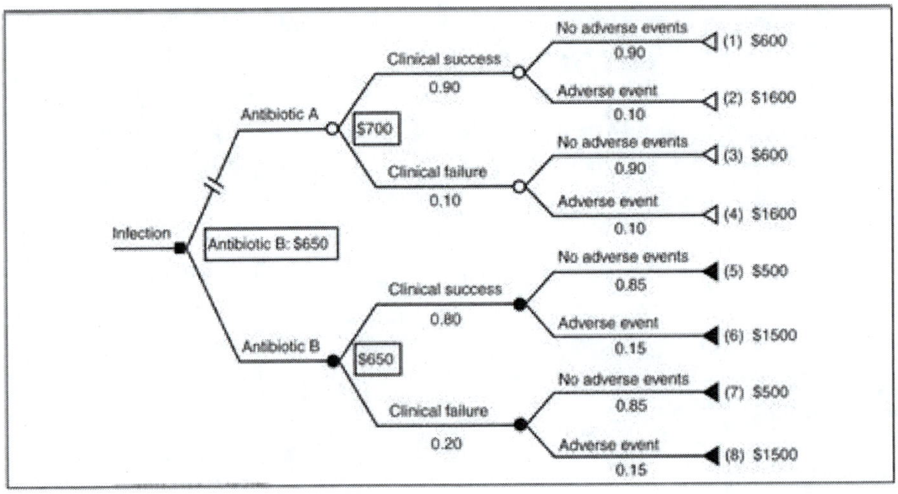

Figure 14. Example on decision tree model.

- The cumulative cost and outcomes for each intervention is calculated for each branch.
- Different interventions then can be compared in terms of their expected costs and outcomes.

Decision tree models are suitable for cost-effectiveness analysis in diseases occurring within a relatively limited time frame (acute conditions).

Markov Models [3, 4]

Markov models are analytical frameworks that represent diseases changing over time and are appropriate to model chronic disease as they can estimate long-term costs and outcomes.

- Markov model use 'health states' to represent all possible consequences of an intervention (Figures 15).

- These health states are mutually exclusive. So each individual in the model can be in only one of these states at a specified period of time.
- Patients move ('transition') between states as their condition changes over time.
- Movements from one state to another are presented as 'transition probabilities.'
- Disease progression is represented by transitions to more severe states, while the treatment effect will either reverse or slow this progression.

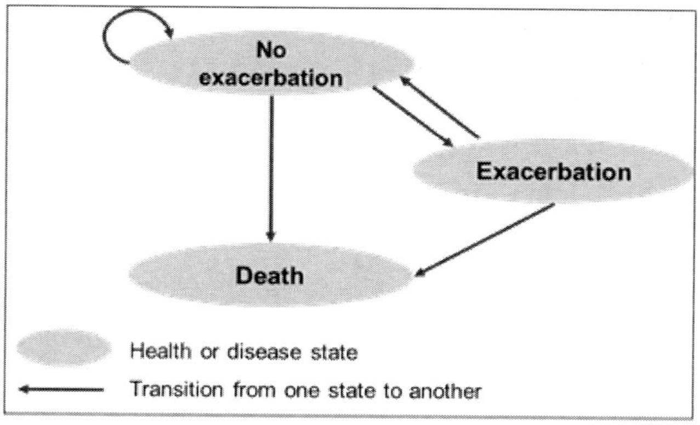

Figure 15. Example on Markov model structure.

- Time itself is measured in fixed periods called 'cycles' (e.g., a week or a month).
- Time spent in each health state for a single model cycle is associated with a cost and a health outcome
- Cumulative outcomes and costs for all patients are calculated at the end of the Markov process.

Advantages of Modelling in Pharmacoeconomics

There are several advantages for using modeling in Pharmacoeconomics, among them:

- Estimating the costs and outcomes on a time frame longer than the study duration. (extrapolation). For example, it is possible to calculate all costs and outcomes associated with using the drug over 20 years while the original clinical trial was only 5 years. This time frame is called "Time Horizon."
- Using evidence from different clinical studies (evidence synthesis).
- Linking surrogate (intermediate) outcomes with the final outcomes. For example, the clinical trial may only measure the effect of the drug on the progression of certain cancer but not on patient survival. It is therefore possible to combine data from another study that measures the effect of progression on death and combine all this information in the model.
- Generalizing results to other categories of patients not included in the clinical trial, such as elderly patients or patients with comorbidities.
- Examining uncertainty around the decision using sensitivity analysis. As certainty in the inputs used in the model never reaches 100%, it is crucial to measure this

uncertainty. For example, it is important to examine how the results of the study will change if the proportion of patients who will develop a certain complication or side effect using the drug was 10% higher or lower in reality than what is used in the study?

Self-Assessment Questions

1. If you are interested to choose between two alternative drugs for the same indication to be added to the hospital formulary and you were asked to provide an economic study to the hospital manager to defend your choice.

   After reviewing the literature, you found that both drugs have similar efficacy and safety. Your objective now is only to select the least costly one, which study type will you use:
   a. Cost-effectiveness analysis
   b. Cost-minimization analysis
   c. Cost-utility analysis
   d. Cost-benefit analysis

2. You are conducting a cost-utility study in 2022 and you are collecting the costs associated with each drug in the study. You found that patients using this drug should perform an ECHO every 6 months from previous literature. The only available official source for the ECHO price was from 2019. What should you do?
   a. Use the same price from 2019 in your study
   b. Apply discounting to change the price to the year 2022
   c. Adjust the price for inflation
   d. Exclude the cost of ECHO from your study.

3. Which of the following is an example of a non-medical direct cost?
   a. The cost of performing a liver function test.
   b. Paying for uber to go to the hospital.
   c. Receives an influenza vaccination at the pharmacy.
   d. An adult daughter misses work to take care of her mother to accompany her mother in chemotherapy sessions.

4. You have conducted a cost-utility study over a time horizon of 5 years to decide whether to replace a currently used antidiabetic drug in the national health insurance drug list with a newer antidiabetic that is more effective, and safer but is also more expensive. From your study, the costs and outcomes of the two drugs were as follows:

   Costs of the new drug = $ 1,500,000
   Outcomes of the new drug = 4 QALYs

   Costs of the old drug = $ 1,300,000
   Outcomes of the old drug = 2.4 QALYs

   Calculate the incremental cost-effectiveness ratio in this study (ICER)?

5. After calculating the ICER in the previous question, you should decide whether to accept the new drug or not. Knowing that the country's cost-effectiveness threshold is $ 50,000 per QALY. What will be your decision?
   a. The ICER is lower than the threshold, the new drug is cost-effective and can be accepted.
   b. The ICER is higher than the threshold, the new drug is not cost-effective and should be rejected.
   c. The ICER is lower than the threshold, the new drug is not cost-effective and should be rejected.
   d. The ICER is higher than the threshold, the new drug is cost-effective and can be accepted.

6. In a cost-utility study, you found that patients receiving the current therapies go through two different stages of the disease before they die. In the early stage, each patient lives on average 4 years with a utility of 0.8. In the advanced stage, each patient lives on average for 6 years with a utility of 0.5. What is the total number of QALYs for each patient in each stage of the disease?
   a. Four QALYs from the early stage and 3 QALYs from the advanced stage.
   b. QALYs from the early stage and 3.5 QALYs from the advanced stage.
   c. QALYs from the early stage and 3 QALYs from the advanced stage.
   d. Four QALYs from the early stage and 3.5 QALYs from the advanced stage.

7. In the following cost-effectiveness plane, the comparator drug is represented on the point (0,0) and the new drug by point (X). According to this graph, what do you consider the new drug compared to the old one?
   a. The new drug has higher costs and benefits and is called "Dominant"
   b. The new drug has lower costs and higher benefits and is called "Dominant".
   c. The new drug has higher costs and lower benefits and is called "Dominated".
   d. The new drug has lower costs and benefits and is called "Dominated".

8. Which of the following is <u>not</u> a characteristic of utility?
   a. It can take a value between zero and one.
   b. It combines the effects of the drug on both mortality and morbidity into a single index.
   c. It provides a generic unit that can be used in any disease area.
   d. It incorporates the physical, social, and emotional aspects of the patient's well-being.

References

[1] Edwards L, Fox A, and Stonier P, editors. *Principles and Practice of Pharmaceutical Medicine.* 3rd Ed. PP: 315-316, Wiley Blackwell Publishing Ltd; Available from: https://onlinelibrary.wiley.com/doi/epub/10.1002/9781444325263

[2] National Information Center on Health Services Research and Health Care Technology (NICHSR). *Health Economics Information Resources* [Internet]. 2016. Available from: https://www.nlm.nih.gov/nichsr/edu/healthecon/03_he_01.html.

[3] Kobelt G. Health Economics, An Introduction to Economic Evaluation [Internet]. 3rd Ed. London: *Office of Health Economics*; 2013. Available from: https://www.ohe.org/publications/health-economics-introduction-economic-evaluation

[4] Cobre A, Garabeli A, Bonetti A. *Evidence-Based Practice and Health Technology Assessment, An Introductory Guideline*. 1st Ed. Fernanda Stumpf Tonin FF-L, editor. Redondela: CIPF; 2021. Available from: http://www.cipf-es.org/book-hta/

[5] Børlum F, Kanavos P, Kalo Z. (2019, September 19). *Introduction to HTA* [PowerPoint presentation]. ISPOR Educational webinar, Dubai, United Arab Emirates. Available from: https://www.ispor.org/docs/default-source/default-document-library/3-sept-19_educational-seminar-introduction-to-hta8ec28fed4b0246089d84e40684dcf2d9.pdf?sfvrsn=62f34682_0.

[6] Turner H, Archer R, Downey L An Introduction to the Main Types of Economic Evaluations Used for Informing Priority Setting and Resource Allocation in Healthcare: Key Features, Uses, and Limitations. *Front Public Heal.* 2021;9:1–17.

[7] Rascati K. *Essentials of Pharmacoeconomics*. 2nd Ed. Lippincott Williams & Wilkins; 2014.

[8] Fasseeh A, Molnar A, Nagy B. *The Role Of Modelling In Economic Evaluations In Health Care.* Balazs Nagy, Jonathan Campbell ZK, editor. Budapest, Eotvos Lorand University; 2019.

Chapter 9

Pharmacovigilance and Medication Safety

Hadir Rostom[1,2,*]
Nada Adel[1]
Yomna Abdelgayed[1]
and Mohamed A. Elhawary[1,3]
[1]International Society of Pharmacovigilance (ISoP), Egypt Chapter, Cairo, Egypt
[2]Faculty of Pharmacy, MSA University, 6th of October City, Giza, Egypt
[3]Egyptian Ministry of Health and Population, Cairo, Egypt

Learning Objectives

After completing this chapter, the reader would be:

- Aware of the science of Pharmacovigilance, scope and activities
- Understand the role of spontaneous reporting in achieving public health and safe use of medicines
- Able to recognize Adverse Drug Reactions (ADRs) during practice and report individual case safety reports as complete as possible.
- Define risk management in pharmacovigilance and understand its aim
- Identify key stakeholders involved with risk management
- Define risk management based on the FDA and EMA definitions
- Identify and characterize safety specifications of medicines
- Understand the risk management framework, including risk management plan and risk minimization measures
- Realize the definition of the medication safety and understand the role of the medication safety officer.
- Identify the medication errors and distinguish between their types.
- Understand the barriers to medication error reporting in the healthcare organization.
- Outline some strategies to prevent medication errors.

---

* Corresponding Author's Email: hadir.rostom@yahoo.com.

In: Clinical Pharmacist Tools to Deliver Rational Medication Use
Editor: Mohamed Emam Abdelmobdy Abdelrahim
ISBN: 979-8-88697-857-5

History of Pharmacovigilance and Global Network

In the late 1950s, a sedative tranquilizer medicine launched in the market called "Thalidomide" and was first marketed by a German Company as an Over the counter sedative; soon after the launch, it was used in a wide range of conditions including cold & flu and was promoted as a "Wonder Drug" as unlike barbiturates, thalidomide induces prolonged sleep but did not cause death, even after an overdose, and later on used off -label for the treatment of nausea in pregnant women especially in the first trimester [1].

In the early 1960s, it became apparent to the public that Thalidomide resulted in a rare irreversible severe birth defect condition that affects the upper and/or lower limbs called "Phocomelia" where the bones of the affected limb are either missing or underdeveloped.

At first, the association between this birth defect and Thalidomide was not recognized, as no teratogenicity was detected prior to launch because teratogenicity tests during medicines development were not mandatory at that time.

The first case series of 33 children born with this malformation was presented in 1961 by German clinicians and then Thalidomide was first withdrawn from the market in Germany in November 1961.

Although reports of Phocomelia had started from 1956/57, thalidomide was first changed from being an Over the counter (OTC) drug to prescription only in Germany after the several complains in April 1961 and then withdrawn from the market in 1961/62. The withdrawal of the thalidomide was not at the same time across the world.

The true numbers of the children affected by this malformation were unknown; as there was no surveillance for either the numbers of women who received Thalidomide or the number of affected children. The number of reported infants affected by phocomelia reached over 10,000 reports.

Only 50% of the affected infants survived as some fetuses with severe defects died before birth or been miscarried or stillborn with severe internal defects of the heart and the kidneys. As a result of the Thalidomide disability epidemic, a wide range of responses took place worldwide; Birth defect surveillance programmes establishment in several countries was a significant response to this epidemic [1].

Among the major consequences was the development of rigorous regulations on the licensing of medicines; Sponsors (mostly pharmaceutical corporations) were required to monitor and report the trial's progress, and investigators were required to keep thorough records that included detailed information on whom received the medication; thus not only a proof to the medicines efficacy but also proof on its safety should be submitted the regulatory authorities prior to medicine authorization and marketing; as for a medicine to be placed in the market its benefits should outweighs its risks.

As a response to this tragedy, was the development of the science of Pharmacovigilance "PV"; with the aim to enhance patient care and safety in relation to the use of medicines; and to support health programmes by providing reliable, balanced information to assess the risk-benefit profile of medicines

In 1964, the "Yellow Card Scheme" was developed in the United Kingdom as a result to the Thalidomide disaster; this scheme was used by healthcare professionals (HCPs) and patients to report any suspected ADR/event from medicines to provide early warning to any possible risk [2].

And then in 1968, the establishment of the WHO Program for International Drug Monitoring "PIDM" counted as one of the major responses to this medical disaster [3].

Currently, Pharmacovigilance is defined according to the World Health Organization (WHO) as "science and activities relating to the detection, assessment, understanding and prevention of adverse effects or any other drug related problems."

WHO Program and Related International Organizations

In 1968, the Program for International Drug Monitoring "PIDM" was created by the WHO to ensure that evidence about harm to patients was collected from as many sources as possible.

Initially, the PIDM started as a pilot project in 10 countries with established national reporting systems for ADRs (pharmacovigilance system) namely Australia, Canada, Czechoslovakia, Federal Republic of Germany, Ireland, Netherlands, New Zealand, Sweden, United Kingdom, and USA.

As of August 2022, 153 members have joined the WHO PIDM, and in addition to 22 associate members are awaiting full membership; thus more than 170 full members and associate members in the programme in 2022, it covers approximately 99% of the world's population.

Uppsala monitoring Center in Sweden "UMC" has been responsible for the technical and operational aspects of the programme since 1978.

Under the WHO guidance, Uppsala monitoring Center "UMC" provides pharmacovigilance tools and services that allow efficient access to information for the member countries throughout "VigiBase"; a WHO's global database of reported potential side effects of medicinal products.

Each Member Country of the programme works nationally and collaborates internationally to monitor and identify the harm caused by medicines; this enables individual countries to be alerted to patterns of risks emerging across the world, which might not be appeared or evident from their local data alone; as of 2022, the number of reports from the member countries exceeds 30 million reports.

The advantage of pooling reports in a large, international database "Vigibase" is that patterns of specific risk may appear from the abundance of data from around the world that may not be obvious in smaller national databases, to find what are known as "Safety Signals" of potential ADRs [4].

In 1986, the Council for International Organizations of Medical Sciences (CIOMS) established its first working group on Pharmacovigilance for international Reporting of ADRs that was limited to post marketing reporting [5]. This working group came up for the first time with a unified standardized method for reporting ADRs by the pharmaceutical companies to the regulatory authorities; this method includes standardized definitions, procedures and format and called "CIOMS reporting form 1", later this form used by many countries as a guide to establish national reporting forms

The Council for International Organizations of Medical Sciences (CIOMS) developed by years and since the 1980s till present, CIOMS launched lots of working groups addressing PV topics [6].

In 1990, the International Council for Harmonization of Technical Requirements for Pharmaceuticals for Human Use (ICH) was established and gradually developed by bringing together the pharmaceutical companies and the regulatory authorities and developed the ICH Guidelines to harmonize the requirements/regulations worldwide to achieve safe, effective and high-quality medicines.

The Pharmacovigilance related Guidelines named from E2A to E2F ICH Guidelines; these guidelines served harmonized clinical safety data management to unify the data elements used in ADRs reporting and other related PV GLs [7]. By time, data analysis was found to be very challenging and difficult to be done using distinct terminologies so a standardized medical terminology was found to be necessary and this issue was identified by the ICH.

In October 1994, the ICH adopted the first version of the standardized medical dictionary for further terminology development.

In 1997, the dictionary released after testing and named the Medical Dictionary for Regulatory Activities "MedDRA" which is a clinically-validated international medical terminology used in the entire regulatory process, from pre-marketing to post-marketing, and for data entry, retrieval, evaluation, and presentation in order to make easier data exchange and facilitate data analysis.

Now MedDRA is available worldwide and widely used by pharmaceutical companies and regulatory authorities and health researchers [8].

The International Society of Pharmacovigilance (ISoP), is a global, independent, professional non-profit society; anyone who is interested in medications safely is welcomed in society [9].

The aim of the society is to improve the science and good understand of Pharmacovigilance all over the world by providing lots of various trainings, meetings and act as an open platform for discussing any new idea regarding medications safety and Pharmacovigilance activities and sharing experiences.

The society was primary founded as the European Society of Pharmacovigilance in 1992 and then developed to ISoP in 2000.

Need for Pharmacovigilance

Before introducing any medicinal product to the market; Clinical development takes place through clinical trials (CTs) [10].

There are phases to be completed in the clinical trial process before a company can submit their treatments to be sold on the market; each stage of a clinical trial has its own purpose in ensuring that a treatment is safe and effective for use by the public as follows:

- Phase I, took place after the preclinical lab studies and usually starts with a small group of healthy volunteers (20-50) to gather preliminary data about the product safety on humans and side effects identification.
- Phase II, the new medication is given to a larger group of volunteers (100-300) to determine its effectiveness in the particular indication and dose recommendations and further study on its safety profile.

- Phase III, the test medicine is then given to a large group of volunteers (1000-3000) for further efficacy and comparative testing with standard or similar treatments and for more expanded view to its safety.
- Phase IV, called the post approval study phase as it took place after the medicine been approved and placed in the market for public use; where the product safety and efficacy tracked after the wide exposure.

Unfortunately, Clinical trials were found to have many limitations like the limited number of studied patients as the number of involved volunteers in the clinical trials did not exceed a few thousand thus rare reactions or chronic toxicities will not be detected until the medication been widely used for a longer period of time.

Among the CTs limitations were the strict inclusion and exclusion criteria of the involved volunteers; as the study performed on a very selective group in relation to age, sex, ethnicity or patients with other comorbidities.

In addition to the previously mentioned limitations special populations such as pediatrics, geriatrics and pregnant women are not studied during the trial.

All these limitation resulted in insufficient data regarding the benefit risk ratio of the approved products as not all actual or potential risks will have been identified at the time of initial authorization.

Risks and benefits of a certain medicine will be more clear and recognized only after its usage by a larger population for a longer time [11].

No medicine is entirely safe for all people in all places at all the times, and Pharmacovigilance can characterize this risk by observation and monitoring the medicines in the real practice helping in the identification of new risks or safety concerns or even a better understand to a known risk.

Through the vigilant monitoring of medicinal products, regulatory actions or decisions may take place by withdrawal, restriction of use or labeling change.

So products recall or withdrawal from the market is not from the aims of PV, because as stated before no medicine is entirely safe for all people at all the times so the aim of PV is to keep the products safer in the market.

One from the under-recognized importance of Pharmacovigilance is that PV can reveal practice issues such as unexpected lack of effect or delayed response of a medicine, quality problems, dependence & abuse, medication errors, misuse and off label use [12].

Self-Assessment Questions

1. PIDM was created by ________ and ________ is responsible for technical and operational aspects
   a. Uppsala Monitoring Center (UMC)
   b. World Health Organization (WHO)
   c. European Medical Agency (EMA)
   d. Council for International Organizations of Medical Sciences (CIOMS)

2. Clinical trials provide adequate information about medications' safety before drug marketing
   a. True
   b. False

The Expanded Scope of Pharmacovigilance

Over the years, the scope of Pharmacovigilance is being expanded in relation to the reported products and the reported information.

In relation to the reported products, the Pharmacovigilance scope widened to include not only Human Medicines but also Biological and Blood products, Vaccines, Medical devices, Vitamins and Herbal products, Veterinary products and Cosmetics.

In relation to the reported information, Pharmacovigilance conducting advanced drug monitoring based on ADRs with the use of medicines including the use in special populations such as pediatric and geriatric populations, exposure during pregnancy, teratogenicity and exposure during lactation [13].

The WHO definition of pharmacovigilance, established in 2002 is "The science and activities relating to the detection, assessment, understanding and prevention of adverse effects or any other drug-related problems". The last part of the definition "...any other drug-related problems." came to confirm on such expanded scope of the reported information. Accordingly, Pharmacovigilance includes not only the reported information from the use of a medicine in its approved indication and dosage but also monitor the reported safety information that arise when the product used in Special situation like Off label use, Medication errors, Overdose, Abuse/ Misuse and Drug Interactions. Adverse events reported from substandard, falsified and counterfeit medicines and reports of lack of therapeutic efficacy or treatment failure are also under the scope of Pharmacovigilance.

In this context, it is important to differentiate between the mentioned above concepts as follow:

Overdose, this refers to the administration of a quantity of a medicine given per administration or cumulatively, which is above the maximum recommended dose according to the authorized product information. Clinical judgement should always be applied of that purpose.

Off-label use, this relates to situations where the medicine is intentionally used for a medical purpose not in accordance with the authorized product information.

Misuse, this refers to situations where the medicine is intentionally and inappropriately used not in accordance with the authorized product information.

Abuse, this corresponds to the persistent or sporadic, intentional excessive use of a medicine, which is accompanied by harmful physical or psychological effects.

Medication Errors, an unintended failure in the drug treatment process that leads to, or has the potential to lead to, harm to the patient.

Occupational exposure, this refers to the exposure to a medicine, as a result of one's professional or non-professional occupation [14].

Accordingly, we can conclude that Pharmacovigilance will help in the following [15]:

- Prevent or reduce the risks aroused from medicines as many ARDs are preventable.
- Improve the public health by protecting patients from unnecessary harms or hazards and this could be achieved after well identification and characterization of a specific risk.
- Continuous monitoring for medicines safety profile to obtain evidence on approved medications safety.
- Avoid the unnecessary use of medicines in special populations (as mentioned before that Geriatrics, pediatrics and pregnant women are excluded during Clinical trials)
- Reveal new potential use/new indication for already approved medicine for further testing by clinical trials; Minoxidil is an example to this as it was originally marketed as antihypertensive medicine, after launch it was noticed that it cause important side effect which is hirsutism (development of excess hair) and ability to slow or stop hair loss and promote hair regrowth, later on it was developed in a topical formula as a treatment for male pattern baldness (androgenic baldness) and for female androgenic alopecia however the mechanism of its ability in hair growth still not fully understood.

Self-Assessment Questions

1. Pharmacovigilance aims to:
   a. Provide safer medicines
   b. Withdrawal of products with severe side effects
   c. Both answers are correct

2. Which of the following is true:
   a. ADRs that may arise from the use of medications used within the labelling specifications should be reported.
   b. Drug exposure during pregnancy without any associated side effect should be reported
   c. ADRs resulted from off label use of medications should not be reported
   d. ADRs affected child whose father was exposed before pregnancy should not be reported
   e. Expected ADRs are not necessary to be reported

Detection and Reporting of AEs

Pharmacovigilance activities are the actions or practices made to ensure the watchful monitoring of medications' safety to guarantee that the benefit-risk balance is favorable towards the medicines for achieving public health by maximizing the benefits and minimizing the risk throughout the appropriate use of medicines.

The primary step in PV activities is collecting information related to medications' safety; to identify new or unrecognized risks or even known risk with increased severity or frequency.

Data collection is done in two ways; First routinely through "Passive surveillance" by collecting Adverse Events (AEs) reports spontaneously reported from Healthcare professionals or patients (medicines' users), monitoring any published risks in press, media and regulatory authorities' websites and also risks discussed in social media [16].

Second through "Active surveillance" by collecting safety information using pre-organized process such as Post authorization safety studies "PASS" and this is done in specific circumstances as this type of surveillance is very high cost-effective when compared to the passive way.

The responsibility of medications' safety monitoring is a shared responsibility between Pharmaceutical Companies by continuous monitoring of their medicines in the market and Health authorities by monitoring the whole market and the companies' performance and also HCPs are responsible for the safe use of medicines and this is done through the timely mannered reporting of any noticed adverse events either to the pharmaceutical company concerned or directly to the Competent authority.

Spontaneous Reporting is a Pharmacovigilance powerful tool in monitoring medications' safety and is defined as an unsolicited (voluntary) communication by a healthcare professional or consumer to a company or regulatory authority that describes one or more ADRs in a patient who was given one or more medicines that does not derive from a study or any organized data collection scheme. Spontaneous Reporting system (SRS) is a fundamental principle in PV since it enables quick identification of potential safety signals related to medicines, and relies mainly on the voluntary reporting of suspected ADRs either from HCPs or from public.

This method is inexpensive and has shown to be very effective in monitoring the ADRs that arise from the medicines as long as they are available in the market [17].

ADRs and Their Classification

Before talking about reporting and how, what and when to report, it's important to understand what are the ADRs and their classification.

An ADR is defined as a noxious and unintended response to a medicine, including lack of efficacy, and which can also result from overdose, misuse or abuse of a medicine in addition to responses that arise during the use of authorized medicines in normal doses. The ADRs may be already known side effect and mentioned in the product's leaflet and may be newly unrecognized risk. Usually, ADRs are classified into two main categories; Type A which refers to dose-related reactions (more severe with higher doses) and mostly expected from the drug Pharmacology and called "Augmented reactions" and this type could be avoided or controlled when doses are adjusted according to the age and condition.

Type B is not dose-related, Uncommon and not Predictable from drug pharmacology and called "Bizarre reactions," these reactions occur in a small percentage of susceptible, intolerant patients, for example, because of an inborn metabolic defect or an acquired enzyme deficit, leading to an abnormal metabolic pathway or production of a toxic metabolite.

The ADRs classification is then widened to include four more types; Type C which is dose and time related and refers to reactions resulted from Chronic or long-term exposure.

Type D refers to Delayed Adverse reactions, Type E resulted from the withdrawal or the end of treatment and Type F refers to the reports of lack of efficacy and failure of treatment.

So, Healthcare professionals should be alert to identify all types of ADRs, whether the medication is given within its authorized dose and indication or used in other circumstances like off-label use and abuse or ADRs that arise as a result of drug interactions, medication errors, occupational exposure, misuse and overdose or even decreased therapeutic response and therapy failure.

ADRs/Adverse Events also classified by seriousness; i.e., the term serious is not a synonym to severe; the term "severe" refers to a reaction's intensity (as in mild, moderate or severe), however the reaction itself might not be of any medical importance (such as severe rash) so a severe reaction is not necessarily to be a serious reaction [18].

The definition of Serious AE/ADR is any untoward medical occurrence associated with the use of a medical product in a patient at any dose, resulted in:

- *Death:* if the direct outcome of the adverse event or reaction is death and this outcome is considered "Fatal"
- *Life-threatening:* this refers to a reaction in which the patient was in immediate possibility of dying at the time reaction, and also refers to situations if the patient may have died as a result of continued usage of the medical product; Anaphylaxis occurred post administration of intravenous antibiotics is famous example to life-threatening events.

Life-threatening does not apply to a reaction that, if it had been more severe, might have actually resulted in death.

- Hospitalization/prolong the existing hospitalization: this outcome when the patient requires inpatient hospitalization as a result of the AE/ADR or had to stay more time in the hospital because of the reaction.

This outcome does not apply to emergency room visits, investigations, or outpatient treatments that do not result in hospital admission and should be assessed for other applicable seriousness criteria.

Example: if shortness of breath and severe hypotension occurred after medicine administration and the patient referred to a hospital and treated immediately then dismissed, this is not considered hospitalization but could be life threatening or medically important condition according to the medical judgment.

- Disabling/incapacitating: refers to cases of permanent/ persistent or significant disability occurred as a result of administration of medicine(s); Tendinopathy and Tendon Rupture because of fluoroquinolones therapy is an example to these criteria.

Inability to walk or move limbs because of transient muscle fatigue, persistent constipation for days are not example for disability as this only used in cases of significant disability.

- Congenital Anomaly/birth defects: this when one of the parents administered a medication before pregnancy or exposure during pregnancy and resulted in abnormal outcome (even if it was not anomaly) on the delivered child; this situation is considered a serious reaction because of the resulted birth defects.

- Important medical events and the events that require intervention to prevent one of the above-mentioned outcomes.

Some ADRs/AEs are considered serious, however, they did not result in any of the above-mentioned criteria and this is considered if intervention or a corrective treatment was required to prevent more consequences or sequelae so medical assessment and judgment are highly required in these situations.

Some events by their nature are considered serious events and named the "Important Medical Event (IME)" such as Thrombocytopenia, Drug dependence and Convulsions.

Transmission of an infectious agent by a medicine and Individual cases with an abnormal outcome following exposure during pregnancy are always classified as serious reports like premature delivery, developmental delay in foetus or child and reports of foetal death or spontaneous abortion.

The EudraVigilance Expert Working Group has developed an important medical event terms list based on the Medical Dictionary for Regulatory Activities "MedDRA" that updated and published periodically in line with the latest MedDRA version on the European Medical Agency (EMA) website. All types of ADRs, serious and non-serious events should be considered by HCPs to be reported in order to achieve the appropriate medication safety monitoring.

Self-Assessment Questions

1. Effective safety monitoring is done mainly through post authorization safety studies
   a. True
   b. False

2. The responsibility of medications' safety monitoring is the responsibility of: (select all applicable)
   a. Pharmaceutical Companies
   b. Health authorities
   c. Healthcare professionals

3. A severe reaction is always a serious reaction
   a. True
   b. False
   c. List the seriousness criteria
   d. __________
   e. __________
   f. __________
   g. __________
   h. __________
   i. __________

ADRs Detection in Clinical Practice

Detection or recognition of ADRs is not an easy process as it's sometimes hard to differentiate between the treated disease and the ADR; thus the detection of ADRs starts with the continuous suspicion of any abnormal response that may appear on patients.

ADRs are not restricted to obvious side effects that appears after a short time from any medicine(s) administration, so HCPs should be alert to any signs or symptoms that shows on the patient; this ADR may be a lab test abnormality, abnormal clinical measurement (example: abnormal pulse, heart rate, temperature, body weight) or may be investigational finding in medical scans.

The following will help HCPs to detect/recognize ADRs:

- Ask the patient if he/she experienced any side effect or abnormality as a part of therapy monitoring because patients usually did not recognize that abnormal response may be from the used medicine, so HCPs have to listen carefully to patients complains and be alert to any hidden described in between words from the patients.
- Verify that the patient actually received the prescribed medicine at the advised dose to detect any treatment noncompliance, dispensing or medication errors, misuse and overdose.
- Patient medical history should be available as some history like previous dependence or abuse, chronic diseases and previously used medicines may explain the resulted ADR
- Refer the patient to the proper specialty physician for proper examination and diagnosis (as appropriate).
- Ask for any medications used concomitantly used medicines to assess drug interactions
- Focus on any abnormal response that may shows on special populations like pediatrics, geriatrics and pregnant women as mentioned before that these population is excluded from clinical trials the safety profile of medicines in special populations could only be recognized through appropriate recognition and reporting of ADRs.

Content of an ADR Report

Back to the Spontaneous reporting, Clinicians and all the HCPs should be aware of the term "Individual case safety reports (ICSRs) which refers to the format and content for the submission of an individual report of suspected adverse reactions in relation to a medicine that occur in a single patient at a specific point of time.

There are four minimum information that should be included in the safety report to constitute a "Valid Report"; one single identifiable patient, at least one reporter, one or more suspected adverse event and at least one medicine. A valid report is the effective and

It's imperative to emphasize that a valid report means a report that contains the minimum information for reporting and to be included in the worldwide database for more data analysis, it does not mean a complete report; to get the most out of the safety report; it should be complete as possible.

The Individual case safety reports (ICSRs) from its name should address reaction(s) that occurred in one single patient; this patient should be identified either by its initials, gender, date of birth, age at the onset of the reaction, age group or by an identification number in a health facility; the patient should be characterized by at least one of the above-mentioned descriptors to prove the patient existence and helps in detecting duplicate reports, however, its preferable to include all the information regarding the patient as data like age and gender are very important during the data analysis and risk assessment.

If the reporter could not remember the exact age of the patient, the age group is enough to identify him.

The ICSR should include information for at least one identifiable reporter; the reporter is characterized by profession or qualifications (e.g., physician, pharmacist, nurse, other healthcare professional, consumer or other non-healthcare professional), name and contact information; its preferred that the reporter is reachable throughout his/her contacts for the possibility of obtaining further information to make the report as complete as possible but the report is still valid if the reporter disagree to provide any contacts.

More than one reporter could report the same ICSR; For example, if a mother reported to the doctor that her son suffered from an ADR, so the mother here considered to be "The primary reporter" and the doctor is the reporter who will deliver the case report either to the pharmaceutical company concerned or to the medicine authority.

Valid ICSR should include at least one suspected medicine to cause the reaction and is characterized by its name (preferred to be the trade name not the generic); this medicine could be dietary supplement or vitamin; interacting medicines should be taken into account too.

The medicine trade name (generics accepted if the reporter did not remember the exact product's name) with the strength and the actually administered dose and frequency, route of administration, exact indication and Duration of usage (Date started and Date end) are the best to describe the suspected product.

Mentioning the other administered medicines concomitantly with the suspected medicine helps in identifying interactions and potentiating medicines effects/side effects.

One or more suspected adverse events/ADRs should be addressed in the safety report; the reporter does not have to be quite sure about the causal relationship between the reaction(s) or the event and the administered medicine, suspicion is enough to report.

When reporting a specific event/reaction; it should be extensively described in details with discussing every symptom, regardless of whether a confirmed diagnosis has been given, and this is crucial since it will aid in the development of a hypothesis to a particular safety signal when the data is being examined globally, in addition to mentioning the time lag between the reaction onset and the medicine administration, date the reaction started and stopped, the seriousness of the reaction (as discussed above), the outcome of the reaction whether recovered, reaction ongoing or resolved with sequelae and the clinical judgment and investigation results (laboratory tests/scans) if any.

Additional data should be taken into consideration in relation to the reported ADR; the data related to the outcome which is the De-challenge and Re-challenge information.

De-Challenge is the withdrawal or dose reduction of the administered medicine; if the ADR decreased or resolved then is called positive de-challenge while Re-Challenge is the re-introduction of a previously administered medicine and if the same ADR re-occurred after re-administration this is called positive re-challenge.

These information will help is the clinical assessment of the relationship between the medicine and the resulted ADR as in cases of positive de-challenge and re-challenge the causal association will increase.

With due consideration of the ADRs that may arise from and special situation like overdose, off-label use, misuse, abuse, medication errors, Occupational exposure, Lack of efficacy and delayed therapeutic effects, Interactions, Quality issues, Poisoning, teratogenicity and exposure during pregnancy and lactation.

ADRs reporting is not limited to serious or newly recognized ADRs, it is very valuable to report already known ADR as this will help in better risk characterization by identifying its frequency and severity and figure out if there is a required risk minimization action.

Overview on ICSRs Processing

ICSRs processing starts once the receipt of the minimum information about an ADR report even if the reporter is not sure that the experienced ADR resulted from the received medicine; only suspicion is enough to trigger reporting. At the healthcare facility level e.g., hospital, the pharmacovigilance officer/medication safety officer, is responsible for processing the ADR reports detected at his healthcare facility. Afterwards, these reports should be sent either to the pharmaceutical company which own the suspected medicine or to the national pharmaco-vigilance center in the country.

Upon receiving the report by the pharmacovigilance officer, it is very important to check for report validity to make sure that the minimum information is reported (One single identifiable patient, one or more reporter, at least one suspected ADR and at least one suspected medicine). Triage of the received cases based on cases validity and seriousness may be needed to prioritize their processing especially when large number of cases were received. In addition, the pharmacovigilance officer needs to check whether the reported ADR is already mentioned in the product information of the suspected medicine "expected ADR", all the reported ADRs should be considered, however, more attention should be given to "unexpected ADRs."

All the received ADR reports should be documented. Those reports which might be received verbally should then be documented by the pharmacovigilance officer. Each safety report should be given a unique ID to facilitate report tracking and the entry of any received updated information of a previously reported case. furthermore, for the ease of detecting case duplications. For this purpose, using safety reports electronic system with structured data elements will be extremely helpful, where all the collected case information is entered in its corresponding data field. All the reported reactions, signs, symptoms and any drug related problems like medications errors and abuse is coded using the MedDRA dictionary to standardize the reported terms and to facilitate the subsequent data presentations and analysis.

Furthermore, such electronic systems always have a free text field where the pharmacovigilance officer can a case narrative, which is a medical story written in a comprehensive way describing all the patient information including the medical history and the reported AE with the reporter's verbatim with the onset of the reaction(s) and the outcome, diagnosis, any interventions or investigations done as a result of the reaction, any concomitant medications and the reporter's opinion or medical judgment should be written (in case the reporter is a HCP). Where the structured data elements are needed to support quantitative analysis, the case narrative is crucial for any subsequent qualitative review of the case.

The pharmacovigilance officer needs to consider whether follow up with the reporter is needed, there are several situations where such follow up will be needed; for example, upon receiving a non-valid case. One other situation is when more details about the case is needed, as mentioned earlier that a valid report does not mean a complete report, accordingly, follow-up with the reporter is done to obtain as much information that will be essential for the scientific evaluation and analysis of the case. Follow-up is not restricted to serious reports only; however, it should be done to any report to complete any essential missing information. When such follow-up is being conducted by contacting, listen carefully to what is said by the reporter or the patient –if the patient himself is the reporter- to characterize the patients' concerns. It is very important also to ask for the special situations according to the expanded scope of Pharmacovigilance e.g., medication error, overdose, off label use…. etc. This can be achieved by requesting details e.g., regarding the exact administered dose and the reason for administering the medicine. Complete the case details as possible according to what mentioned above in the section "Components of ADR report" and any related supportive information.

In case of the reported complain is a syndrome or a specific medical condition (example: Guillain-Barré syndrome, Toxic epidermal necrosis), description of the event and the associated sign and symptoms should be requested to be included in the case report.

Table 1. WHO-UMC causality categories

Causality term	Assessment Criteria
Certain	• Event or laboratory test abnormality, with plausible time relationship to drug intake • Cannot be explained by disease or other drugs • Response to withdrawal plausible (pharmacologically, pathologically) • Event definitive pharmacologically or phenomenologically (i.e., an objective and specific medical disorder or a recognized pharmacological phenomenon (example: (for instance 'grey baby syndrome' and chloramphenicol, or anaphylaxis immediately after the administration of a drug that had been given previously) • Rechallenge satisfactory, if necessary
Probable/Likely	• Event or laboratory test abnormality, with reasonable time relationship to drug intake • Unlikely to be attributed to disease or other drugs • Response to withdrawal clinically reasonable • Rechallenge not required
Possible	• Event or laboratory test abnormality, with reasonable time relationship to drug intake • Could also be explained by disease or other drugs • Information on drug withdrawal may be lacking or unclear
Unlikely	• Event or laboratory test abnormality, with a time to drug intake that makes a relationship improbable (but not impossible) • Disease or other drugs provide plausible explanations
Conditional/ Unclassified	Event or laboratory test abnormality: 1. More data for proper assessment needed, or 2. Additional data under examination
Unassessable/ Unclassified	Report suggesting an adverse reaction: 3. Cannot be judged because information is insufficient or contradictory 4. Data cannot be supplemented or verified

If not mentioned in the primary report, the outcome of the reported ADR should be requested to assess for the seriousness; it is preferable not to question directly the reporter on the reaction seriousness but rather to ask whether one of the seriousness criteria detailed previously applicable with the reported reaction. If the suspected product is biological medicinal product or vaccine, batch number is extremely important information to ask about.

Follow-up should be tailored to each case and should be done in a way to encourage the reporter to submit new information or further safety reports submission; this could be achieved by not asking about information already mentioned in the primary report and requesting further information without raising any worries or insecurity feeling to the reporter.

After making sure that all the needed information about the case is made available, medical review and Causality assessment of the case can be carried out trying to answer the question "Is there a possibility that the reported ADR has been caused by the medicine administered by the patient?". Trying to answer this question is a process named "Causality assessment" which is defined as standardized/harmonized process used to find the causal relationship between and medicine and the reported reaction using scales or algorithms. There are some widely used methods for the causality assessment, but the most well-established commonly used method and adopted by many countries is the WHO-UMC scale and the categories are "certain", "probable", "possible", "unlikely", "unclassifiable or conditional", and "unclassified" (Table 1). Causality assessment methods will not prove the association between the medicine and the reported reaction but it will improve the scientific evaluation and Classify relationship likelihood, as in clinical practice it's rare to be able to tell that this ADR is Certain or unlikely to be caused by the medicine.

Data Analysis

As mentioned earlier, that the primary step in Pharmacovigilance activities is collecting information related to medications' safety either spontaneously or via conducting safety studies. The information obtained from such ADR reports will be used to promote safe use of medicines in the local, national and international levels. The collected reports will be entered into the national PV database - and sent also to the global database "Vigibase"- to be analyzed on a regular basis for signal detection.

The signal management process is defined as the set of activities performed to determine whether there are new risks associated with an active substance or a medicine or whether known risks have changed in its characterization.

The outcome of the analysis is then communicated and could be a recommendation to HCPs or to the public to change practice/ behavior or could be a regulatory action, for example one or more of the following actions may be taken:

- Changes or warnings in the product information or on the package label
- Changing the information on how the medicine should be used
- Changes in the specified dose of the medicine
- Restricting the indications for use of a medicine, for example advising that it should not be used by particular groups of patients
- Changing the legal status of a medicine, for example, from over-the-counter to prescription only
- Additional investigations into the use of the medicine
- Enhancing educational initiatives to improve the safe use of that medicine

- In rare circumstances, removal of the medicine from the market, if the risks of a medicine are found to outweigh the benefits

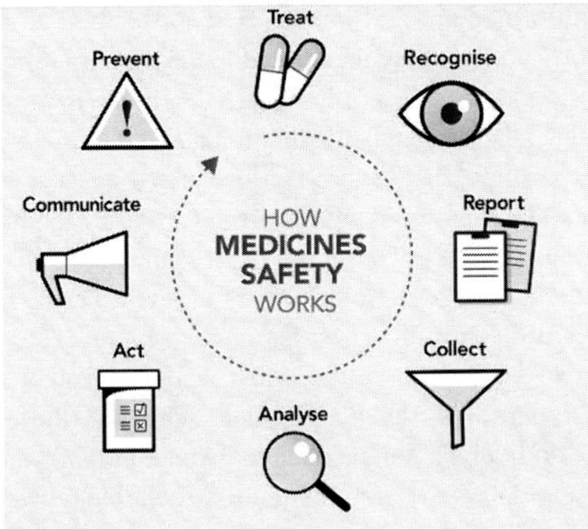

Source Uppsala Monitoring Centre.

Figure 1. Diagram illustrating the cycle for medicines safety.

Medications' safety through ADRs collection, data management and analysis is the cornerstone pharmacovigilance activity and a dynamic cycle for the safe use of medicines and achieving public health [19] (Figure 1).

Self-Assessment Questions

1. The ICSR is considered invalid and doesn't qualified for reporting until the following information is collected: (choose as many as applicable)
   a. Suspected ADR/AE
   b. The full name of the patient
   c. Batch number of the suspected medicine
   d. Reporter's information

2. For an ICSR to be reported the patient's exact age should be known and age group is not enough
   a. True
   b. False

3. ADRs reporting is restricted to new/ unrecognized AE.
   a. True
   b. False

4. Follow-up of reports is not restricted to serious reports only.
   a. True
   b. False

5. Causality assessment methods will prove whether is there any association between the medicine and the reported reaction
   a. True
   b. False

6. In the WHO-UMC causality assessment scale, the following should be fulfilled to choose the category "Possible": (choose as many as applicable)
   a. Reasonable time relationship between the ADR and the medicine intake.
   b. The ADR could be explained by underlying disease
   c. Positive de-challenge
   d. Re-challenge is not required

Safety Communications

Safety/Risk communication to Healthcare professionals and public is a fundamental necessity for achieving the goals of pharmacovigilance, including promoting the rational safe effective use of medicines, preventing harm from adverse reactions, minimizing risks, and helping to the protection of patients' and public health.

As mentioned earlier that the responsibility of medications' safety monitoring is a shared responsibility between Pharmaceutical Companies, Regulatory Authorities and HCP; Safety communication is a public health responsibility of these three stakeholders and there should be a coordination between then while communicating any new safety information; accordingly, safety communication that is generated by pharmaceutical companies should be approved by the regulatory authority before being distributed to HCPs.

Effective safety communication should be done using clear understandable terms and language to the targeted audience to:

- Deliver accurate and precise information at the appropriate time for them to take adequate action (as applicable) without raising any unnecessary concerns.
- Promoting modifications to medical practices.
- Support the risk minimization procedures.
- Modulate perceptions and attitudes concerning the use of medicines.

Safety communications should be customized according to targeted audiences; as communication to HCPs will definitely differs from public communication talking into consideration the level of knowledge and accordingly the level of communicated details in a way that does not affect the accuracy of the information and message needed to be delivered.

Safety communications include all the information of the medicines from the approved information routinely mentioned in the medicines' insert leaflets or summary of product characteristics (SmPCs) or on the outer package of the medicine to any additional way to communicate additional information on a new or already known risk that may affect the safety profile of a medicine.

Among the additional ways of safety communications:

- Direct healthcare professional communications (DHPCs)
- Publications on regulatory authorities websites
- Press release
- Social media communications (Official)
- Newsletters

Safety communications should include relevant background information with all the information needed to be delivered objectively in a non-misleading way in addition to recommendations to the audiences and how to deal with safety concern and contact information for reporting any related safety issue. The effectiveness of these communications should be measured to evaluate that the target message delivered properly and understood to the targeted audiences [20].

Medicines Risk Management in Pharmacovigilance

Definition of Risk Management

Medicines are assessed by regulatory authorities to ensure that the benefits outweigh the risks before granting the medicine authorization. However, not all side effects and adverse events are identifiable in the clinical trials phase or at the time of authorization. For this purpose, marketing authorization holders are required to prepare and submit risk management plans (RMPs) for the medicine during its authorization procedure, this plan provide data regarding the uncertainties in the safety profile of the medicine, the means to minimize those risks and the measure of effectiveness of those measures [21].

The interventions that are put in place to minimize the product's risks and maximize the benefits are called minimization interventions (RMIs)or risk minimization measures (RMMs). These interventions are ranging from routine risk communication messages included in the medicine's label, to additional risk minimization measure Examples of those intervention include but are not limited to communication materials such as prescribers guide and patient education cards, patient informed consent, registries for patient tracking and many more [22].

The RMP is a dynamic document that should be updated throughout the life cycle of the medicine. This includes the addition of safety concerns where required, but also, as the safety profile is further characterized, the removal or reclassification of safety concerns.

The Aim Behind Risk Management

The safety data available at the time of approval is based on animal studies during the pre-clinical trial phase and clinical trial data. Clinical trial data derived from randomized clinical trials have some drawbacks compared to "real life" understanding or observational studies. Table 2 outlines some of those differences which trigger the need for risk management post-marketing.

While RCTs have many advantages, including easier patient follow-up, it however is too restricted and selective to draw a comprehensive conclusion on the safety of the medicine in the real-world setting in all sub-groups.

Table 2. Some of the differences which trigger the need for risk management post-marketing

Risk	Definition	RMP focus	RMP requirement
Identified Risk	risks that are undesirable clinical outcomes and for which there is sufficient scientific evidence that they are caused by the medicine	important identified risks	Further evaluation as part of the pharmacovigilance plan (e.g., to investigate frequency, severity, seriousness and outcome of this risk under normal conditions of use, which populations are particularly at risk) Risk minimization activities (Routine or additional)
Potential risk	risks that are undesirable clinical outcomes and for which there is scientific evidence to suspect the possibility of acausal relationship with the medicine, but where there is currently insufficient evidence to conclude that this association is causal	important potential risks	require further evaluation as part of the pharmacovigilance plan
Missing information	refers to gaps in knowledge about the safety of a medicine for certain anticipated utilization (e.g., long-term use) or for use in patient populations, for which there is insufficient knowledge to determine whether the safety profile differs from that characterized so far	The absence of data itself (e.g., exclusion of a population from clinical studies) does not automatically constitute a safety concern. Instead, the risk management planning should focus on situations that might differ from the known safety profile	A scientific rationale is needed for the inclusion of that population as missing information in the RMP

Spontaneous reports for instance, provide a pool of safety-related information from the real-life setting. For example, a few cases of high blood pressure may be observed during phase 3 of clinical trials through safety testing of a medicine, with the data being retrieved from 3000 patients. Hypertension would therefore be classified as a potential risk of the medicine in the product label, covering all sub-groups and indications. With further data collection post-marketing through spontaneous reporting for example, the identification of this risk for specific age groups or in specific doses can be confirmed or denied. Previously, regulatory authorities would postpone medicine authorization until further clinical trials were conducted, but this delayed patient and societal benefit from the product. On the other hand, selling the medicine with gaps in certain risk areas like hypertension in certain age groups will only show up after some time post-marketing. The risk minimization strategy of adding a potential risk of hypertension in the product label post marketing would provide a safe and beneficial option to patients [23].

"The overall aim of risk management is to ensure that the benefits of a particular medicine exceed the risks by the greatest achievable margin. The primary aim and focus of the RMP remains that of appropriate risk management planning throughout a medicine's life cycle. The risk management system shall be proportionate to the identified risks and the potential risks of the medicine, and the need for post-authorization safety data" [24].

Stakeholders Involved in Risk Management

As previously mentioned, the risk management process starts at the pre-authorization stage and monitoring of the product's benefit/risk profile extends beyond medicine authorization. This therefore would involve many stakeholders such as medicine manufacturers, regulatory authority, health care professionals, patients, and marketing authorization holders. The framework followed by pharmaceutical companies to achieve risk management and minimization is provided through guidance created and published by two main regulators: the American Food and Drug Administration (FDA) and the European Medicines Agency (EMA). These come in the form of legislations and other regulatory authorities across the world have done the same and published their own based on the FDA and EMA guidance legislations. In the US, Risk management interventions are called Risk Evaluation and Mitigation Strategies (REMS) while the EU refers to it as Risk Management Plan (RMP).

FDA and EMA Guidelines and Definitions on Risk Management

The first officially published guidance targeting post-marketing surveillance was the FDA Draft Guidance Document in March 2005 [25].

This was then followed by the EMA guidelines on Pharmacovigilance for Medicinal Products for Human Use. Within these guidelines, Volume 9A provided a template for risk management plan, and marketing authorization holders were required to present them at product authorization step and in other occasions post-marketing. This volume was then replaced with the GVP guidelines with Module V on Risk management systems [21, 24].

According to EMA, risk management is "A set of pharmacovigilance activities and interventions designed to identify, characterize, prevent, or minimize risks relating to a medicine, including the assessment of the effectiveness of those interventions" [26].

According to the FDA, "Risk Management is an iterative process of:1. assessing a product's benefit-risk balance, 2. developing and implementing tools to minimize its risks while preserving its benefits, 3. evaluating tool effectiveness and reassessing the benefit-risk balance, and 4. making adjustments, as appropriate, to the risk minimization tools to further improve the benefit risk balance."

Terminology Based on Good Pharmacovigilance Practice (GVP) Guidelines

In the EU risk management plan, previously Volume 9A and later the EU Pharmacovigilance Legislation (2012), a classification of identified risks, potential risks, and missing information are the reasons for conducting a risk management strategy post-marketing [23].

With reference to the Module V of the GVP guidelines, listed below are the types or risks and what the RMP should focus on in relation to those risks [24].

The Risk Management Framework

Now that we have defined the basic definitions of risk management and how to classify risks, a strategy for risk management is required. Risk management would therefore fall under Risk assessment or risk minimization.

Risk assessment is based on safety specifications and require PV methods to address issues identified. It includes routine PV, Additional actions, and an action plan with milestones. Risk minimization is a set of activities used to reduce the Risk(s), and these could be routine such as labeling, additional activities and involves effectiveness measurements. The below risk management framework composes the three pillars of an RMP, which are safety specification previously discussed in terms of terminology, pharmacovigilance plan, and risk minimization plan [23] (Figure 2).

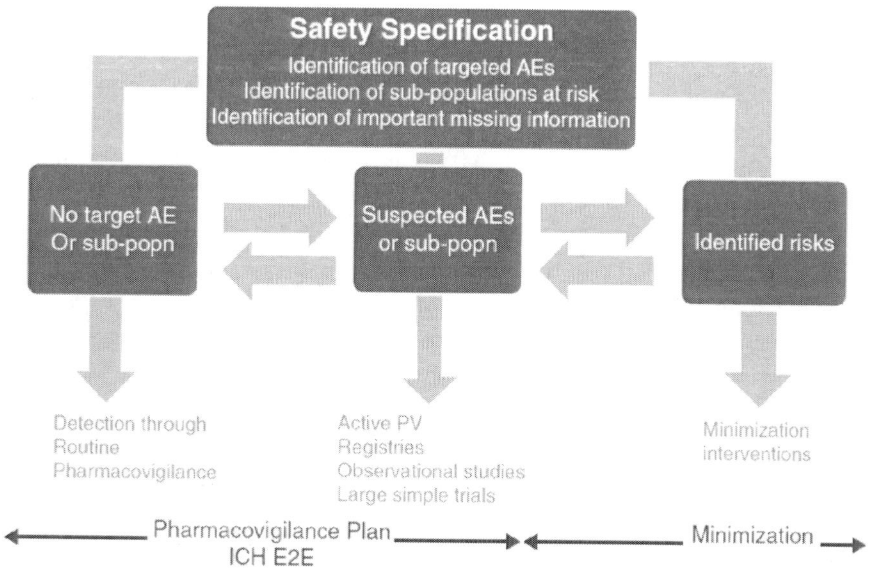

Figure 2. The iterative process and methodological strategies of risk management are illustrated.

Pharmacovigilance Plan

The aim of the pharmacovigilance plan is to identify and characterize known and unknown risks and to set up an action plan for each safety concern. For products with no special concerns, standard pharmacovigilance may be sufficient such as collection of ADRs, signal detections and Periodic Safety Update Reports (PSURs). For important safety concerns, Additional pharmacovigilance activities should be considered, such as observational studies or randomized controlled trials. Routine and additional pharmacovigilance activities will make up the pharmacovigilance plan [27].

According to EMA, "A Risk Minimization Plan details the risk minimization activities which will be taken to reduce the risks associated with an individual safety concern. They can be both routine (labeling) or additional minimization activities" [27].

According to the FDA, "A REMS is a strategic safety program designed to meet specific goals and objectives in minimizing product risks while preserving its benefits, and it goes beyond routine risk minimization strategies (e.g., labeling)" [22].

When a safety concern is observed, an evaluation for the need of risk minimization is first conducted. If required, the risk minimization will either be classified as routine or additional.

Examples of routine risk minimization are update to product information or pack size limitations. Examples of additional risk minimization are HCP educational program, controlling distribution, and patient education program. Routine and additional risk minimization will make up the risk minimization plan.

Practical Example on Risk Minimization

To demonstrate the risk management plan including risk communications and risk minimization strategies, the safety profile of Tysabri® will be considered.

Tysabri is indicated for use as a single disease modifying therapy (DMT) in adult patients with highly active relapsing remitting multiple sclerosis (RRMS) and rapidly evolving severe. It contains natalizumab as the active substance, and it is given by either intravenous infusion or subcutaneous injection, according to the SmPC of the product [28].

Two cases of progressive multifocal leukoencephalopathy (PML) in patients with multiple sclerosis were reported for Tysabri, and one case was treated in the clinical trial already suffering from Crohn's disease also reported PML. The drug was therefore suspended from the market on 28 February 2005 and the risk management plan was updated after performing a proper safety analysis and re-submitted to the regulatory authority [29].

The Table 3 outlines the summary of ongoing safety concerns that was discovered for natalizumab.

Table 3. Summary of ongoing safety concerns [30]

Important identified risks	Risk 1 • Progressive Multifocal Leukoencephalopathy (PML)
	Risk 2
	• Serious herpes infections
Important potential risks	Risk 1 • Malignancies
Missing information	Risk 1 • PML risk following switch from disease modifying therapies with immunosuppressant effect
	Risk 2 • Immunogenicity potential of subcutaneously administered Tysabri (anti-natalizumab antibody formation resulting in a potential adverse clinical consequence of serious hypersensitivity reactions including anaphylaxis)

Below is an example of the patient Alert card and continuation form created as an additional risk minimization activity as shown in Table 4 [30] [31].

Table 4. The actions taken for safety reasons to minimize the outlined risks, along with the classification of each activity

Safety concern	Proposed pharmacovigilance activities (routine and additional)	Proposed risk minimization activities (routine and additional)
Important identified risks		
Progressive multifocal leukoencephalopathy (PML)	Additional PV activities: • Study IMA-06-02 - Tysabri Observational Programme – An observational study using real world data to assess long-term safety in patients with RRMS. • Study 101MS411 – An observational cohort study utilising data from the United States natalizumab TOUCH prescribing program and select European Union MS Registries.	Routine risk minimization measures: • Information in SmPC added • Legal status: Restricted medical prescription - Tysabri is prescribed and continuously supervised by specialized physicians experienced in the diagnosis and treatment of neurological conditions with timely access to MRI. Additional risk minimization measures: • Educational tools for healthcare professionals (HCPs; Physician Information and Management Guideline) • Educational tools for patients/carers (Patient alert card, Tysabri treatment initiation form, Tysabri treatment continuation form and Tysabri discontinuation form)
Important potential risks		
Malignancies	Additional PV activities: • Study IMA-06-02 - Tysabri Observational Programme – An observational study using real world data to assess long-term safety in patients with RRMS.	Routine risk minimization activities: • Information in SmPC added • Legal status: Restricted medical prescription - Tysabri is prescribed and continuously supervised by specialized physicians experienced in the diagnosis and treatment of neurological conditions with timely access to MRI.
Important missing information		
Immunogenicity potential of subcutaneously administered Tysabri (anti-natalizumab antibody formation resulting in a potential adverse clinical consequence of serious hypersensitivity reactions, including anaphylaxis)	Additional PV Activities: • PASS to investigate the immunogenic potential of SC administration (Following study approval)	Routine risk minimization activities: • Information in SmPC added • Legal status: Restricted medical prescription - Tysabri is prescribed and continuously supervised by specialized physicians experienced in the diagnosis and treatment of neurological conditions with timely access to MRI.

Self-Assessment Questions

1. What are risks that are undesirable clinical outcomes and for which there is scientific evidence to suspect the possibility of a causal relationship with the medicinal product, but where there is currently insufficient evidence to conclude that this association is causal?

   a. Identified risks
   b. Potential risks
   c. Missing information

2. The document that outlines the risk minimization strategies according to EMA is called
   a. A Risk Minimization Plan
   b. A REMS
   c. A safety concerns document

3. Who are the stakeholders involved in risk management?
   a. drug manufacturers
   b. regulatory agencies,
   c. health care professionals,
   d. patients
   e. All of the above
   f.
4. Risk minimization measures are interventions that are present in the product label and are product and risk specific.
   a. True
   b. False

Medication Safety in the Healthcare Setting

Globally, medicines are the most prevalent treatment intervention used in healthcare. They are generally safe when used properly as prescribed or as directed on the label. According to Institute of Safe Medicine Practice (ISMP) medication safety is defined as freedom from preventable harm with medication use [32]. Actually, medication safety should be started with the first step which is the prescribing. Where a thorough risk–benefit analysis of each medicine should be initiated in this step. In fact, the medication errors considered the most common type of unsafe medication practices [33].

Medication Errors

According to the National Coordinating Council for Medication Error Reporting and Prevention the medication errors is defined as "any preventable event that may cause or lead to inappropriate medication use or patient harm while the medication is in the control of the healthcare professional, patient, or consumer," [34].

Generally, medication errors usually occur at one of these points:

- Ordering/prescribing
- Documenting
- Transcribing
- Dispensing

- Administering
- Monitoring

The first stage (Ordering/prescribing) include the large bulk of the medication errors as typing errors in conjunction with the ordering errors account for almost 50% of medication errors [35].

Fortunately, many studies reveal that nurses and pharmacists identify anywhere from 30% to 70% of typing and ordering errors. It is clear that it's a widespread problem, but the problem is avoidable in the most cases [36].

Various Taxonomies Behold the Sources of the Error [37]

- Prescribing
- Omission
- Wrong time
- Unauthorized medicine
- Improper dose
- Wrong dose prescription/wrong dose preparation
- Administration errors include the incorrect route of administration, giving the medicine to the wrong patient, extra dose, or wrong rate
- Monitoring errors such as failing to take into account patient liver and renal function, failing to document allergy or potential for drug interaction
- Compliance errors such as not following protocol or rules established for dispensing and prescribing medicines

Types of Medication Errors [38, 39, 40]

- *Expired Product*
  Appears due to inappropriate storage of the pharmaceutical products resulting in deterioration or utilizing of expired products.
- *Counterfeit medication*
  Misleading HCPs about the correct diagnosis through the side effects of the falsified medicines.
- *Incorrect Duration*
  Appears when medication is administered for a longer or shorter period of time than prescribed.
- *Incorrect Preparation*
  Appears with combining or some other type of preparation before the administration. (e.g., mistaken diluent to reconstitute)
- *Incorrect Strength*
  Appear at several stages of the healthcare process. It often appears due to human error (e.g., when similar bottles or syringes with the incorrect strength is picked).
- *Incorrect Timing*

Appears even in home or hospital settings. It is not easy to be strict with scheduled doses. The concern is that some pharmaceutical product's bioavailability is remarkably modified if taken with or without food. As such, it is vital to adhere to times as commonly; this may lead to under or overdosing.

- *Incorrect Dose*
  Appears as overdose, underdose, and an extra dose when an improper or different dose is given other than what was ordered. It also occurs when there is an error in the surveillance when a scheduled dose is not given, and when a medicine is given through an incorrect route.
- *Incorrect route*
  Appears due to indeterminate labeling or tubing that is adaptive to multiple connectors/lines of access. It often results in considerable morbidity and mortality.
- *Incorrect Dosage Form*
  Appears when a patient dispensed a dosage form different than prescribed (e.g., immediate-release instead of controlled-release).
- *Known Allergen*
  Appears when there is a poor communication between the patient and the HCPs via dispensing a medication that the patient has an allergy.
- *Incorrect Patient Action*
  Appears when a patient takes a medication improperly.
- *Known Contraindication*
  Appears when medicines are not vigilantly checked for drug-drug, drug-disease, or drug-nutrient interactions.
- *Distractions*
  Appears due to the HCPs have many duties in the hospital setting. and in the midst of these duties, they are often asked to write or dispense or administers the prescriptions. In the rush to do their work under the unlimited stress a medication error occurs.
- *Deteriorated storage*
  Appears when the pharmaceutical products stored under inappropriate conditions especially the thermosensitive products (e.g., vaccines, hormones. etc.)

The Nccessity for a Leader Positioned to Transform Medication Safety

To manage all these potential risks a committed position directly responsible and empowered to lead health system medication safety strategies and implementation is necessary: the Medication Safety Officer (MSO).

According to the American Society of Health-System Pharmacists (ASHP) the MSO is "a clinical practitioner designated by a healthcare organization to serve as the authoritative expert in safe medication use." There are other titles to represent this position include medication safety leader, medication safety manager, medication safety coordinator, medication safety clinical specialist, medication safety pharmacist, and director of medication safety [41].

Medication Safety Officers Society (MSOS) at the ISMP has Described the Characteristics of the MSO [42]

- An intense grasp of the facility's internal systems, healthcare processes, medication-use procedures including procurement, prescribing, transcribing, preparation, distribution, administration, documentation, and monitoring.
- Clinical experience and a wide understanding of health care systems and processes to facilitate precise interpretation of clinical events.
- Potent analytical skills and a comprehension of statistics, population data, and the notions of risk and prioritization.
- leadership skills.
- Presentation skills and accomplished oral communication skills, specifically the ability to communicate to all the categories of HCPs, as individuals as well as in small and large groups.
- Believing that addressing the problem of medication errors is a systems issue and not a personage health care provider issue.
- Capacity to be proactive.
- Understanding the aspects of the risk, applying the safety strategies, continuous quality improvement, and human factors engineering.
- The MSO should be assertive.
- Can work with multidisciplinary teams and engaging different stakeholders. As the MSO expected to collaborate with other departments (e.g., pharmacy, infection control and quality control), hospital senior leadership, frontline staff, and nursing and medical staff leadership to recognize and prioritize safety issues and improve risk-minimization strategies.
- Enthusiasm to learn from events outside one's own facility to apply learning about what went wrong in order to be proactive and building capacities for addressing any potential risks to ensure the patient safety.

Scope of Practice

The MSO role includes responsibility for leadership, medication safety expertise, influencing practice change, research, and education.

Leadership

Whether there is an authority or not for the MSO over the many disciplines and departments participating in the medication-use process among the healthcare organization, as the MSO cannot simply "order" a transformation, and anticipate it to happen. The MSO must combine the leadership skills, medication safety expertise, experience in performance improvement methods, and teamwork to implement an impact among the practice to make a change and improve the safety.

The MSO have to:

- Create a vision of an ideal safe medication-use system for the organization.
- Empower the risk minimization and error-prevention strategies based on practice standards, literature review, medication safety tools, and analysis of the organization's medication safety data.
- Engage in the planning, design, and applying of the organization's medication-use technology and automation systems (e.g., replacement the paper-based system by an electronic based system).
- Amend the risk communication strategies.
- Establish a culture of safety through "lesson learned" education and communication across the entire organization. This culture admit that humans make errors, so when we design processes around medication use, we build in redundancies, countermeasures, and safeguards to prevent errors from happening. In addition, it's very essential that the organization encourages reporting errors that have appeared.
- Monitor the process of collecting the data on the organization's medication errors and system failures to ensure that they are detected and obstacles to reporting are addressed.

Medication Safety Expertise

The MSO have to:

- Act as an authoritative resource on medication safety for the organization.
- Participate in development the medication safety perspective for technology initiatives.
- Participate in the medication safety overview of the internal and external emergency preparedness planning.
- Act as an internal consultant to investigate medication safety events or issues and develop recommendations for action.
- Update the policies of the organization according to the what ensure the patient safety, setting the agenda, reviewing general and specific error reports, and examining the progress of projects and initiatives.
- Keep the organization updated with the new trends in the patient safety field through continuous professional development: reading articles, journals, and related material; attending appropriate seminars, conferences, or educational programs.

Impacting Practice Change

To impact practice change, the MSO have to:

- Updates risk communication templates and support for capacity-building and surge capacity, as well as for monitoring and evaluation.

- Create a framework with the other departments participating in the medication-use process among organization ensure the medication safety.
- Involve patients and family member.
- Give more attention on those at higher risk of safety incidents.
- Encourage the use of medication reconciliation by physicians and ensure that pharmacists actively review prescriptions.

Research and Education

To enhance the research and education among the organization, the MSO have to:

- Educate HCPs about common causes of medication errors.
- Provide information about actual or potential medication errors with safety organizations such as ISMP.
- Lead medication-use safety research through well designed, externally validated studies and implement evidence-based practices for medication safety.
- Conduct more research for a better understanding of the medication errors causes and generate evidence for interventions impacting on adverse outcomes.

Medication Error Risk Factors [43]

Factors associated with health care professionals

- Inadequate medication knowledge and clinical experience
- Unclear handwriting

Factors associated with patients

- Complex cases
- Patient characteristics (e.g., personality, literacy and language barriers)

Factors associated with the work environment

- High volume (Distractions and interruptions)
- Shift work
- Reluctance in policy enforcement
- Workplace culture

Factors associated with medicines

- Doses needing calculations

Factors associated with tasks

- Absence of follow-up
- Absence of appropriate surveillance

Factors associated with communication

- Oral orders
- Poor communication between the primary and secondary care

The Barriers to Medication Error Reporting in the Hospital Setting [44]

It seems that the main obstacle within health organizations to report medication errors is a set of psychological barriers consisting of fear and anxiety. Where workers may fear that this will affect performance evaluation and career progression paths, or worry about the impact of work relationships

The appearance of medication errors in hospitals is recognized a common and potentially serious threat to patient safety. Adopting a computerized system in all medication-use processes is the most effective intervention to prevent medication errors due to the paper-based system is a real and major source of errors, as it depends on the handwriting being readable or clear in order to implement the instructions in it accurately.

In addition, depending on an Electronic Health Record (EHR) system for collecting the patient's health information (e.g., medical history, medication orders, vital signs, laboratory results, radiology reports, and physician and nurse note, etc.) could be an ideal solution for the follow-up and monitoring problems due to it will help to improve the accuracy and quality of data recorded in a health record. Furthermore, enhance physicians'' access to a patient's healthcare information enabling it to be shared by all for the present and continuing care of that patient [45].

It's very important in the organization to promote the "No blaming" culture which acknowledges that humans make errors, this will cultivate a suitable environment encouraging the HCPs and other to reports any medication errors or ADRs.

Here, some strategies to minimize the technical medication errors [43, 46]:

- Handling every prescription with caution.
- Write the accurate dosage in a clear form.
- Utilize metric measures.
- Avoid drug abbreviations when writing orders.
- Taking the patient age into account.
- Provide supplemental instructions.
- Indorse a reporting system.
- Regular check for the liver and kidney functions before ordering any medication.
- Keep vigilant with high-risk medications.
- Document conversation and decision.
- Confirm understanding.

References

[1] Kar, Anita. "Thalidomide: Understanding the Responsibilities of a Birth Defects Service," in *Birth Defects in India*, Singapore: Springer, 2021, pp. 75–93. doi: https://doi.org/10.1007/978-981-16-1554-2_3.

[2] Medicines and Healthcare products Regulatory Agency, "*Yellow Card Scheme.*" https://www.gov.uk/guidance/the-yellow-card-scheme-guidance-for-healthcare-professionals (accessed Nov. 01, 2022).

[3] World Health Organization, *"The WHO Programme for International Drug Monitoring."* https://www.who.int/teams/regulation-prequalification/regulation-and-safety/pharmacovigilance/health-professionals-info/pidm (accessed Oct. 06, 2022).

[4] Uppsala Monitoring Center, "*About the WHO PIDM - A global collaboration for patient safety.*" https://who-umc.org/about-the-who-programme-for-international-drug-monitoring/about-the-who-pidm/ (accessed Oct. 06, 2022).

[5] Council for International Organizations of Medical Sciences, "*CIOMS History.*" https://cioms.ch/history/ (accessed Oct. 06, 2022).

[6] Council for International Organizations of Medical Sciences., "*CIOMS - Pharmacovigilance.*" https://cioms.ch/pharmacovigilance/ (accessed Oct. 06, 2022).

[7] International Council for Harmonization of Technical Requirements for Pharmaceuticals for Human Use, *"ICH."* https://www.ich.org/ (accessed Oct. 06, 2022).

[8] MedDRA, "*Medical Dictionary for Regulatory Activities (MedDRA).*" https://www.meddra.org/ (accessed Nov. 01, 2022).

[9] International Society of Pharmacovigilance, "*ISoP.*" https://isoponline.org/ (accessed Oct. 06, 2022).

[10] National Institute of Health (NIH), "*NIH clinical research trials and you.*" https://www.nih.gov/health-information/nih-clinical-research-trials-you (accessed Oct. 06, 2022).

[11] Prakash B. and G. Singh, *"Pharmacovigilance: scope for a dermatologist,"* Accessed: Oct. 06, 2022. [Online]. Available: doi: 10.4103/0019-5154.87121

[12] Jose, J., M. H. al Rubaie, H. al Ramimmy, and S. S. Varughese, "Pharmacovigilance basic concepts and an overview of the system in oman," *Sultan Qaboos Univ Med J,* vol. 21, no. 2, pp. e161–e163, Jun. 2021, doi: 10.18295/squmj.2021.21.02.001.

[13] Eugène P. van Puijenbroek and Linda Harmark, "Broadening the Scope of Pharmacovigilance," in *Pharmacovigilance, Adis, Cham: Adis*, 2016, pp. 131–144. doi: https://doi.org/10.1007/978-3-319-40400-4_13.

[14] European Medicine Agency (EMA) and Heads of Medicines Agencies, "*Guideline on good pharmacovigilance practices (GVP) - Annex I - Definitions (Rev 4),*" Oct. 2017. Accessed: Nov. 01, 2022. [Online]. Available:https://www.ema.europa.eu/en/documents/scientific-guideline/guideline-good-pharmacovigilance-practices-annex-i-definitions-rev-4_en.pdf.

[15] Rossi, A., C. Cantisani, L. Melis, A. Iorio, E. Scali, and S. Calvieri, *"Minoxidil Use in Dermatology, Side Effects and Recent Patents,"* 2012. doi: doi: 10.2174/187221312800166859.

[16] Coleman J. J. and S. K. Pontefract, "Adverse drug reactions," *Clinical Medicine,* doi: doi: 10.7861/clinmedicine.16-5-481.

[17] European Commission, *"Pharmacovigilance."* https://health.ec.europa.eu/medicinal-products/pharmacovigilance_en (accessed Oct. 06, 2022).

[18] European Medicine Agency (EMA), "*Guideline on good pharmacovigilance practices (GVP).*" Accessed: Oct. 06, 2022. [Online]. Available: https://www.ema.europa.eu/en/documents/regulatory-procedural-guideline/guideline-good-pharmacovigilance-practices-gvp-module-vi-collection-management-submission-reports_en.pdf.

[19] Uppsala Monitoring Center (UMC), "*The use of the WHO-UMC system for standardised case causality assessment,*" Apr. 2018. Accessed: Nov. 01, 2022. [Online]. Available: https://who-umc.org/media/164200/who-umc-causality-assessment_new-logo.pdf

[20] European Medicines Agency (EMA) and Heads of Medicines Agencies (HMA), "*Guideline on good pharmacovigilance practices (GVP) - Module XV - Safety communication (Rev 1),*" Oct. 2017. Accessed: Nov. 01, 2022. [Online]. Available: https://www.ema.europa.eu/en/documents/scientific-

guideline/guideline-good-pharmacovigilance-practices-module-xv-safety-communication-rev-1_en.pdf.

[21] European Medicine Agency (EMA), "Guideline on good pharmacovigilance practices (GVP) Module VIII - *Post Authorisation Safety Studies* (Rev 3)," 2017. Accessed: Oct. 06, 2022. [Online]. Available: https://www.ema.europa.eu/en/documents/scientific-guideline/guideline-good-pharmacovigilance-practices-gvp-module-viii-post-authorisation-safety-studies-rev-3_en.pdf.

[22] Food and Drug Administration (FDA), "*Guidance for Industry - Development and Use of Risk Minimization Action Plans,*" 2005. Accessed: Oct. 06, 2022. [Online]. Available: https://www.fda.gov/media/71268/download.

[23] Moride, Y. "Risk Management and Minimization: Clinical and Quantitative Aspects," in *Evidence-Based Pharmacovigilance*, New York: Humana Press, pp. 217–232. doi: https://doi.org/10.1007/978-1-4939-8818-1_12.

[24] European Medicine Agency (EMA), "*Guideline on good pharmacovigilance practices (GVP) Module V – Risk management systems,*" 2017. Accessed: Oct. 08, 2022. [Online]. Available: https://www.ema.europa.eu/en/documents/scientific-guideline/guideline-good-pharmacovigilance-practices-module-v-risk-management-systems-rev-2_en.pdf.

[25] Food and Drug Administration (FDA), "*Guidance for Industry Good Pharmacovigilance Practices and Pharmacoepidemiologic Assessment,*" 2005. Accessed: Oct. 08, 2022. [Online]. Available: https://www.fda.gov/media/71546/download.

[26] European Commission, "Directive 2001/83/Ec Of The European Parliament and of the Council of 6 November 2001," 2001. Accessed: Oct. 08, 2022. [Online]. Available: https://health.ec.europa.eu/system/files/2016-11/dir_2001_83_cons_2012_en_0.pdf.

[27] European Medicine Agency, *"Guideline on Risk Management Systems for Medicinal Products for Human Use,"* 2005. Accessed: Oct. 08, 2022. [Online]. Available: https://www.emwa.org/Documents/Freelancer/riskmanagement/rmp%20guidelines.pdf.

[28] Stüve O. and J. L. Bennett, *"Pharmacological Properties, Toxicology and Scientific Rationale for the use of Natalizumab (Tysabri) in Inflammatory Diseases,"* Blackwell Publishing Inc, 2007. [Online]. Available: http://www.ingentaconnect.com/content/maney/nres.

[29] Gert Van Assche, "*Progressive Multifocal Leukoencephalopathy after Natalizumab Therapy for Crohn's Disease*." doi: doi: 10.1056/NEJMoa051586.

[30] European Medicines Agency (EMA), "*Risk management plans.*" https://www.ema.europa.eu/en/human-regulatory/marketing-authorisation/pharmacovigilance/risk-management/risk-management-plans (accessed Nov. 01, 2022).

[31] The electronic medicines compendium (emc), "*Risk Minimisation Materials.*" https://www.medicines.org.uk/emc/rmm-directory#gref (accessed Nov. 01, 2022).

[32] Institute of Safe Medicine Practice (ISMP) Canada, "*ISMP Canada Definitions of Terms.*" https://www.ismp-canada.org/definitions.htm (accessed Oct. 08, 2022).

[33] World Health Organization (WHO), *Technical Series on Safer Primary Care: Medication errors*. 2016. Accessed: Oct. 08, 2022. [Online]. Available: https://www.who.int/publications/i/item/9789241511643.

[34] Food and Drug Administration (FDA), "*Working to Reduce Medication Errors.*" https://www.fda.gov/drugs/information-consumers-and-patients-drugs/working-reduce-medication-errors (accessed Oct. 08, 2022).

[35] Tariq, R. A., R. Vashisht, A. Sinha, and Y. Scherbak, M*edication Dispensing Errors and Prevention.* 2022. Accessed: Oct. 08, 2022. [Online]. Available: https://www.ncbi.nlm.nih.gov/books/NBK519065/.

[36] Röhsig, V. "Near-miss analysis in a large hospital in southern Brazil: A 5-year retrospective study," *International Journal of Risk and Safety in Medicine*, vol. 31, no. 4, pp. 247–258, 2020, doi: 10.3233/JRS-194050.

[37] N. Y. Loskutova, C. Lutgen, C. Smail, E. W. Staton, S. D. Nichols, and R. G. Pinckney, "Stimulant Prescribing Error Assessment Rubric Development," *J Patient Saf,* doi: https://doi.org/10.1097/PTS.0000000000000775.

[38] Hoyle, J. D., R. P. Crowe, M. A. Bentley, G. Beltran, and W. Fales, "Pediatric Prehospital Medication Dosing Errors: A National Survey of Paramedics," *Prehospital Emergency Care*, vol. 21, no. 2, pp. 185–191, Mar. 2017, doi: 10.1080/10903127.2016.1227001.

[39] Payne, R., S. Slight, B. D. Franklin, A. J. (Anthony J. Avery, World Health Organization, and World Health Organization. Department of Service Delivery and Safety., *Medication errors.*

[40] Leahy, I. C., M. Lavoie, D. Zurakowski, A. W. Baier, and R. M. Brustowicz, "Medication errors in a pediatric anesthesia setting: Incidence, etiologies, and error reduction strategies," *J Clin Anesth*, vol. 49, pp. 107–111, Sep. 2018, doi: 10.1016/j.jclinane.2018.05.011.

[41] Saine D. and C. M. Larson, *Medication Safety Officer: Getting Started* - American Society of Health-System Pharmacists (ASHP). Accessed: Oct. 08, 2022. [Online]. Available: https://www.ashp.org/-/media/store-files/p2104-sample-chapter-1.

[42] Bonner, L. "*ISMP defines roles, value of medication safety officer*," doi: https://doi.org/10.1016/j.ptdy.2018.10.033.

[43] Stewart, D. "Exploring facilitators and barriers to medication error reporting among healthcare professionals in Qatar using the theoretical domains framework: A mixed-methods approach," *PLoS One*, vol. 13, no. 10, Oct. 2018, doi: 10.1371/journal.pone.0204987.

[44] Salim Aljabari and Zuhal Kadhim, "Common Barriers to Reporting Medical Errors," *The Scientific World Journal*, 2021, doi: https://doi.org/10.1155/2021/6494889.

[45] Jungreithmayr, V. "The impact of a computerized physician order entry system implementation on 20 different criteria of medication documentation—a before-and-after study," *BMC Med Inform Decis Mak*, vol. 21, no. 1, Dec. 2021, doi: 10.1186/s12911-021-01607-6.

[46] Gillani, S. W. "Role and Services of a Pharmacist in the Prevention of Medication Errors: A Systematic Review," *Curr Drug Saf,* vol. 16, no. 3, 2021, doi: doi: 10.2174/1574886315666201002124713.

Chapter 10

Conclusion

Hadeer Harb*
and Mohamed Emam Abdelmobdy Abdelrahim
Clinical Pharmacy Department, Faculty of Pharmacy,
Beni-Suef University, Beni Suef, Egypt

Learning Objectives

After completing this chapter, the reader would be able to:

- Be aware of the various difficulties that clinical pharmacy practice faces all across the world.
- Identify and value current advancements in Egypt's clinical pharmacy practice.
- Recognize how potential future developments might assist in overcoming the numerous difficulties faced by clinical pharmacy practice.
- Affect the health of the patient and the wider public by promoting and strictly upholding future pharmacist obligations.

Clinical Pharmacy's Expectations for the Future

In the upcoming years, it is anticipated that both the function of the pharmacist and medical care practices would change more quickly. There are numerous obstacles that the clinical pharmacy profession must continually grow and update to overcome. Despite the encouraging advancements made in clinical pharmacy practice over the past several years, several difficulties need to be taken into account. These include establishing clinical pharmacy departments in hospitals, reaffirming the need for pharmacists to continue their education to adopt the professional clinical practice, raising the number of clinical pharmacists working in the private sector, recognizing pharmacists as healthcare professionals, removing doctors' resistance to pharmacist's role in providing medical care, and establishing highly specialized neighborhood pharmacies that offer more than just prescription filling services. Future

* Corresponding Author's Email: Hadeersafwat@pharm.bsu.edu.eg.

In: Clinical Pharmacist Tools to Deliver Rational Medication Use
Editor: Mohamed Emam Abdelmobdy Abdelrahim
ISBN: 979-8-88697-857-5

pharmacists are anticipated to play a variety of important roles in delivering the best possible medical care by helping to make wise judgments regarding patients and medications. These consist of leadership, scientific, and patient-facing jobs in medical development and hospitals or communities.

Operations of Pharmacists

Pharmacists work in a setting that is always changing. In the upcoming years, it is anticipated that both the function of the pharmacist and medical care practices will change more quickly. However, there has not been any standardization of pharmacy methods worldwide up to this point [1]. Clinical pharmacy practice is faced with many challenges worldwide, which require continuous development and updates to be overcome [2, 3]. The healthcare system faces several challenges, including an insufficient number of healthcare services, the high cost of drugs, and the complexity of medicines. The pharmaceutical market provides several prescription and non-prescription drugs including dietary supplements, and herbal medicines. Therefore, it is difficult for healthcare practitioners to be fully aware of all medications in the patient's regimen when taking decisions about treatment. Furthermore, the established medical malpractice and knowledge of drug-related morbidity/mortality have confirmed the importance of pharmacists' role in patient safety [4]. Clinical pharmacy practice within ward rounds has been shown to minimize adverse drug reactions (ADRs) and treatment complications [5]. Many future directions are suggested to overcome these challenges and that will be discussed in this chapter.

Recent Developments in Clinical Pharmacy Practice in Egypt

There is a continuous need for the development of clinical pharmacy services in hospitals and this creates extra demands on healthcare practitioners due to the great importance of the clinical pharmacists' roles in the healthcare system. The government has taken significant steps toward the implementation and application of clinical pharmacy. The first step includes the introduction of a clinical pharmacy fellowship program to consider the pharmacist as an active member of the healthcare team and develop pharmacists' sharing in pharmacy education and training. The introduction of clinical pharmacy centers is a priority to grow clinical pharmacy services. In 2012, the Egyptian government considered drug information centers for the practice of clinical pharmacy in hospitals as a prerequisite for hospital licensing according to the latest ministerial decree. The Egyptian ministry of health (MOH) mandated that all hospitals must implement clinical pharmacy practices before July 2013. In 2014, the Hospital Pharmacy Administration and Central Administration of Pharmaceutical Affairs introduced standards and guidelines for clinical pharmacy practice in hospitals. A ministerial decree was also issued in 2014 to extend the duration of the pharmacy study from five to six years. This sixth year includes student training in communities, hospitals, and industrial institutions to ensure that pharmacy graduates have obtained the required competencies for professional pharmaceutical and clinical practice [3].

Clinical Pharmacy Practice Challenges and Future Directions

Clinical pharmacy practice is faced with several challenges. Clinical pharmacy practice has been recently introduced in some Egyptian hospitals in obstetrics wards, pediatrics units, intensive care units, and cancer institutes. However, most Egyptian hospitals employ pharmacists who largely deal with medication supply, procurement, and distribution. The majority of hospitals were established in the past with no proper clinical pharmacy units for providing appropriate clinical pharmacy services. Therefore, there is a current trend towards the establishment of clinical pharmacy units and drug information centers to help in practicing all clinical pharmacy services in a professional manner [3]. Also, geographical distribution is another challenge. Clinical pharmacy practices are more comprehensive in large institutions in major cities. Healthcare facilities in rural areas have a limited clinical pharmacy service if it even exists. This challenge is more extensive in the private sector, which did not recognize clinical pharmacy as one of the core specialties. Fortunately, the number of clinical pharmacists in the private sector is expected to increase in the future as a result of mandating their presence [2].

Another major challenge for clinical pharmacy practice in hospitals is the lack of well-trained clinical pharmacists to provide clinical pharmacy services and train pharmacy students on clinical skills across different clinical rotations. This may be due to the relatively short history of clinical pharmacy training and is expected to improve over the next 5 to 10 years as new graduates are educated and trained to be qualified to meet the requested competencies of work. Other challenges for clinical pharmacists include gaining the acceptance of other healthcare team members and being trusted to modify drug therapy and provide medical care. The physician-pharmacist relationship is complex, and not all physicians are comfortable with pharmacists providing direct medical care [6-8]. Inter-professional Physician– pharmacist communication is essential during providing medical care to enhance medication safety and outcomes and minimize treatment errors and adverse drug reactions [9]. Several studies have reported a physician-pharmacist communication gap [10, 11]. Despite physicians' awareness of the availability of clinical pharmacy services, they did not utilize them [12]. These challenges are not only in Egypt but also in other Arabic countries including Saudi Arabia, Jordan, Kuwait, United Arab Emirates, and Sudan [2, 13-17].

There is a major future direction toward introducing clinical pharmacy practice in community settings in the next few years, as it is currently not introduced there. This is important to provide comprehensive medication therapy management services in community settings in which pharmacists can provide direct patient care in community pharmacies. This could be achieved in a separate patient care area where pharmacists can provide counseling, check vital signs, and even administer vaccines [18]. However, there is a public perception that specialized pharmaceutical care is delivered in the hospital setting and not in the community. Introducing highly specialized community pharmacies that provide more than dispensing services can help in overcoming this challenge. Lastly, there is a need to unify clinical pharmacists' competencies and job requirements worldwide. In the meantime, position statements are needed for outlining the clinical pharmacy's role in providing direct patient care and in the management of different disease states besides a statement of clinical pharmacists' roles and responsibilities as well as competency assessment and job requirements [2].

Future Pharmacist Responsibilities

No matter where the future pharmacist's work (within the community or hospital) or to what specialist area they belong, their roles will impact the patient and public health generally. These roles include [19]:

- Providing expert healthcare with a leading role in the clinical interactions with patients and the decisions surrounding the patient.
- Being the pharmaceutical scientist within healthcare provides the team with the knowledge and skills surrounding medicines and their use, to provide information and evidence in support of decisions surrounding medicines.
- Providing primary care and public health role through high skills, knowledge, and expertise in patient consultation, and medicines optimization, to minimize referrals to general practice, hospital re-admissions, and secondary care referrals.
- Advising other healthcare professionals in complex cases of diagnosis, in cases of initial medicine failure, and about newly available therapies.
- Led the development of new medicines and their approval, distribution, and optimization in the use.
- Taking a leading role in the training of prescribers.
- Being recognized within the pharmaceutical industry- related sciences and the international regulatory governance of medicines, as a patient-focused leader of pharmaceutical research and drug development.
- Being recognized in workforce planning for their positive contributions and skills and cost-effective impact on healthcare delivery and the economics surrounding medicines.

In general, the future pharmacist is expected to have multiple efficient roles in providing optimal medical care through a contribution to making adequate decisions surrounding both the patient and the medicines. These include patient-facing roles (within the community or hospital) or in medicine development, scientific, and leadership positions.

References

[1] Inoue, Y., Future expectations for Japanese pharmacists as compared to the rest of the world. *Research in Social and Administrative Pharmacy,* 2015. 11(3): p. 448-458.

[2] Badreldin, H. A., S. Alosaimy, and A. Al-jedai, Clinical pharmacy practice in Saudi Arabia: Historical evolution and future perspective. *Journal of the American College of Clinical Pharmacy,* 2020. 3(5): p. 920-929.

[3] Abdel-Latif, M. M. and K. Sabra, Clinical pharmacy practice in Egyptian hospitals. *American Journal of Health-System Pharmacy,* 2016. 73(1): p. e63-e66.

[4] Edbril, S. D. and R. S. Lagasse, Relationship between malpractice litigation and human errors. *The Journal of the American Society of Anesthesiologists,* 1999. 91(3): p. 848-848.

[5] Leape, L. L., Pharmacist participation on physician rounds and adverse drug events in the intensive care unit. *Jama,* 1999. 282(3): p. 267-270.

[6] Ranelli, P. L. and J. Biss, Physicians' perceptions of communication with and responsibilities of pharmacists. *Journal of the American Pharmaceutical Association* (1996), 2000. 40(5): p. 625-630.

[7] Tanskanen, P., Counselling patients on psychotropic medication: physicians' opinions on the role of community pharmacists. *Pharmacy World and Science,* 2000. 22(2): p. 59-61.

[8] Hughes, C. M. and S. McCann, Perceived interprofessional barriers between community pharmacists and general practitioners: a qualitative assessment. *British Journal of General Practice*, 2003. 53(493): p. 600-606.

[9] Worley, M. M., Pharmacists' and patients 'roles in the pharmacist-patient relationship: are pharmacists and patients reading from the same relationship script? *Research in Social and Administrative Pharmacy,* 2007. 3(1): p. 47-69.

[10] Bradshaw, S. J. and W. R. Doucette, Community pharmacists as patient advocates: physician attitudes. *Journal of the American Pharmaceutical Association* (1996), 1998. 38(5): p. 598-602.

[11] Nesbit, F., Counseling of patients by pharmacists. Blessing or curse? *North Carolina medical journal*, 1995. 56(2): p. 115-1..18

[12] Sabry, N. A. and S. F. Farid, The role of clinical pharmacists as perceived by Egyptian physicians. *International Journal of Pharmacy Practice,* 2014. 22(5): p. 354-359.

[13] Matowe, L., Physicians' perceptions and expectations of pharmacists 'professional duties in government hospitals in Kuwait. *Medical Principles and practice,* 2006. 15(3): p. 185-189.

[14] Fahmy, S., B. Rasool, and S. Abdu, Health-care professionals' perceptions and expectations of pharmacists' role in the emergency department, United Arab Emirates. *East Mediterr Health J,* 2013. 19(9): p. 794-801.

[15] Francis, J. and S. Abraham, Clinical pharmacists: Bridging the gap between patients and physicians. *Saudi Pharmaceutical Journal*, 2014. 22(6): p. 600-602.

[16] Tahaineh, L. M., Perceptions, experiences, and expectations of physicians in hospital settings in Jordan regarding the role of the pharmacist. *Research in social and administrative pharmacy*, 2009. 5(1): p. 63-70.

[17] Awad, A., L. Matowe, and P. Capps, Medical doctors' perceptions and expectations of the role of hospital pharmacists in Sudan. *Pharmacy World & Science,* 2007. 29(5): p. 557-564.

[18] Abdel-Latif, M. M., S. B. Hassan, and K. Sabra, The status of community pharmacy in egypt: are community pharmacies ready to deliver clinical pharmacy services at the national level? *Bulletin of Pharmaceutical Sciences.* Assiut, 2021. 44(1): p. 99-110.

[19] Council, T. P. S. *The future role of the pharmacist* 2018 [cited 2022; Available from: https://www.pharmacyschoolscouncil.ac.uk/features/the-future-role-of-the-pharmacis/.

Index

F

G

H

I

K

L

M

N

O

P

R

S

T

U

V

About the Editors

Editor

Prof. Mohamed Emam Abdelmobdy Abdelrahim, is a Professor in Department of Clinical Pharmacy, Faculty of Pharmacy, at the Beni-Suef University in Egypt. Prof. Abdelrahim has published 2 books, 6 book chapters, over 200 papers, and more than 100 conference presentations. His main area of expertise is clinical pharmacy and aerosol therapy.

Email: Mohamedemam9@yahoo.com.

Co-Editors

Dr. Mohammed Almeziny, PhD, is a Consultant Clinical Pharmacist, Prince Sultan Military Medical City (PSMMC), Riyadh, KSA. He holds essential skills in Medical Education (ESME) certificate, Association for Medical Education in Europe, Dundee, UK and International Medication Safety Mentorship, Institute for Safe Medication Practices (ISMP), Horsham PA, USA. He is an Adjunct Clinical Assistant Professor, College of Pharmacy, King Saud University, Riyadh, Saudi Arabia, Princess Nourah Bint Abdul Rahman University. He published 1 book and a number of manuscripts in several peer-reviewed journals.

Email: meziny@hotmail.com.

Dr. Haitham Saeed, PhD, is a Lecturer in Department of Clinical Pharmacy, Faculty of Pharmacy, Beni-Suef University, Egypt. His main research interests are clinical pharmacy and aerosols, and he has published 2 books, approximately 20 book chapters, over 45 papers, and 10 conference papers. His main area of expertise is clinical pharmacy and aerosol therapy.

Email: haitham.sd1@gmail.com.

Dr. Hasnaa Osama, PhD, is a Lecturer in Department of Clinical Pharmacy, Faculty of Pharmacy, Beni-Suef University, Egypt. Her main research interests are clinical pharmacy, and she has published 1 book, 2 book chapters, over 30 papers and 10 conference papers. Her main area of expertise is clinical pharmacy.

Email: hasnaa011137@pharm.bsu.edu.eg.